Speech, Language, and Communication

Handbook of Perception and Cognition
2nd Edition

Series Editors
Edward C. Carterette
and **Morton P. Friedman**

Speech, Language, and Communication

Edited by
Joanne L. Miller

Department of Psychology
Northeastern University
Boston, Massachusetts

Peter D. Eimas

Department of Cognitive and Linguistic Sciences
Brown University
Providence, Rhode Island

Academic Press
San Diego   New York   Boston
London   Sydney   Tokyo   Toronto

Academic Press, Inc.
A Division of Harcourt Brace & Company
525 B Street, Suite 1900, San Diego, California 92101-4495

United Kingdom Edition published by
Academic Press Limited
24-28 Oval Road, London NW1 7DX

Library of Congress Cataloging-in-Publication Data

Speech, language, and communication / edited by Joanne L. Miller,
    Peter D. Eimas.
        p.   cm. -- (Handbook of perception and cognition, 2nd ed. : v. 11)
    Includes index.
    ISBN 0-12-497770-7
        1. Psycholinguistics.   2. Speech perception.   3. Language
    acquisition.   I. Miller, Joanne L.   II. Eimas, Peter D.
    III. Series: Handbook of perception and cognition series : 11.
    BF455.S58   1995
    401'.9--dc20   94-39355
                                                                CIP

PRINTED IN THE UNITED STATES OF AMERICA
95   96   97   98   99   00   BC   9   8   7   6   5   4   3   2   1

Contents

2   *Speech Production*

Carol A. Fowler

3   *Speech Perception: New Directions in Research and Theory*

Lynne C. Nygaard and David B. Pisoni

7 Sentence Comprehension

Michael K. Tanenhaus and John C. Trueswell

8 Language Acquisition: Speech Sounds and the Beginning of Phonology

Peter W. Jusczyk

Contributors

Numbers in parentheses indicate the pages on which the authors' contributions begin.

Sheila E. Blumstein (339)
Department of Cognitive and
  Linguistic Sciences
Brown University
Providence, Rhode Island 02912

Bridget Bly (371)
Department of Psychology
Stanford University
Stanford, California 94305

Kathryn Bock (181)
Department of Psychology
Beckman Institute
University of Illinois
Champaign, Illinois 61820

Eve V. Clark (303)
Department of Linguistics
Stanford University
Stanford, California 94305

Herbert H. Clark (371)
Department of Psychology
Stanford University
Stanford, California 94305

Anne Cutler (97)
Max–Planck–Institut für
  Psycholinguistik
6525 XD Nijmegen,
The Netherlands

Carol A. Fowler (30)
Haskins Laboratories
270 Crown Street
New Haven, Connecticut 06511

Lyn Frazier (1)
Linguistics Department
University of Massachusetts
Amherst, Massachusetts 01003

Peter W. Jusczyk (263)
Department of Psychology
State University of New York
  at Buffalo
Buffalo, New York 14260

Lynne C. Nygaard (63)
Speech Research Laboratory
Department of Psychology
Indiana University
Bloomington, Indiana 47405

David B. Pisoni (63)
Speech Research Laboratory
Department of Psychology
Indiana University
Bloomington, Indiana 47405

Mark S. Seidenberg (138)
Program in Neural, Informational,
  and Behavioral Sciences
University of Southern California
Los Angeles, California 90089

Michael K. Tanenhaus (217)
Department of Psychology
University of Rochester
Rochester, New York 14627

John C. Trueswell (217)
Department of Psychology
University of Pennsylvania
Philadelphia, Pennsylvania 19104

Foreword

The problem of perception and cognition is in understanding how the organism transforms, organizes, stores, and uses information arising from the world in sense data or memory. With this definition of perception and cognition in mind, this handbook is designed to bring together the essential aspects of this very large, diverse, and scattered literature to give a précis of the state of knowledge in every area of perception and cognition. The work is aimed at the psychologist and the cognitive scientist in particular and at the natural scientist in general. Topics are covered in comprehensive surveys in which fundamental facts and concepts are presented, and important leads to journals and monographs of the specialized literature are provided. Perception and cognition are considered in the widest sense. Therefore, the work will treat a wide range of experimental and theoretical work.

The *Handbook of Perception and Cognition* should serve as a basic source and reference work for all in the arts or sciences, indeed for all who are interested in human perception, action, and cognition.

Edward C. Carterette and Morton P. Friedman

Preface

Since the Chomskyan revolution in linguistics in the late 1950s and early 1960s, experimental and theoretical studies of language have become major endeavors in a number of diverse disciplines ranging from cognitive and brain science to computer and engineering science. Authors and editors of books reporting on these studies have lauded the seemingly ever-increasing progress in the scientific study of language, and we are no exception. We need only to compare the present volume with its predecessor of nearly two decades ago to see the almost quantal increase in our knowledge of the processes of language comprehension, production, and acquisition. It is also clear that the gains in knowledge have continued to reveal even deeper levels of complexity that await investigation. This is not, we suggest, to be taken as a point for despair. Rather, we see exemplified in these chapters the progress of a young science, one that with gains in maturity not only adds to a repertoire of facts and testable theories but also yields insights into the issues of the future. The opening contribution by Lyn Frazier shows the increasing sophistication in our understanding of the nature of language as a formal entity and its relation in the form of linguistic theory to psycho-linguistic theory—a relationship that Frazier shows rests on the presumed representations of language at its various levels of analysis.

The next two contributions review research and theory in speech. Carol Fowler surveys the domain of speech production, which she takes as the endeavor to describe "how a linguistic message can be conveyed by vocal tract activity." Although recognizing that a complete understanding of speech production must include the production of connected discourse, Fowler confines her contribution to processes of production at the segmental level. Her exposition argues for phonological primitives of a gestural nature and shows how they provide a match between linguistic (phonological) theory and vocal tract activity—a clear demonstration of how the representational format deeply constrains and illuminates psycholinguistic phenomena. Lynne Nygaard and David Pisoni provide a review of selected topics that aim to explain how listeners derive the speaker's intended phonetic message from the acoustic signal of speech. They provide summaries of recent research, focusing on the role of systematic variability in the signal. As they note, this research raises serious questions about the nature of the initial representations of speech. Nygaard and Pisoni also discuss organizational processes in the perception of speech, work that has become particularly important because the organization of speech appears governed by principles inherent to speech.

Anne Cutler and Mark Seidenberg, in the next two chapters, discuss the recognition and production of spoken words and visual word recognition, respectively. It is at the level of the word that form and meaning make contact; that is, we see the intersection between the vehicle of language and the message it is to convey. Cutler's review describes many of the major issues in the perception and production of spoken words and provides a review of current methodologies. She likewise presents an overview of current theories of recognition and production and a discussion of the commonalities and differences underlying the two processes. Seidenberg's discussion offers a comprehensive review of data and theory, noting in particular how visual word recognition, despite its reliance on inventions perceived by the eye, helps to inform our understanding of language in particular and of perception in general. His discussion also shows how the increasing use of connectionist models has begun to alter our conceptions of recent controversies in the domain of word recognition.

The next two chapters move from the level of the word to that of the sentence. Kathryn Bock provides a summary of work on sentence production—that is, on "how speakers turn messages into utterances." What is made most clear is that the path from communicative intent to speech is one marked by a number of substages or levels of processing, which if not fully modular are sufficiently encapsulated such that their individual contributions are readily measurable. Bock concludes with caveats that production is not simply perception turned in direction and offers reasons for this state of affairs. Michael Tanenhaus and John Trueswell discuss sentence comprehension, focusing on the relation between language structure and language processing at this level of analysis. The chapter presents a history of sentence comprehension over the past 35 years that reviews now classic experiments and theories that drove these research efforts. Tanenhaus and Trueswell also summarize recent experimental efforts and the evolving theories and metatheories that have driven these experimental investigations; this discussion includes a consideration of the important evolving notions of the lexical/syntactic interface.

The acquisition of language is the focus of the next two chapters. In the first, Peter Jusczyk reviews experiments on the abilities of young infants to perceive the sounds of speech. The task for the infant is, as Jusczyk notes, not trivial given the lack of acoustic invariance and absence of explicit acoustic segmentation for linguistically significant units. What is apparent from these studies is the proficiency of the young infant in processing speech and in acquiring knowledge of the specific segmental and prosodic characteristics of the native language—a proficiency that would appear to provide the bootstraps necessary for full linguistic competence. In her chapter, Eve Clark describes the acquisition process in terms of the developing lexicon and early syntax. She provides a review of early lexical development and proposes that the syntax of children "emerges as part and parcel of their lexical knowledge." On this view, children learn the syntactic forms that go with specific lexical items and with time build sets of words that are syntactically equivalent. Syntactic competence is thus the result of a gradual process of acquisition that is lexically based.

In the penultimate contribution, Sheila Blumstein discusses developments in the neurobiology of language, describing the current state of our understanding of how language is organized and processed in the brain—an understanding that has been constrained by the fact that much of the research in this domain has been performed on brain-damaged individuals. Despite this limitation, however, progress continues and, as Blumstein notes, the coming decades should produce even greater advances as imaging methodologies that enable us to examine on-line language processing in the normal brain gain in sophistication.

In the final contribution, Herbert Clark and Bridget Bly describe their view of language as a means of communication. Their concerns are with communicative acts—that is, with the elements necessary to describe the everyday use of language. Clark and Bly discuss the multiple levels at which communication occurs, the units of communication, and the principles that govern conversation, noting in particular the cooperative nature that exists between speaker and listener. They make clear, above all, that the use of language is a social phenomenon and that to understand language as communication requires understanding the role of psychological principles over and above those of traditional psycholinguistic theory and experimentation.

It was our intention in planning this volume to provide an overview of human language from the perception and production of the spoken signal at the segmental level to the comprehension and production of sentences and the processes underlying communicative acts. We believe that our objectives were well met by our contributors and we wish to express our appreciation to them for their efforts and for their forbearance with our editorial concerns.

Joanne L. Miller and Peter D. Eimas

CHAPTER 1

Issues of Representation in Psycholinguistics

Lyn Frazier

I. INTRODUCTION

There is at present no fully general consensus about where the line falls between linguistic and nonlinguistic representations or between symbolic and subsymbolic representations. There is no agreement about whether, or which, representations are localist versus distributed. However, no one today is making progress in the study of the acquisition, mental representation or processing of language without making assumptions about the nature of linguistic representations. Given that any research on language must make assumptions about these representations, it makes sense to rely on reasonable assumptions, that is, assumptions that are explicit, descriptively valid, and cast in a form that makes psycholinguistic and cross-language generalizations perspicuous.

Fortunately, the days are past when a serious researcher may invoke notions like *sentence, subject,* or *spoken word,* and then mumble something incoherent or indefensible concerning what these notions mean, such as "a string of words separated by pauses" (for sentence); "the first noun phrase in a sentence," "the noun phrase immediately preceding the(?) verb" or "agent" (for subject); or, "the sounds corresponding to a string of adjacent characters set off by spaces in conventional written language" (for spoken word). Such superficial and downright sloppy assumptions (hypotheses)

Speech, Language, and Communication

about linguistic representations are trivially falsified[1] and certainly merit no serious attention today, given that tenable, well-articulated, empirically motivated alternative hypotheses exist.

Linguistic theory is a theory of native speakers' underlying knowledge of their language. The general theory of language (Universal Grammar) includes a representational system and constraints on the well-formedness of linguistic representations. In phonology, for example, this might include a set of universally available distinctive features, together with constraints of several varieties, such as one allowing, in principle, specification of a secondary place of articulation of a sound but not a ternary one. Turning to syntax, the theory might specify a set of categorial features and basic syntactic relations as well as specific constraints such as one requiring a thematic role to be assigned to one and only one syntactic position; for example, the Patient role cannot be assigned to both the subject and object of a verb or to both the direct and indirect object. The theory of an individual language will also characterize the particular structures found in that language. Hence, the grammar of English and many other Indo-European languages will allow structures containing a questioned constituent at the beginning of the sentence (*Who did Max marry?*), whereas languages like Turkish or Japanese will not. Instead, they will contain structures in which a question particle appears after the questioned constituent.

The precise characterization of a structure provided by any particular hypothesized representational system can have far-reaching consequences for a theory of language processing. For example, are structures defined in terms of relations like *precedence* (A precedes B) and *dominance* (A dominates B; roughly going from B to the root node in a tree structure one must pass through A), or in terms like *immediate dominance* (A immediately dominates B, hence A is the first node above B)?

If dominance, not immediate dominance, is available for characterizing structures, then A immediately dominates B amounts to the statement that (1) A dominates B and (2) there is no node C such that C dominates B but does not dominate A. For parsing sentence structure, the difference between these characterizations of structural prominence can matter (Gorrell, 1992; Marcus, Hindle, & Fleck, 1983). If the parser can analyze a phrase B stating only that A dominates B, without committing itself to whether A immediately dominates B, then it will be possible later to postulate some new node D that intervenes between A and B without revising a prior (immediate dominance) decision. Instead, the postulation of D will be only an addition of new information consistent with all previously postulated structure. This illustrates an important point for present purposes, namely, that a representational system must not only describe the structures in a language but also be fully explicit about the exact representational vocabulary for defining or describing those structures.

The relation between linguistic theory and psycholinguistic theory thus comes down to issues concerning the way linguistic knowledge is mentally represented and the role it plays in particular language performance systems. The goal of linguistic theory is to provide the characterization of the structures found in any particular language using the most restrictive descriptive means consistent with the richness and variety of the languages of the world. The goal of psycholinguistics is to explain how linguistic knowledge is acquired and how it is mentally represented and used to actually produce and perceive language.

Any valid linguistic generalizations are likely to play a role in at least one of the performance systems: production, perception, or acquisition. Typically, generalizations that are not simply historical relics play an active role in all three systems (for discussion, see the Consistent Realization Hypothesis in Frazier, 1986).

Linguistic theory is in a state of flux like all growing sciences. It thus corresponds to an empirical hypothesis, or web of hypotheses, subject to repeated disconfirmation as new facts and generalizations are discovered. At any one time, linguistic theory may encompass a broad range of specific hypotheses, or even competing grammatical frameworks, being developed in detail and tested. This is a healthy state of affairs. It may, however, prove frustrating to specialists in another discipline who want to exploit a set of fixed unchanging linguistic assumptions in their own work. But to condemn or eschew linguistic theory because it develops over time is patently absurd and amounts to a demand that linguistics be a rigid dogma or religion.

But what is the nonlinguist to do? How may one develop a theory based on a developing theory? One solution is to "freeze" linguistic theory, choosing whatever explicit defensible framework researchers find most suited to their own area of inquiry and to proceed on the basis of that linguistic hypothesis. The only trick is to remember that the linguistic assumptions constitute a scientific hypothesis and therefore are open to subsequent revision based on new findings. Will this revision invalidate psycholinguistic studies based on those assumptions? Typically not. It simply means that the researcher's original conclusions may need to be reinterpreted or modified in light of new evidence, as in any scientific endeavor.

Making explicit assumptions about language structure and linguistic representation is necessary in psycholinguistic investigation, and it may turn out that these representational assumptions carry much of the explanatory burden in psycholinguistic theories, determining, for example, how language is acquired and mentally represented, why it is processed in the particular way it is, and even why the human language processing mechanism assumes the particular shape it does. The nature of the basic representational system for natural languages, along with the linguistic representations it defines, may explain many of the mysteries of the human language ability. Taken together with a few simple general processing assumptions, it may explain many of the characteristics of actual language performance systems as well. Put differently, the idiosyncratic characteristics of the language system(s) that distinguish them from, say, the visual system(s) may stem in large part from the characteristics of the representations that the language system(s) manipulate and not necessarily from the processing principles themselves.

II. THE REPRESENTATIONAL APPROACH: LET THE REPRESENTATIONS DO THE WORK

In order to illustrate this representational view of the language systems, I turn now to some actual examples. The examples are taken, in the first instance, from the area of syntactic or sentence processing, the area with which I am most familiar. The goals of a theory of syntactic processing are to explain how humans manage to assign an appropriate syntactic description to an input sentence in real time, and why the processor exhibits the particular properties it does. Given the restricted immediate memory capacity of humans and the existence of pervasive temporary ambiguity in natural language, the parsing problem is not trivial. For example, how can the perceiver know in advance how the string in (1) will continue?

(1) *John told the girl that Bill liked* . . .
   a. *John told the girl [that Bill liked the story].*
   b. *John told the girl that Bill liked the eggplant.*
   c. *John told [the girl that Bill liked] the story.*
   d. *John told the girl that Bill liked.*

With luck, it will continue as indicated in (1a), where *that Bill liked the story* forms a unit. This complement clause analysis is the analysis that the reader probably assigned. Hence, the reader probably has no difficulty processing the disambiguated complement clause sentence in (1b). Alternatively, the fragment in (1) might contain a relative clause (*the girl that Bill liked*), as indicated in (1c). If the fragment ends after *liked,* as in the disambiguated (1d), *the girl that Bill liked* must be interpreted as a relative clause. In contrast to (1c), where told takes two objects, in (1d), told takes only one. Thus, even figuring out verb structure requires disambiguation of the syntactic structure of the sentence.

Given unlimited immediate memory, the human perceiver could simply compute all analyses of a fragment and later throw out the disconfirmed ones. Or, perhaps the perceiver could just hold the entire string of words in memory and wait to assign a structure until disambiguating information was found. But the human perceiver does not have unlimited memory and there is no guarantee that disambiguating information will arrive, when it will arrive (if it does), or what shape the disambiguating information will take.

Much evidence (Frazier, 1987a, for review) suggests that human perceivers assign a syntactic structure to a sentence as each word is encountered, as illustrated in (2) for the string in (1):

(2)

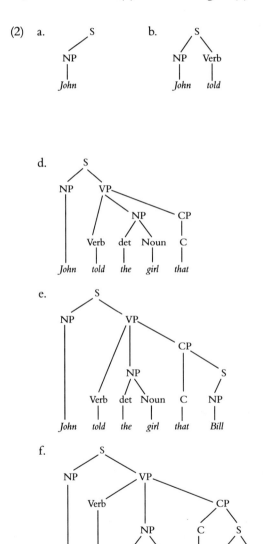

At each point the new word is connected into the developing sentence structure according to the Minimal Attachment Principle, which instructs the processor to postulate only as many nodes (phrases) as are required by the grammar of the language, in this case the grammar of English. Example (2c) shows the state of the representation after *the girl* is minimally attached into the structure. Given the structure in (2c), the complement clause analysis in (1a, 1b) naturally emerges as the preferred structure of a sentence like (1), since the alternative [the relative clause in (1c) and (1d)] requires a revision of existing relations. This revision involves the addition of a new N̄ node, circled in (3b):[2]

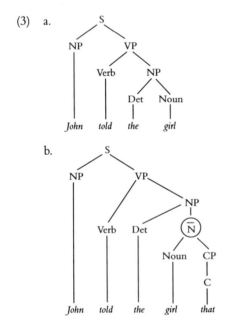

(3) a.

b.

Thus, according to the Minimal Attachment Principle, it is the direct attachment of *the girl* into VP that results in the complement clause preference in (1).

Direct attachment of a phrase without postulating potentially unnecessary nodes appears to be the source of many syntactic processing preferences. Considerable research shows that revisions of the first (simple) syntactic structure take extra processing time, and that revisions to the first analysis are not made unless necessary. Indeed, the Minimal Revisions Principle specifies that revisions of already-assigned structure or interpretation are made only when necessary, and even then revisions retain as much of the existing structure and interpretation as possible. Some revisions are not very costly in perceptual terms, but others may be and thus they may induce regressive eye movements in reading, for example (Frazier & Rayner, 1982; see Altmann, 1989, for an overview).

Notice that the general simplicity principles of Minimal Attachment and Minimal Revisions make empirical predictions about processing complexity across a range of disparate syntactic structures because of the property of those syntactic structures, for example, how many nodes they contain. Thus, it is the representational assumptions that determine which structures are postulated first, and which are easy to process and which are difficult.

Below, several additional examples are discussed in which an understanding of language processing is directly dependent on the assumptions made about the linguistic representation of the structure being processed. The purpose of the examples is to illustrate how a processing theory is dependent on an explicit theory of representation.

How does the language processing mechanism know what is a possible sentence structure? This is where the grammar of the language comes in. In a phrase-structure grammar, the notion of well-formed sentence is captured in a series of phrase-structure rules, shown in (4a), which are equivalent to the definitions in (4b):

(4) a. i. S $\rightarrow$ NP $-$ VP   b. S   = NP $-$ VP
    ii. NP $\rightarrow$ Det $-$ (Adj) $-$ Noun   NP = Det (Adj) Noun
    iii. VP $\rightarrow$ Verb $-$ (NP) $-$ (CP)   VP = Verb $-$ (NP)(CP)
    iv. CP $\rightarrow$ Complementizer $-$ S   CP = Complementizer $-$ S

These rules must be embellished to capture the full range of English sentences. Also, the rules might look slightly different for another language. For example, the verb phrase rule in (4aiii) would have the verb at the end, instead of the beginning, if this were the grammar of Dutch, German, Turkish, or Japanese, where objects precede the verb.

In the principles and parameters framework of Chomsky (1981) and much subsequent work, universal principles of grammar are parameterized, meaning that they have open positions where languages may exhibit variation within some limited range of options. In the ideal case, an entire host of superficially unrelated properties might follow from the setting of one parameter. (Note that for theories of language acquisition, this could be important in essentially clueing in the child about the language type being acquired: evidence about any one characteristic of the language would suffice; evidence about other consequences of the parameter would be unnecessary.)

Take the rules in (4), for example. They may be decomposed into invariant principles and parameterized principles. The invariant principles are fully universal, for example, each phrase of type X must contain a word of type X (the *head*), which determines the properties of the phrase; any object of the head (e.g., the direct object of the verb) must appear adjacent to the head of the phrase.

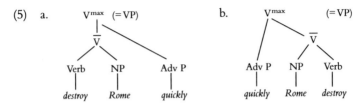

(5) a. V^{max} (=VP)
Verb NP Adv P
destroy Rome quickly

b. V^{max} (=VP)
Adv P NP Verb
quickly Rome destroy

The parameterized principles contain an option, fixed by language-specific data; for example, any object of the head must precede?/follow? the head. The resulting structures are illustrated in (5) for verb phrases. In (5), V^{max}, the maximal projection of the verb (called the *verb phrase*), dominates some nonargument (adverb) phrase Adv P and $\bar{V}$. $\bar{V}$ is the verbal projection that dominates the verb and its internal (object) arguments.[3] Since the principles do not mention specific syntactic categories, they also permit the noun, adjectival, and pre-/postposition to project phrases, as in (6).

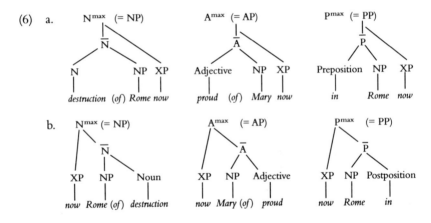

(6) a. N^{max} (= NP)
N NP XP
destruction (of) Rome now

A^{max} (= AP)
Adjective NP XP
proud (of) Mary now

P^{max} (= PP)
Preposition NP XP
in Rome now

b. N^{max} (= NP)
XP NP Noun
now Rome (of) destruction

A^{max} (= AP)
XP NP Adjective
now Mary (of) proud

P^{max} (= PP)
XP NP Postposition
now Rome in

In capturing crosslinguistic generalizations, this approach has been quite successful in two respects. First, it appears that languages do tend to order heads of phrases systematically before or systematically after the object within a given language. In English, heads regularly precede objects as shown in (5a) and (6a); whereas, in Japanese and Turkish, heads systematically follow their objects, as in (5b) and (6b), in NPs, APs, PPs, and VPs. Mixed languages do also occur, however. For example, in Dutch the VP is head-final, as in (5b) but other phrases are usually head-initial, as in (6a). The mixed case is claimed to be *marked* or exceptional. Second, and perhaps more important than its empirical success, however, the principles and parameters view has defined one extremely productive approach to linguistic investigation, prompting linguists to search for potential correlations corresponding to the consequences of setting some particular parameter of language variation.

Often the analysis of a construction is murky looking only at the one construction in just one language. But relating the construction to other structures within the language and to other languages often renders the analysis transparent. For example, *of* appears superficially to be a preposition in a phrase like *destruction of Rome*. However, deeper linguistic analysis suggests it is simply a casemarker for the object of a noun or adjective, and does not assign a thematic role such as Patient or project to a syntactic phrase, that is, a prepositional phrase. Notice, for example, that there is no PP dominating *of* in (6a). The correct linguistic analysis becomes obvious once a phrase like *of Rome,* the postnominal object in (6a), is compared to *Rome* in (5a), where *Rome* again appears after the head (the verb) and serves as object of the head (verb). Similar remarks apply to the prenominal object in (6b) and the preverbal object in (5b). The expected position of an object in English, the position after its head, reinforces the notion that *Rome* is the object of *destruction* in (6a) and *of* is just a casemarker. It is quite commonly the case that the analysis of an isolated phrase is unclear but becomes transparent once the phrase is related to other phrases of the language and to the expected situation in other languages.

The above linguistic analysis of *of* is confirmed by a psycholinguistic study of relative clause interpretation preferences in Spanish and English. Consider the ambiguous phrases in (7):

(7) a. *the table of wood that had been destroyed*
   [*the* **table** *of* [*wood*$_{NP}$]$_{NP}$]
   b. *the photograph of the tree that had been destroyed*
   [*the* **photograph** *of* [*the tree*$_{NP}$]$_{NP}$]
   c. *the car near the tree that had been destroyed*
   the car [**near** [*the tree*$_{NP}$]$_{PP}$]

The relative clause *that had been destroyed* is usually interpreted by subjects as modifying the second noun (*tree*) in (7c), whereas subjects allow the relative clause to modify either the second or the first noun in (7a) and (7b) (Gilboy, Sopena, Clifton, & Frazier, in press).

What is the difference between (7c) and (7a,7b)? In (7c) the last head of a phrase that assigns a thematic role is the preposition *near*. By contrast, in (7a,7b) the last thematic role assigner is the first noun [*table* in (7a), *photograph* in (7b)]. By hypothesis, the phrasal projection of the last thematic role assigner [the entire noun phrase in (7a,7b), the PP in (7c)] defines the current processing domain. The relative clause simply associates into the current processing domain in all cases. Only in (7c) does this result in a systematic preference, that is, for the second noun (*tree*) to be the head of the relative clause. The same processing assumptions (roughly, relate adjuncts like relative clauses to material within the current thematic processing domain) explain several other preferences, too. But the point, again, is that the underlying representational assumptions bear the weight of the empirical predictions of the processing hypothesis. In the particular case at hand, it is only because *of* is treated as a casemarker, rather than a thematic role assigner, that (7a,7b) are distinguished from (7c). Indeed, in examples where *of* does assign a thematic role, the Possessor role in cases of alienable possession, *of* like *near* in (7c), projects to a full PP. As predicted, in this case subjects will interpret a following relative clause to modify the second noun just as in (7c), as in *the car of the man that was on the corner.*

Adult psycholinguistic evidence also provides support for the analysis linguistic theory provides for the relation between questioned constituents (e.g., *who* and *what*) and the position where they receive their thematic role, indicated by a dash in (8):

(8) a. *Who did John see ___?*
$$|\rule{4cm}{0.4pt}|$$

  b. *What did John see ___?*
$$|\rule{4cm}{0.4pt}|$$

In cases where this syntactic dependency spans more than one grammatical domain (for simplicity, more than one clause), many linguists analyze the dependency as a series of local dependencies (Chomsky, 1973, 1977, 1981), as illustrated in (9):

(9) *Who did you think [that John saw ___]?*
$$|\rule{3cm}{0.4pt}|\ |\rule{3cm}{0.4pt}|$$

This conclusion, too, has received psycholinguistic support in terms of increases in processing complexity correlated with the complexity of the grammatical composition of a long dependency (Frazier & Clifton, 1989). Such psycholinguistic support is striking, since it exists despite the fact that no superficially apparent observation about a sentence forces a long syntactic dependency to be broken up into a series of local dependencies.

Much recent attention has focused on the typology of empty categories in natural language, that is, what kinds of phonetically empty phrases exist in syntactic representations. Considerable evidence from reading-time studies (e.g., Clifton & Frazier, 1989; de Vincenzi, 1991; Frazier & Flores d'Arcais, 1989), secondary-load studies (Wanner & Maratsos, 1978), priming studies (e.g., Nicol, 1988; Swinney, Nicol, Ford, Frauenfelder, & Bresnan, 1987; Tanenhaus, Carlson, & Seidenberg, 1985), and probe recognition studies (e.g., Bever & McElree, 1988; Foder, 1989) shows that perceivers postulate an empty object following the verb *see* in questions like (8) and (9) and immediately relate this empty object to the question words that determine its interpretation. In priming studies, for example, investigators exploit the already-established facilitation effect that emerges when naming (or making a lexical decision on) a target semantically associated to a word that appeared immediately before the target. In studies of the relation between a questioned phrase and its gap (e.g., the relation between *which girl* and the position following *see* in *Which girl do you think the principal wanted to see ____ before scheduling the conference?*), investigators have demonstrated priming for *boy* immediately following *see,* but no priming for *boy* when it appears in positions intervening between *girl* and the position of the gap following *see*. This suggests that processing of the relation between the questioned phrase and its gap reactivates the questioned phrase *which girl,* which then acts as if it occurred immediately before the target (*boy*). (I give this example only as an illustration of the type of study that has been done. Investigators have actually tested an array of different structures.)

Current debate focuses on issues such as whether empty pronominals (e.g., the "missing" subject in Italian) are treated like the empty phrases involved in question formation [e.g., in (8) and (9)], how the obligatorily empty object in a passive [see (10)] is processed, and the like.

(10)   a.   *The table was built ___ by John.*
             | _____ |

       b.   **The table was built the house by John.*

In each of these cases, our understanding of how the syntactic structure of the sentence is processed depends directly on our representational assumptions. Where linguistic theories differ, competing psycholinguistic hypotheses are often developed. Choosing between them may in turn contribute to the resolution of the linguistic debate.[4]

III. OPEN ISSUES IN SYNTACTIC AND SEMANTIC REPRESENTATION

I turn now to discussion of several open issues that confront what I have called the representational approach to language processing and begin by examining the area of syntax and, to a lesser extent, semantics.

A. Precompilation of Grammatical Knowledge

To this point in the chapter discussion of psycholinguistic results has illustrated the dependence of processing hypotheses on the linguistic representations assigned to particular sentences. Now as I take up issues of precompilation, I look instead at the mental representation of the grammar itself, that is, at the format in which humans store the grammatical knowledge that permits a well-formed representation to be assigned to a (novel) word, phrase, or sentence.

Are grammatical principles precompiled? For purposes of sentence production, it might be simplest to project phrasal structure directly from the word that heads the phrase, at least in cases where the speaker can specify this information first, before the speaker can specify the nature of any dependent items. Thus, grammatical principles may not need to be precompiled in an efficient sentence production device. But what about the case of sentence comprehension, where the processor is clearly not in control of the temporal order of input items? Consider syntactic rules such as those shown in (4). They essentially provide a template that may be matched against a (lexically analyzed) input sentence. More abstract principles like those requiring a head for each phrase, or those requiring a match between the syntactic features of the head and the features of its phrasal projection, do not directly constrain the properties of the input string of words. The precompilation issue amounts to the question of whether, and if so, how, the joint consequences of distinct principles of grammar are computed or precompiled to form templates or generalizations about the superficial or surface properties of the input.

Though the precompilation issue is also relevant to language acquisition, I address it only in the case of adult language processing, since this is where my competence lies. Imagine that the adult sentence processor (at least) operates directly with the principle requiring each phrase to be headed, without precompiling the effect of this principle together with the principle determining head–object order or the principle requiring the head and its projection (the phrase node) to bear matching syntactic category features. In this system, a phrasal node should be postulated only once the head has been encountered (except maybe in contexts where the existence of a particular syntactic category can be predicted in advance). In English, the VP node, for example, could be projected immediately as soon as the verb occurred. But in a verb-final language, such as Dutch, Japanese, or Turkish, the processor would need to wait to postulate the VP until after its objects appeared, since the verb (the head) follows them. Do such delays in node postulation actually occur in the processing of a head-final language? Little evidence exists at present. (See Frazier, 1987b, for evidence that such delays do not occur in head-final Dutch VPs. This evidence suggests that the grammar is used in precompiled form.) The point here is simply that one may empirically address issues about the form in which grammatical knowledge is mentally represented by forming detailed hypotheses about how that information is exploited during actual language performance. The form in which the grammatical knowledge is stored will then determine what grammatical decisions must be made on-line by the language processor, and determine when in principle they may be made (as in the Dutch example).

B. The Architecture of the Language Processing System

A related set of questions concerns the architecture of the language processing system. How is it organized into subsystems that may perform simple coherent tasks? It seems likely to me that this is accomplished on the basis of the type of vocabulary needed for linguistic representation. The vocabulary of phonology (e.g., notions like *syllable* or features like *consonantal*) for the most part does not overlap with the vocabulary of the syntax (V, VP, A, AP, etc., *sisterhood, c-command, coindexation, government,* and the like). Further, even within the sentence syntax, the syntax of phrases (discussed above) seems largely independent from the syntax governing nonlocal dependencies between two widely separated phrases or positions [e.g., the dependency between *who* in (8) and (9) and its gap, the empty phrase following *see* and *saw* in (8) and (9)].

Perhaps the decomposition of the language processing system into subsystems is determined by clusters of rules or principles that share with each other the same theoretical vocabulary (e.g., mentioning terms like verbs and verb phrases, not consonants and vowels) and the same definitions of, say, "local domain" (e.g., requiring codependents to be in the same phrase vs. in the same syllable). On this view, the language processing system may have natural fractures or divisions emerging from the nature of the represented knowledge itself. Clear divisions that suggest themselves include divisions between the phrasal syntax and the phonology, for example, but also the division within the syntax between local dependencies between sisters (two nodes immediately dominated by the same node) and (potentially) nonlocal dependencies, involving structurally dominant versus subordinate phrases (e.g., the dependency between *who* and its associated gap).

A competing but similar hypothesis might imply that distinct levels of grammatical representation (e.g., deep structure, surface structure, logical form, phonetic form) serve as the basis for defining processing subsystems. On any such account linguistic representation will play a fundamental descriptive and explanatory role in specifying and understanding the language processor. And it will largely determine what information will be available to resolve grammatical decisions, assuming priority of within-module information. For example, a processor with distinct syntactic versus semantic modules predicts that syntactic analysis itself will be unaffected by the presence of semantic anomalies in the input sentence. Hence, even with anomalous sentences, syntactically well-formed strings of words, for example, *The bee sued,* should be processed more quickly and accurately than syntactically ill-formed ones, *Bee the sued* (Marslen-Wilson & Tyler, 1980, for empirical evidence). This follows, since disruptions in processing due to the anomaly are predicted to lie outside the syntactic processing module. In a model with distinct modules for local (constituent structure) versus nonlocal (binding) syntactic dependencies, similar predictions obtain, for example, binding ill-formedness should not interfere with constituent structure processing if binding lies outside the constituent structure module (see Freedman & Forster, 1985, for discussion, but also Crain & Fodor, 1987). Put concretely, in *Bill liked herself* or in *Herself liked Mary* the violation in the binding of the reflexive (*herself*) is predicted not to interfere with phrase postulation, for example, with identification of *Bill* as subject or of *Mary* as the direct object. Given the hypothesis of separate modules for necessarily local versus possibly long-distance dependencies, the reflexive binding and phrase postulation are simply separate tasks, treated as being distinct from each other in advance of any particular input sentence.

C. The Interface between (Sub)Systems

The interface between distinct grammatical processing subsystems, whatever they may turn out to be, must involve some (limited) sharing of representational vocabulary or else no communication between subsystems would be possible. Identifying this overlapping vocabulary would place strong constraints on the type of processing hypotheses that could be considered.

The interface issue also arises with respect to grammatical versus non-grammatical processing systems. In syntax, thematic roles play a purely formal role regulated by the Theta criterion, which specifies that a given role may be assigned to only one position (see Chomsky, 1981). Several investigators have proposed that thematic roles (agent, patient, instrument, etc.) provide the vocabulary shared by the syntax and by the system for representing nonlinguistic knowledge about the properties of actual objects. Carlson and Tanenhaus (1989) develop this view and propose a system of explicit principles for determining the thematic roles of verbs in particular. They argue that the thematic roles of a verb are entered into the discourse representation, even if the roles are not syntactically expressed. The open or unexpressed roles may be used to integrate subsequent items into the discourse representation. For example, in (11a) *unloaded* has a theme role, the thing unloaded, which remains unexpressed.

(11) a. *John unloaded his car. The suitcase was very heavy.*
b. *John ran to catch his plane. The suitcase was very heavy.*

When the second sentence in (11a) occurs, *the suitcase* may be taken to instantiate this open thematic role, facilitating comprehension of the second sentence. Indeed, Tanenhaus and Carlson present comprehension time evidence suggesting that the second sentence of (11a) is understood more quickly by readers than the second sentence in (11b). This supports the idea that the representations themselves, in the present instance open thematic roles, may mediate the relation between subsystems. In the present example, the representations constructed by the sentence subsystem guide the operations of the subsystem responsible for integrating individual sentences into a structured discourse representation.

D. Representation of Unexpressed Arguments

Another series of extremely fundamental issues concerns the representation of unexpressed roles (see previous section) and unexpressed or implicit variables. A word like *son* or *enemy* contains an implicit variable, since each inherently entails a relation to an unexpressed entity (*son of X* or *enemy of X*). Is this implicit variable represented in the grammatical representation of a sentence or is it simply something the perceiver can infer given the meaning of the words? (See Partee, 1989.) A similar example is the implicit variable in a perspectival word like *local* (*near X*) in (12), in which X may be bound by either *Max, Penny,* or the speaker (see Mitchell, 1986). Is this implicit variable represented in the grammatical representation of (12)?

(12) *Max thought Penny went to the local bar.*

Understanding what inferences are drawn under what conditions during language comprehension will depend in part on the answer to these currently open representational questions. It is important to know which representations always contain variables and to figure out what types of variables may or must be bound under what conditions during language processing. Given well-motivated answers to questions about the representation of implicit arguments and variables, language processing may reduce to the task of selecting a legitimate grammatical representation of the input from a highly circumscribed set of possibilities, and then integrating that representation with context, maintaining coherence. To the extent that the representations are rich in guiding interpretation and to the extent that the set of possible representations to choose from is narrowly circumscribed, the processing task itself may be trivialized, like the task of following a well-designed map with all important points of destination clearly marked.

E. Definition of the Search Space: How Many Representations?

Fundamental to the success of the representational approach is resolving the issue of vagueness versus ambiguity in linguistic representation. Wherever vagueness is permitted in the representation manipulated by one subsystem, there is room for later specification by another subsystem. An immediate choice between possibilities is unnecessary. By contrast, where ambiguity (multiple representations) is involved, either revision of a single representation will be needed at times, whenever the unpreferred structure is correct, or multiple analyses must be assigned. Delay in the sense of resolution by a distinct processing system is not a possibility, assuming that the constraints needed to define the well-formedness of linguistic representation are not (redundantly) represented in more than one processing subsystem.

To take a concrete example, how many meanings does a word like *head* or *turn* have? When is a word ambiguous?; when is it vague? The difficulty of distinguishing ambiguity from vagueness arises not only with respect to implicit variables and the representation of word meanings, but also in decisions about what underspecification grammatical theory permits in syntactic, and phonological, representations. For example, linguistic arguments (Culicover & Rochemont, 1990) and psycholinguistic evidence (Frazier & Clifton, in press) indicate that certain adjuncts may receive a syntactic analysis that is underspecified, that is, their syntactic representation in effect does not specify whether the phrase is a sister of the associated VP or a sister of the S dominating that VP. From this it almost immediately follows that the purely structural parsing principles responsible for quick syntactic analysis do not govern interpretation preference in this case. The parser simply has no need to make an early commitment.

In logical form and discourse representation, the issue of vagueness arises in terms of what must obligatorily be specified. For example, is the resolution of quantifier scope in (13) representationally dictated in the sense that no well-formed logical form exists unless the quantifiers have been assigned determinate scope relations?

(13) *Everybody loves somebody sometime.*

In some theories, yes, in some theories, no. Barbara Partee (personal communication) suggests that the surface syntactic representation of the sentence may itself constitute a vague or underspecified representation of scope relations (which may later be determinately specified when biasing semantic, discourse, or world knowledge is supplied). These issues remain open to date. But what decisions the processor must make depend on the resolution of questions of this type.

In discourse representation, a related matter arises, namely, what parameters of discourse are always specified and thus automatically available? Indexicals (*here, now*) suggest that speech time and place must be represented. The obligatory choice of first, second, or third person forms (P1–P3) suggest that speaker(s) (P1), hearer(s) (P2), and others (P3) must be distinguished, possibly along with number and other grammatical features that are obligatorily marked in the language.

In English, tense marking is obligatory (past vs. nonpast) but evidential markers (distinguishing firsthand report from inferred or secondhand reports) are not. In Turkish, both tense and evidential markers are obligatory. How do cross-language differences in the obligatoriness of grammatical markers influence the structure or parameterization of the discourse model?

IV. ISSUES IN PHONOLOGICAL REPRESENTATION

I turn now to issues in phonological representation. With respect to precompilation, modularity, and the interface of distinct representation types, they parallel those issues already discussed. When it comes to determining the target representation of phonological processes, however, several new representational questions arise that do not directly parallel issues in syntactic representation. These concern the nature and status of underlying phonological representations. In syntax, the underlying (deep structure) representation of a sentence presumably must be recovered by the perceiver in order to determine the argument structure of the sentence, for example, to figure out which phrases correspond to which argument of the verb. By contrast, in phonology, it would be possible in principle for the perceiver to store (a family of) surface phonological representations of a word and to contact these, at least on occasions when the input consists of a familiar or already-encountered word of the language.

A. The Target Representations: Surface Representations or Underlying Ones?

The possible role of underlying representations in phonological processing depends on the assumptions made about the nature of these representations. In phonology, it is quite generally accepted (e.g., Archangeli, 1984) that underlying representations are underspecified and contain only contrastive or unpredictable information. For example, the nasality of vowels need not be represented if vowels are always (and only) nasalized when they occur before nasal consonants. In the surface representation, all feature values are specified, both the predictable and the unpredictable ones. If an under-specified underlying representation is the only phonological representation of a morpheme or word that is stored in memory, then an enormous amount of computation will be required during speech perception or production. Alternatively, surface representations might also be stored for all words or for only some, for example, complex words derived from relatively unproductive Level 1 affixation, the affixes like -*ion* or -*ity,* which in principle may alter the stress pattern of a word.

Lahiri and Marslen-Wilson (1991) present evidence that only under-specified underlying representations are involved in speech recognition. Bengali speakers were presented with homophonous words containing nasal vowels. Bengali has contrastive nasal vowels, specified as nasal in underlying representation. It also contains vowels that are nasalized due to the operation of a phonological rule. In the Bengali experiment, the ambiguous word had two analyses. On one analysis (14a) the nasal vowel was specified as [+nasal] in the underlying representation because this specification was contrastive or unpredictable:

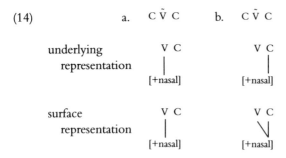

(14)   a. C Ṽ C   b. C Ṽ C

On the other analysis (14b) the nasal vowel was unspecified for nasality in the underlying representation because the nasality was predictable from the occurrence of a following nasal consonant (vowels before nasal consonants are always nasalized in Bengali). Bengali listeners showed a systematic preference to perceive and report the nasalization as evidence of an underlying nasal vowel, not as surface nasalization due to the presence of a following nasal consonant. This supports the idea that listeners try to match spoken words to their underlying phonological representations that thus receive priority in accounting for surface features of the input. Why this would occur if stored surface representations were available to the listeners is unclear.

The issue of what phonological representation (surface or underlying) is stored is difficult to resolve, precisely because in principle, at least, fully specified surface phonological representations for listed morphemes and words could be already present in the perceiver's lexicon. (This contrasts with the phrasal phonology that captures phonological regularities concerning the way a word is altered depending on the phonological properties of the larger syntactic and semantic context in which it occurs.) Storing the many surface forms of a word might be costly in some respects, especially given the numerous dialectal and social-register variants of words. High storage costs and access costs, because of large search sets, might thus be imposed. However, this option would also save on the computational cost imposed by the derivation from underlying form to surface form. Surprisingly little decisive psycholinguistic evidence exists that would help choose between the various possibilities (though see the discussion of Lahiri & Marslen-Wilson, 1991, above).

B. Precompilation

Precompilation issues arise concerning phonological representation regardless of whether it is a surface or an underlying representation that is at stake. The question is whether information of distinct types is already integrated into a complex representation where each element bears a determinate relation to each other element. For example, in current phonological theory, tone is represented autosegmentally, that is, on a different tier from information about the segmental makeup of a word (Goldsmith, 1976). The segmental composition is itself represented on distinct planes (McCarthy, 1989) with consonants on one plane and vowels on another. This separation onto distinct tiers or planes allows phonologists to capture well-attested locality effects whereby only adjacent segments influence each other. But the adjacency that matters is adjacency on a plane. For example, in (15) A and C are adjacent in the relevant respect but A and D are not:

(15) a. A B C D   (where A, C, and D = consonants, B = vowel)

    b. A   C D
        | | |
      x x x x
        |
        B

With respect to speech perception, it is unclear whether only the representation of the individual planes is available, as in (15b), or whether the precompiled representation in (15a), matching the surface input, is available. To exploit phonological regularities, (15b) might be more useful, since it transparently captures crucial notions of phonological locality. But for purposes of exploiting coarticulation effects, perhaps (15a) more perspicuously captures the dependence of C on B. Thus, it is difficult to argue on a priori grounds whether (15a), (15b), or both are represented mentally.

C. Architectural Issues: Modularity

Issues of modularity arise with respect to the processing of prosody. The temporal patterning of an utterance and its intonation (pitch contours) may perhaps be represented and processed separately from each other and probably are represented and processed separately from segmental information.[5] Take, for example, a simple case like the noun *convict* or the verb *convict*. Are they represented and processed, as implied by (16b), with the prosody separate from the segmental makeup, or with the two together, as in (16a)?

(16) W (= word)   O = onset   () = appendix
      σ (= syllable)   R = rime   N = nucleus
      σ$_s$ (= strong syllable) C = coda

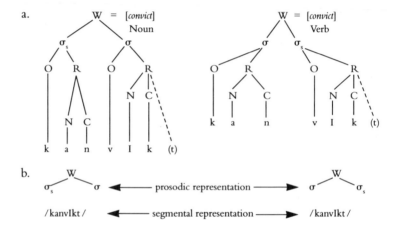

(16a) contains not only the unpredictable aspects of prosodic structure (whether it is the first or the second syllable that is stressed, here represented by assignment of a strong syllable) but also a lot of predictable information concerning the structure of an English syllable. All syllables must have a nucleus and the nucleus must be the most sonorous segment in the syllable (the vowels in the examples), with a decrease in sonority as one proceeds from the nucleus to either the beginning or the end of the syllable. Hence, the syllabic parsing of the segmental representation in (16b) is fully predictable. Given only the information in (16b), together with general constraints on the possible syllables of English, the representations in (16a) are fully predictable. One question is whether this predictable information is mentally represented in a fully specified representation like that in (16a). Another question, particularly salient if the actual mental representation is more like (16b), is whether the two parts of the representation are used by the same processing subsystem? One possibility is that the prosodic representation might primarily be used to inform whatever subsystem of the processor constructs metrical representations of phrases and sentences; another is that segmental representation might inform the auditory word recognition device.

D. Interface Issues

The interface between phonology and phonetics, on one hand, and between these and general (not specifically linguistic) auditory and motor systems, on the other, is an issue of central concern to contemporary phoneticians and phonologists (e.g., see Kingston & Beckman, 1990). In both phonetics and phonology, the relation between different features, *feature geometry,* is currently receiving considerable attention (Sagey, 1986; Selkirk, 1992). Feature geometry specifies the general relations between different features, determining which ones predominate over which others. For example, the features for *backness* and *rounding* are highly correlated in natural languages. Does the specification for backness determine that for rounding, or vice versa? As it turns out, the vocalic feature for backness typically determines the vocalic feature for rounding in most languages.

Apparently feature geometry is part of the phonology, though the phonetic implementation rules of the language must also make reference to it. It is unclear at present precisely how the formal representation of this and other aspects of sound structure influences processing. It would be extremely surprising if they had no effect, for example, if the processor were insensitive to which feature values are contrastive in a language and to which features determine the values of which other features. To assume this would be to assume that the perceiver places equal perceptual weight on important features and on predictable consequences of those features. Similar remarks apply to the language producer. One may speculate that the influence of a particular language on the motor control programs for articulation is mediated by the dominance relations of the native language feature geometry. If so, there may be subtle motor program consequences of the particular native language a person speaks reflecting the dominance hierarchy of the feature geometry of the language.

Before leaving this section, it should be admitted that here and throughout I have brushed aside suggestions that phonology is fundamentally different from syntax in requiring rules and rule ordering (Bromberger & Halle, 1989). I have also ignored ongoing debates about the explicit representation of rules, as such, which is particularly relevant to the area of phonology and morphology (Pinker & Prince, 1988; Prince & Smolensky, 1991, 1992; Rumelhart and McClelland, 1986; Seidenberg, 1991). Instead, certain aspects of these issues have been handled indirectly. The issue of explicit representation of rules here falls under the rubric of precompilation of principles, since in the most extreme case the consequences of all rules are precompiled into actual stored forms of particular items. This is perhaps possible in at least some domains of phonology and morphology, such as inflectional morphology (see references above).

V. ISSUES OF LEXICAL REPRESENTATION

Many issues of lexical representation exist. As in the representation of phonological and syntactic knowledge, questions arise about whether predictable information is explicitly represented, and about whether lexical items formed by general derivational and inflectional morphology are stored at all and, if so, whether they are stored as surface or underlying phonological forms. What is special about the lexicon, however, is that it establishes a connection between the various representations within the grammatical representational systems. It captures arbitrary pairings of phonological forms and semantic forms, for example. Lexical representations may also connect linguistic representations of words to nonlinguistic representations, for example, ones in semantic memory. Hence, the lexicon may serve as an interface between subsystems. However, given evidence for, say, the distinctness of phonological versus syntactic representational and processing subsystems, one interesting question is whether the lexicon itself is modular or whether it is, so to speak, the translation center, thus directly mediating between distinct vocabulary types. It is this question that I pursue here.

Is there a nontrivial notion of *lexical entry* corresponding to the notion of a dictionary entry, that is, a package of all grammatical information concerning a particular word or morpheme? This possibility is illustrated in (17):[6]

(17) *Kill*
    phonological representation   /kIl/
    syntactic representation   Verb: [__NP]
    thematic representation   (Agent, Patient)
    semantic representation   X CAUSE (Y DIE)

The assumption underlying this representation is that the entire package coheres. To access *kill* is to recover this bundle of information.[7]

Alternatively, the notion of a lexical entry may be misleading. Perhaps the human mind really contains a lexicon of phonological forms, organized according to phonological principles, and a lexicon of semantic forms, organized according to semantic principles, as is often assumed in language production studies (Levelt, 1989). Of course, since the lexical pairing of sound and meaning is arbitrary, it would be necessary to assume the existence of a pointer indicating the correspondence between a phonological form and its semantic form.

These two hypotheses about lexical organization seem to make distinct predictions about the role of frequency. On the lexical entry theory, each entry should have its own characteristic frequency of occurrence. The frequency of its homophone, if it has one, should be irrelevant. This contrasts with the view in which the phonological lexicon simply contains phonological forms. If two words have the same phonological form, then this form should be accessed more often than it would be for either word alone. Hence, a homophonous word should be recognized *more* quickly than an otherwise similar unambiguous word, for example, one of comparable length and frequency as measured by the occurrence of form-meaning pairs. The empirical evidence seems to favor the view that homophones are recognized more quickly than are unambiguous words (see discussion in Millis & Button, 1989).

Yet another possibility is proposed by Schmauder (1992). She suggests that neither lexical entries nor forms are organized. Instead, the features contained in lexical entries inherently define dimensions that implicitly organize the lexicon. Indeed, she suggests that two feature types exist: grammatical features, with consequences in the grammatical subsystems, and conceptual features, which also have consequences outside the grammatical representation system. She uses this distinction to capture differential effects of sentential context on the processing of words composed primarily of grammatical features versus those with substantial conceptual features. Put crudely, those items lacking substantial, conceptually interpretable features (roughly, closed-class terms and can't-stand-alone open-class items) benefit more from presentation in a sentential context (which invokes the interpretive system for grammatical features) than do items ladened with conceptually interpretable features, which can be interpreted by using general conceptual knowledge (see also Shillcock & Bard, 1991; Taft, 1990).

VI. CONCLUSIONS

The need for explicit, well-motivated linguistic representations in psycholinguistics has been discussed, along with the possibility that much of the predictive and explanatory work of psycholinguistic theories may derive from the properties of these representations and from the (theoretical) vocabulary and constraints needed to generate or describe them. Natural classes of representations emerge and in my view these probably offer the rationale for the particular way the language processor is modularized, determining the overall architecture of the system and the relation between subsystems. On this approach, it is essentially the representations that define the (sub)tasks of language comprehension and regulate the interplay between subsystems.

Open questions remain about whether distinct principles are precompiled into a form matching surface properties of the input. Extremely important questions also remain concerning what aspects of structure or meaning must obligatorily be specified within each subsystem or representation type. But to attempt to conduct psycholinguistic investigation without explicit representational assumptions is to leave the search space of possible solutions undefined, whether this be in the area of language acquisition, production, or perception. By contrast, an explicit representational theory equips the investigator, and the language performance system, with a relatively precise map indicating just where a decision must be made and the information necessary to make it.

Acknowledgments

This work was supported by Grant HD18708 to Charles Clifton and the author. I am extremely grateful to the editors of this volume and to Charles Clifton for extensive comments on the initial draft of this chapter. I would also like to thank Lisa Selkirk and John McCarthy for discussion of phonology.

Endnotes

1. Pauses typically occur at phonological and intonational phrase boundaries, not just at sentence boundaries, falsifying the pausal definition of sentence. Furthermore, native speakers of a language hear a pause at sentence boundaries whether a period of acoustic silence occurs or not. As for the definition of subject, in a sentence like *Last night the stadium near the beltline collapsed,* the subject is the noun phrase *the stadium near the beltline.* This is neither the first noun phrase in the sentence, the last noun phrase before the verb (which is the phrase *the beltline*), nor an Agent. Therefore, the example disconfirms each of the facile definitions of subject considered in the text. Turning to the definition of the problematic notion of *word,* one must be more precise about whether, for example, it is a phonological [e.g., *corner's* in (i)] or a syntactic notion of word [e.g., *corner* in (i)] that one is trying to define.

   (i) $[[[$ *The boy on the* $[corner_N]'_{NP}]_{S_{Det}}]hat_{NP}]$ *has blown off*

   The conventional written words do not correspond directly to either, as (i) shows. *Corner's* is not a syntactic word; *has* is not a phonological word (except perhaps in the speech of airline attendants, where the auxiliary may be treated as a phonological word).

2. Some theories of phrase structure require three levels of structure to always be present in a phrase, regardless of whether the middle level is distinct from the highest phrasal node itself. By contrast, I assume that a nonbranching $\bar{X}$ node, an $\bar{N}$ node between N and NP in (3a), is not syntactically required and thus is not postulated until or unless it must dominate two constituents.

3. It is really $\bar{V}$ that was defined in (4).

4. The principles and parameters approach has been quite successful in stimulating linguistic research and turning up generalizations and analyses confirmed by psycholinguistic studies of sentence comprehension. However, in my opinion the particular idea of parameters as

the description of possible variation across languages and the representational underpinnings for the language acquisition device, has been successful in only limited domains, null subject phenomena (Hyams, 1986, 1992) and binding theory (Manzini & Wexler, 1987), for example. Few actual parameters have been worked out in detail in a manner consistent with all known language and dialect variation. The conclusion I would draw from this is that we need a richer but perhaps slightly different set of representational assumptions to characterize the means available to children for representing the speech in their environment. My own bias is that a few general minimality and uniqueness preference principles (Borer & Wexler, 1987; Wexler, 1990), together with subset principles requiring cautious generalizations (Berwick, 1985; Crain, Drozd, Philip, & Roeper, 1992; Manzini & Wexler, 1987) may do considerable work in guiding the acquisition process (much on par with the approach to adult processing advocated above), but only if the child is assumed to be equipped with a rich and well-articulated system for representing utterances.

5. The mere existence of drum-and-whistle speech, which preserves only prosodic properties of utterances, suggests at the very least that it is possible to process prosody in the absence of segmental information.

6. The representation in (17) uses standard notation where [__NP] indicates the verb is transitive, requiring a following NP, and the external (subject) argument is distinguished by underlining it.

7. Balota (1990) discusses the assumption that there is a "magic moment" when the correct phonological or orthographic form of a word has been identified, granting access to all information stored with the word. Viewing things this way, the form of a word might be considered the name of the lexical entry—in essence, a distinguished property of the entry itself.

References

Altmann, G. T. M. (1989). Parsing and interpretation: An introduction. In G. T. M. Altmann (Ed.), *Language and cognitive processes: Special issue on parsing and interpretation* (pp. 1–20). Hove, UK: Lawrence Erlbaum Associates Ltd.

Archangeli, D. (1984). *Underspecification in Yawelmani phonology and morphology.* Doctoral dissertation, MIT, Cambridge, MA.

Balota, D. A. (1990). The role of meaning in word recognition. In D. A. Balota, G. B. Flores d'Arcais, & K. Rayner (Eds.), *Comprehension processes in reading.* Hillsdale, NJ: Erlbaum.

Berwick, R. C. (1985). *The acquisition of syntactic knowledge.* Cambridge, MA: MIT Press.

Bever, T. G., & McElree, B. (1988). Empty categories access their antecedents during comprehension. *Linguistic Inquiry, 19,* 35–44.

Borer, H., & Wexler, K. (1987). The maturation of syntax. In T. Roeper & E. Williams (Eds.), *Parameter setting.* Dordrecht: Reidel.

Bromberger, S., & Halle, M. (1989). Why phonology is different. *Linguistic Inquiry, 20,* 51–70.

Carlson, G. N., & Tanenhaus, M. K. (1989). Thematic roles and language comprehension. In W. Wilkins (Ed.), *Automatic natural language processing.* West Sussex, UK: Ellis Horwood.

Chomsky, N. (1973). Conditions on transformation. In S. Anderson & P. Kiparsky (Eds.), *A festschrift for Morris Halle.* New York: Holt, Rinehart & Winston.

Chomsky, N. (1977). On *wh*-movement. In P. Culicover, T. Wasow, & A. Akmajian (Eds.), *Formal syntax.* London & San Diego: Academic Press.

Chomsky, N. (1981). *Lectures on government and binding: The Pisa lectures.* Dordrecht: Foris.

Clifton, C., & Frazier, L. (1989). Comprehending sentences with long-distance dependencies. In M. Tanenhaus & G. Carlson (Eds.), *Linguistic structure in language processing,* Dordrecht: Kluwer.

Crain, S., Drozd, K., Philip, W., & Roeper, T. (1992, June 8–9). *The semantic subset principle in the acquisition of quantification.* Presented at the Second Workshop on Acquisition and Wh-Movement, University of Massachusetts, Amherst.

Crain, S., & Fodor, J. D. (1987). Sentence matching and overgeneration. *Cognition, 26,* 123–169.

Culicover, P., & Rochemont, M. (1990). Extraposition and the complement principle. *Linguistic Inquiry, 21,* 23–47.

de Vincenzi, M. (1991). *Syntactic parsing strategies in Italian.* Dordrecht: Kluwer.

Fodor, J. D. (1989). Empty categories in sentence processing. In G. T. M. Altmann (Ed.), *Language and cognitive processes: Special issue on parsing and interpretation* (pp. 155–210). Hove, UK: Lawrence Erlbaum Associates Ltd.

Frazier, L. (1986). The mapping between grammar and processor. In I. Gopnik & M. Gopnik (Eds.), *From models to modules: Studies in cognitive science* (pp. 117–134). Norwood, Nd: Ablex.

Frazier, L. (1987a). Sentence processing: A tutorial review. In M. Coltheart (Ed.), *Attention and performance XII: The psychology of reading* (pp. 559–586). Hillsdale, NJ: Erlbaum.

Frazier, L. (1987b). Syntactic processing: Evidence from Dutch. *Natural Language and Linguistic Theory, 5,* 519–560.

Frazier, L., & Clifton, C. (1989). Successive cyclicity in the grammar and the parser. *Language and Cognitive Processes, 4*(2), 93–126.

Frazier, L., & Clifton, C. (in press). *Construal.* Cambridge: MIT Press.

Frazier, L., & Flores d'Arcais, G. B. (1989). Filler driven parsing: A study of gap filling in Dutch. *Journal of Memory and Language, 28,* 331–344.

Frazier, L., & Rayner, K. (1982). Making and correcting errors during sentence comprehension: Eye movements in the analysis of structurally ambiguous sentences. *Cognitive Psychology, 14,* 178–210.

Freedman, S. A., & Forster, K. I. (1985). The psychological status of overgenerated sentences. *Cognition, 19,* 101–131.

Gilboy, E., Sopena, J. M., Clifton, C., & Frazier, L. (in press). Argument structure and association preference in complex noun phrases in Spanish and English. *Cognition.*

Goldsmith, J. (1976). *Autosegmental phonology.* Doctoral dissertation, MIT, Cambridge, MA.

Gorrell, P. (1992). *The parser as tree builder.* Manuscript, University of Maryland, College Park.

Hyams, N. (1986). *Language acquisition and the theory of parameters.* Dordrecht: Reidel.

Hyams, N. (1992, October). *Null subjects across child languages.* Presented at the Boston University Conference on Language Development, Boston.

Kingston, J., & Beckman, M. (1990). *Papers in laboratory phonology: I. Between the grammar and physics of speech.* Cambridge, UK: Cambridge University Press.

Lahiri, A., & Marslen-Wilson, W. (1991). The mental representation of lexical form: A phonological approach to the recognition lexicon. *Cognition, 38,* 245–294.

Levelt, P. (1989). *Speaking: From intention to articulation.* Cambridge, MA: MIT Press.

Manzini, R., & Wexler, K. (1987). Parameters, binding theory, and learnability. *Linguistic Inquiry, 18,* 413–444.

Marcus, M., Hindle, D., & Fleck, M. (1983). D-theory: Talking about talking about trees. *Association for Computational Linguistics, 21,* 129–136.

Marslen-Wilson, W., & Tyler, L. (1980). The temporal structure of spoken language understanding. *Cognition, 8,* 1–71.

McCarthy, J. J. (1989). Linear order in phonological representation. *Linguistic Inquiry, 20,* 71–99.

Millis, M. L., & Button, S. C. B. (1989). The effect of polysemy on lexical decision time: Now you see it, now you don't. *Memory & Cognition, 17,* 141–147.

Mitchell, J. (1986). *The formal semantics of point of view.* Doctoral dissertation, University of Massachusetts, Amherst.

Nicol, J. (1988). *Coreference processing during sentence comprehension.* Doctoral dissertation, MIT, Cambridge, MA.

Partee, B. H. (1989). Binding implicit variables in quantified contexts. In C. Wittshire, B. Music, & R. Garczyk (Eds.), *Papers from the 25th regional meeting of the Chicago Linguistic Society* (pp. 342–365). Chicago: Chicago Linguistics Society.

Pinker, S., & Prince, A. (1988). On language and connectionism: Analysis of a parallel distributed processing model of language acquisition. *Cognition, 28,* 73–194.

Prince, A., & Smolensky, P. (1991). *Connectionism and Harmony theory in linguistics.* Manuscript. Brandeis University, Waltham, MA.

Prince, A., & Smolensky, P. (1992). *Optimality: Constraint interaction in generative grammar.* Manuscript, Brandeis University, Waltham, MA.

Rumelhart, D., & McClelland, J. L. (1986). On learning the past tenses of English verbs. In J. McClelland & D. Rumelhart (Eds.), *Parallel distributed processing* (Vol. 2). Cambridge, MA: MIT Press.

Sagey, E. (1986). *The representation of features and relations in nonlinear phonology.* Doctoral dissertation, MIT, Cambridge, MA.

Schmauder, A. R. (1992). *Grammatical and conceptual features in the mental lexicon: Processing in isolation and in context.* Doctoral dissertation, University of Massachusetts, Amherst.

Seidenberg, M. S. (1991). Connectionism without tears. In S. David (Ed.), *Connectionism: Theory and practice.* Oxford: Oxford University Press.

Selkirk, E. O. (1992). [Labial] relations. Manuscript, University of Massachusetts, Amherst.

Shillcock, R. C., & Bard, E. G. (1993). Modularity and the processing of closed-class words. In G. T. M. Altmann & R. C. Shillcock (Eds.), *Cognitive models of speech processing: The second Sperlonga meeting.* Hillsdale, NJ: Erlbaum.

Swinney, D. A., Nicol, J., Ford, M., Frauenfelder, U., & Bresnan, J. (1987, November). *The time course of co-indexation during sentence comprehension.* Paper presented at the Psychonomics Society, Seattle, WA.

Taft, M. (1990). Lexical processing of functionally constrained words. *Journal of Memory and Language, 29,* 245–257.

Tanenhaus, M. K., Carlson, G. N., & Seidenberg, M. S. (1985). Do listeners compute linguistic representations? In D. Dowty, L. Karttunen, & A. M. Zwicky (Eds.), *Natural language parsing: Psychological, computational and theoretical perspectives.* Cambridge, UK: Cambridge University Press.

Wanner, E., & Maratsos, M. (1978). An ATN approach to comprehension. In M. Halle, J. Bresnan, & G. A. Miller (Eds.), *Linguistic theory and psychological reality.* Cambridge, MA: MIT Press.

Wexler, K. (1990). On unparsable input in language acquisition. In L. Frazier & J. deVilliers (Eds.), *Language processing and language acquisition* (pp. 105–118). Dordrecht: Kluwer Academic Publishers.

CHAPTER 2

Speech Production

Carol A. Fowler

This chapter addresses the question of how a linguistic message can be conveyed by vocal-tract activity. I make my job easier by considering linguistic messages only in their phonological aspect. So the question is not how linguistically structured *meanings* can be conveyed by vocal-tract activity, but rather, how language *forms* can be conveyed. Further, I do not discuss production of prosodic structure in speech, including its intonational and stress patterning. Despite these considerable simplifications, many difficulties remain in finding an answer.

A fundamental issue to confront right away concerns the extent of the mutual compatibilities among the different levels of description of the message that talkers, in one sense or another, embody as they speak. I consider three levels of description, those of the phonological forms of *linguistic competence* (language users' knowledge of their language), forms in a speaker's plan for an utterance, and forms in vocal-tract activity. It will become clear that a theory of speech production is profoundly shaped by the theorist's view of the compatibilities or incompatibilities among these levels (see Bock, Chapter 6, and Frazier, Chapter 1, this volume).

Speech, Language, and Communication

I. PHONOLOGICAL FORMS OF LINGUISTIC COMPETENCE

Phonological theories are intended to describe part of speakers' linguistic competence. The particular domain of a phonological theory includes an appropriate description of the sound inventories of languages and of the patterning of phonological segments in words. Before the mid-seventies, phonological theories generally took one fundamental form, now known as *linear*. These theories described phonological segments in a way that implied a poor fit between consonants and vowels as known to the language user and as implemented in articulation. Since the mid-seventies, *nonlinear* phonologies have been proposed. In some implementations, nonlinear theories have considerably improved the apparent fit between phonological segments as known and as produced.

A. A Linear Phonology

The most prominent, relatively recent, linear theory is generative phonology (Chomsky & Halle, 1968). In that class of theory (see Kenstowicz & Kisseberth, 1979, for a tutorial presentation), lexical entries for words include a specification of the word's phonological form represented as a (linear) sequence of consonants and vowels. Consonants and vowels themselves are represented as columns of feature values. For example, *bag* would have the following featural representation:

Phonological segments

Features	b	æ	g
vocalic	−	+	−
high	−	−	+
back	−	−	+
low	−	+	+
anterior	+	−	−
coronal	−	−	−
voice	+		+
continuant	−		−
nasal	−		−
strident	−		−
round		−	
tense		−	

(Vowels are not specified for the features voice, continuant, nasal, or strident; contextual influences aside, being vocalic implies +voice, +continuant, −nasal, and −strident. Consonants are not specified for rounding and tenseness.)

Features represent articulatory and acoustic attributes of phonological segments. However, for at least two reasons, the articulatory specification that they provide is abstracted away from, or is just plain unlike, the articulations that convey the segments to a listener. One reason for the abstraction has to do with a fundamental goal of most phonological theories, that of expressing as rules systematicities in the distribution of phonological properties in words. In English, syllable-initial voiceless stop consonants (/p, t, k/) are aspirated (breathy). Compare the /k/ sounds in *key,* where /k/ is syllable-initial, to the /g/-like /k/ in *ski,* where the /k/ is syllable-internal. However, the lexical entry for *key* will not include the information that the /k/ is aspirated, because aspiration is predictable by rule. In general, lexical entries for words indicate only properties of the phonological segment that are idiosyncratic to that word. Rules fill in the systematic properties of words. In articulation, of course, actions implementing all feature values of a word, whether lexically distinctive or not, must be provided.

Kenstowicz and Kisseberth (1979) offer some indications that the distinction between systematic and idiosyncratic properties of words is part of a language user's knowledge. Two such indications are speech errors and foreign accents. The authors report a speech error in which *tail spin* (phonetically, [tʰeyl spIn]) became *pail stin,* pronounced [pʰeyl stIn]. This is an exchange error, in which, apparently, /p/ and /t/ exchanged places, but aspiration (indicated by the raised [h] in the phonetic representation) remained appropriate to its context. One interpretation of this outcome is that /p/ and /t/ were exchanged before the aspiration rule was applied by the speaker. Had the exchange occurred between the pronounced forms of /p/ and /t/, the result would have been [peyl stʰIn]. As for foreign accents, they can be described as the inappropriate application of the phonological systematicities of the speaker's native language to utterances in the foreign language. For example, native English speakers producing French, find it difficult to avoid aspirating syllable-initial voiceless stops in French words, even though French does not have an aspiration rule. (Accordingly, they erroneously pronounce French *pas* as [pʰa] rather than [pa].) It has not proven a straightforward matter to decide what properties of a language are sufficiently regular that they should count as systematic properties to be abstracted from lexical entries and later applied as rules. Chomsky and Halle (1968) had a rather low threshold for acceptance of a property as regular and therefore had many rules and quite abstract lexical entries.

A different reason why the lexical entries of a linear phonology provide phonological segments that are far from their articulatory implementations concerns their representation of consonants and vowels as distinct feature columns. In the lexical entry, the columns are discrete one from the other (in that they do not overlap along the abstract time axis), the features are static (i.e., they represent states of the vocal tract or of the consequent acoustic signal), and the featural representation for a segment in a feature column is context free. However, in speech production, actions relating to distinct consonants and vowels overlap in time, the vocal tract is in continuous motion, and, at least at some levels of description, its manner of implementing a given feature of a consonant or vowel is context sensitive.

B. Nonlinear Phonologies

Development of nonlinear phonologies was not spurred by concern over this apparent mismatch between phonological competence and articulatory performance. It was fostered by failures of the linear phonologies to handle certain characteristics of some phonological systems. In particular, Goldsmith (1976) argued that an implicit assumption of linear phonologies (which he termed the *absolute slicing hypothesis*) is refuted by data from many languages. The absolute slicing assumption is that every feature's domain is the same as every other feature's domain, namely, one feature column's width. However, in fact, the domain of a feature can be less or more than one column.

In some languages, there are *complex segments,* such as pre- or post-nasalized stops that behave in most respects like one segment, but they undergo a feature change (from [+nasal] to [−nasal] or vice versa) in mid-segment. In other languages, nasality may span more than one column. Van der Hulst and Smith (1982) describe work of Bendor-Samuel (1960) on a language, Terena, in which the first-person possessive of a noun is expressed in a word by addition of a nasality feature to the word. The feature spans every segment beginning at the left edge of the word up to the first stop or fricative. That segment becomes a prenasalized obstruent. So, for example, /ʻowoku/ (*his house*) becomes /ʻõw̃õŋgu/ (*my house;* ˜ represents nasalization, and /ŋg/ is a prenasalized velar stop).

There is another way in which some features may participate in the phonological system differently from others. In particular, they may be differentially likely to undergo a phonological process in which other features participate. For example, some features evade deletion when other features of a segment are deleted. In another example from van der Hulst and Smith (taken from Elimelech, 1976), in the language Etsako there is a reduplication rule so that a noun X becomes each X by undergoing reduplication. For example, ówà (*house*), becomes ówǒwà (*each house;* ´ is a high tone on the vowel, ` is a low tone, and ˇ is a rising tone analyzed as a low followed by a high tone.) The first /a/ is dropped in the reduplication process, but its tone is not deleted. The tone attaches to the following /o/ forming a rising tone with the high tone already on the vowel.

These phenomena suggest that the feature column metaphor does not provide an accurate reflection of phonological competence. As an alternative, Goldsmith (1976; also see Goldsmith, 1990) proposed an analysis in which some features are represented as occupying different tiers from others; features on one tier become associated with those on others by rule. A prenasalized stop might be represented as follows (from van der Hulst & Smith, 1982) with the nasality feature occupying its own tier:

[+nas]   [−nas]
    −syll
    +cons
    −high, etc.

Compatibly, the analysis of reduplication would be represented as follows (with H and L representing high and low tones, respectively). Notice that tonal features occupy a separate tier from segmental features (indicated jointly by the symbols for each consonant or vowel):

```
H    L    H    L  H    L    H    LH L
|    |  → |    |  |    |  → |    \|  |
o  w  a    o  w     o  w  a    o  w   o  w a
```

In both of these examples, features that distinguish themselves from others (in the size of their domain and in their surviving application of a deletion rule, respectively) occupy tiers distinct from those that do not distinguish themselves from others. Examination of phonological processes reveals a patterning in this regard. Some features commonly participate jointly in a phonological process. Some appear never to do so. As Clements (1985) points out, this observation reveals another insufficiency of the feature column notion. The column has no internal organization; however, the set of features does. Clements' examination of the relative tendencies for subsets of features to participate jointly or not in phonological processes suggested a hierarchical organization of featural tiers. Features separating lower down in the hierarchy were those that participated jointly in more phonological processes than features that separated early in the hierarchy. To a remarkable degree, the organization of featural tiers in Clements' hierarchy mirrored patterns of anatomical independence and dependence in the vocal tract, and it is important, therefore, to realize that the model was not developed in order to mirror those patterns. Rather, as noted, it was designed to mirror patterns of featural cohesion as reflected in the features' joint participation or not in phonological processes. The fact that an organization derived this way does reflect vocal-tract organization suggests a considerably better fit between elements of the phonology and capabilities of the vocal tract than linear phonology, a matter of importance to us here. In addition and more fundamentally, perhaps, it suggests a major impact of the performance capabilities and dispositions of the vocal tract on the historical development of phonological systems.

Articulatory phonology (Browman & Goldstein, 1986b, 1989, 1990a,

1992) constitutes an even more radical movement away from linear phonologies and toward a phonology that should be fully compatible with vocal-tract capabilities. This phonology is articulatory in two major senses. First, its primitives are neither features of consonants and vowels nor phonemes, but, rather, gestures of the vocal tract and constellations of gestures. Gestures are "characteristic patterns of movement of vocal tract articulators or articulatory systems" (Browman & Goldstein, 1986b, p. 223). They are, in addition, like features of a linear phonology, units of contrast (i.e., a change of one feature in a linear theory or a change of one gesture in articulatory phonology can change one word of the language to another word). Phonology itself is defined (Browman & Goldstein, 1992, p. 56) as "a set of relations among physically real events, a characterization of the systems and patterns that these events, the gestures, enter into."

Articulatory phonology is explicitly articulatory in a second sense as well. Browman and Goldstein (1989) proposed the hierarchy of anatomical subsystems in Figure 1 based entirely on patterns of anatomical dependence or independence in the vocal tract, not, as Clements had, on patterns of featural cohesion in phonological processes. Browman and Goldstein's hierarchy, therefore, should constitute a language universal base on which individual languages may elaborate, but which they cannot reorganize because the dependencies are grounded in the anatomy of the speech production system.

In Figure 2, the hierarchy of Figure 1 has been rotated 90 degrees so that

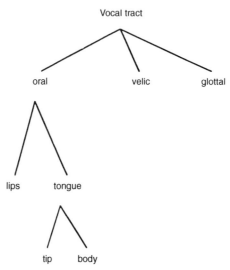

FIGURE 1   Browman and Goldstein's hierarchy of gestural subsystems. (Redrawn from Browman & Goldstein, 1989.)

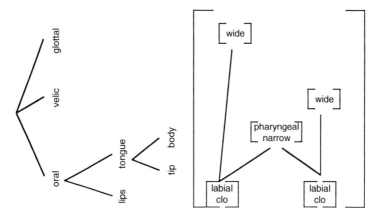

FIGURE 2   A gestural score for the word *palm*. (Redrawn from Browman & Goldstein, 1989.)

its terminal nodes face the gestural score for the word *palm* (from Browman & Goldstein, 1989). The gestural score provides parameterizations for dynamical gestures associated with the articulatory subsystems involved in producing *palm*. In the figure, parameter values (in brackets) in the gestural score lie to the right of the corresponding parameterized articulatory subsystems in the rotated hierarchy. Thus, the parameter value [wide] to the right of the glottal subsystem signifies that, initially in the word *palm*, the glottis is open. Below that, the parameter values [labial] and [clo] opposite the lips subsystem provide the constriction location (labial) and degree (clo, for closed) of the word-initial consonant /p/. [Pharyngeal] and [narrow] characterize the constriction location and degree, respectively, of the tongue body during /a/ in *palm*. For the final consonant, /m/, the velum is lowered [wide], and the lip subsystem is parameterized as it was for /p/. In general, the gestural score for a word indicates the relative timing of successive gestures in a word; the association lines in the figure indicate gestures that are explicitly phased with respect to the others.

It is not necessary to achieve a deeper understanding of articulatory phonology to appreciate that it provides a good fit to the capabilities of the vocal tract in both central respects in which it is an articulatory phonology. First, the primitives of the phonological theory are dynamical actions, not static attributes of idealized abstract categories. Indeed, they are the patterns of movement in which the vocal tract engages during speech production. Second, articulatory phonology provides patterns of dependency among features (now gestures) that are wholly natural in reflecting patterns of anatomical dependency.

We must ask, however, whether there is any cost associated with this apparent benefit. Can the theory in fact characterize "the systems and patterns that these events, the gestures, enter into" (Browman & Goldstein, 1992)? For example, can the theory make the distinction that Kenstowicz and Kisseberth consider fundamental to a phonological theory between systematic and idiosyncratic properties of words?

Articulatory phonology does identify some systematic properties of words, for example, in rules that phase gestures one with respect to the other. To pursue the aspiration example, English voiceless stops are aspirated syllable-initially because of the way that the glottal opening gesture is phased with respect to release of the consonantal constriction. (Regulated phasings are indicated by association lines in the gestural score of Figure 2.) However, these systematic properties are not abstracted from the lexical entries for words. Accordingly, there is no distinction in the theory between words as represented lexically and as pronounced. It is fair to ask, then, how, if at all, articulatory phonology explains the two phenomena alluded to earlier, and mentioned by Kenstowicz and Kisseberth as evidence for the psychological reality of rule application by speakers, namely, errors such as [pʰeyl stɪn] and foreign accents that preserve the systematic properties of the speaker's native language.

Articulatory phonology has an account of errors such as [pʰeyl stɪn] that does not require an inference that a rule is applied to an abstract lexical entry: the exchange occurred between two constriction gestures (or just their location parameters) not between two phonemes. As for foreign accents, the theory has not explicitly addressed the question. However, there are at least two accounts that it could invoke. An unappealing possibility is to suppose that systematic properties are represented explicitly as rules and are represented implicitly across the set of lexical entries, and these explicit rules are applied to novel forms. An alternative account is to suppose that novel forms are pronounced by analogy with similar existing forms in the lexicon.

Clearly, theories of speech production will differ significantly depending on the theory of phonology they adopt; at the extremes, a linear theory in which phonological features of consonants and vowels cannot be implemented in a literal or analogical way in the vocal tract, or articulatory phonology in which phonological primitives *are* vocal-tract actions.

II. PLANNING UNITS IN SPEECH PRODUCTION

A. Speech Errors as Evidence for Planning Units

Some planning must occur in language production, because the nature of syntax is such that dependencies (e.g., subject–verb agreement) may be established between words that are far apart in the sentence to be produced.

The occurrence of anticipatory speech errors such as "we have a laboratory in our own computer" (from Fromkin, 1971) verifies the occurrence of advance planning. For the present, our interest is in the nature of the units used to represent the planned utterance. The most straightforward assumption, and the one generally made, is that they are the units of linguistic competence. Indeed, investigators have used evidence about planning units as revealed in speech errors as a way to assess the psychological reality of proposed units of linguistic competence. For example, according to Stemberger (1983, p. 43): "Speech error data argue for the psychological reality of many basic phonological units."

Salient kinds of speech errors are those in which a unit moves from an intended slot in an utterance to another slot. Anticipatory, perseverative, and exchange movement errors are illustrated, respectively, in (1)–(3) below using the phonological segment as the sampled moved unit (errors below are from Fromkin, 1973):

(1) *a reading list* → *a leading list*
(2) *leaflets written* → *leaflets litten*
(3) *left hemisphere* → *heft lemisphere*

Another common error type is a substitution of one unit for another of the same size, where the substituting segment does not appear to originate in the planned string. An example of a phonemic substitution is given in (4):

(4) *what Malcolm said* → *what balcolm said*

Phonemes and words are reported to participate frequently in speech errors, whereas syllables and, more controversially, features are reported to participate rarely. Syllables and features do serve a role in speech production planning as revealed by errors, however, even if not as planning units. Generally phonemes involved in movement errors move to the same part of a syllable as that they would have occupied in the intended utterance. Accordingly, the syllable may be seen as a frame into which planned units, syllable-position-sensitive phonemes (e.g., Dell, 1986) are inserted. As for features, increased featural similarity of two segments increases the likelihood that they will interact in an error.

However, the foregoing observation is, in part, why the claim that feature errors are rare is controversial. Compare and contrast:

> Single distinctive features rarely appear as exchange errors, even though many pairs of exchanged segments differ by one feature. (Shattuck-Hufnagel, 1983, p. 112)

> The feature paradox . . . First there is the rarity of feature errors, which, like the case with syllables, signifies a very limited role for the feature as a unit (Shattuck-Hufnagel & Klatt, 1979). However, again like the syllable, features

play an important role in determining which phonemes can slip with which. (Dell, 1986, p. 294)

[Feature] errors are less rare than has been suggested. (Fromkin, 1973, p. 17)

It has been repeatedly observed that most speech production errors are single feature errors. (Browman & Goldstein, 1990b, p. 419)

When a talker produces an error such as *vactive verb* (intending *factive verb*), we cannot be sure that the error is a whole phoneme anticipation; it might be a voicing feature anticipation. (Recall also the two interpretations of [pʰeyl stIn] above.) The response to this has been that clear cases of feature errors, in which the identity of interacting phonemes is not pre-served [as in Fromkin's (1971) much-cited example of *glear plue sky* for *clear blue sky*] occur rarely. In their corpus of 70 exchange errors in which inter-acting word-initial consonants differed by at least two features (so that feature and phoneme errors could be distinguished), Shattuck-Hufnagel and Klatt (1979) found just three errors in which the identity of the interacting consonants was not preserved.

Despite some uncertainties, speech errors generally support the claim that planning units are elementary units of linguistic competence. That is, the units that either participate actively in errors (move or substitute one for the other) or constrain the form that errors take are consistent with units proposed by linguistic theories.

Can we ask more of the errors, however? In particular, can we ask whether they can help distinguish among competing views of linguistic competence? For example, can they help determine whether phonological primitives are phonemes with featural attributes represented in competence as feature columns or else on featural tiers? Can they distinguish either of these alternatives from Browman and Goldstein's proposal that primitives are gestures and gestural constellations? Finally, can they help determine to what extent lexical representations are abstract or, alternatively, close to surface pronunciations?

The answer to all these questions is that they probably can help to address these issues, but they have not yet been used to do so to any significant extent. Consider the issue of whether primitives are featurally specified phonemes or gestures. The issue is difficult to adjudicate, because descrip-tions in terms of features and gestures are redundant. Thus, in an error in which interacting segments differ by a single feature (as in *vactive verb* above), the segments generally also differ by a single gesture (voicing in the example) or a parameter of a gesture (e.g., constriction location in *taddle tennis* for *paddle tennis*). Some interacting segments that differ in two features (*Fillmore's face* from the intended *Fillmore's case*) differ in both parameters, location and degree, of a single constriction gesture. Despite the redundancy, it is likely that distinctive predictions can be made about error patterns from the featural/phonemic and gestural perspectives. For example, one prediction distinguishing a gestural account from most others is that errors involving both parameters of a single constriction gesture (location and degree) will be more common, other things being equal, than errors involving one of those parameters and another gesture (constriction location and devoicing, e.g.). Such predictions have yet to be proposed and tested, however.

As for the issue of the abstraction of planned units, two interesting recent findings appear to tug the preponderance of evidence in opposite directions. Findings by Stemberger (1991a, 1991b) suggest that planned units are abstract; findings by Mowrey and MacKay (1990) suggest to them that "errors which have been consigned to the phonemic, segmental, or featural levels could be reinterpreted as errors at the motor output level" (p. 1311).

B. Stemberger: Radical Underspecification

Generally in speech errors there is a bias for more frequent units to substitute for, or move to slots of, less frequent ones. Stemberger (1991a) pointed out two "antifrequency biases." In one, an error more frequently creates a consonant cluster than a singleton. For example, in attempts to produce sequences such as *puck plump* or *pluck pump,* speakers are more likely to produce *pluck plump* than *puck pump.* This addition bias is antifrequency because clusters are less frequent than are singletons. The second antifrequency bias, the palatal bias, was first noted by Shattuck-Hufnagel and Klatt (1979). It is a tendency for /s/ and /t/ to be replaced in errors by /š/ and /č/, respectively, even though /s/ and /t/ are the more frequent consonants in the language.

Stemberger's account of the addition bias derives from an interactive activation model of speech production. In those models, units are activated in advance of being uttered, and activated units compete. In particular, word-initial consonants compete with word-initial consonants, vowels compete with vowels, and so on. Competition may take the form of mutual inhibition. In the case of *puck plump,* the /l/ in *plump* will be active during planned production of *puck*. The /l/ will be in competition, however, with no segment in *puck*. (There is supposed to be an empty slot in *puck;* henceforth a C_2 slot, after the word-initial consonant and before the vowel signifying the phonotactic legality of a cluster in that position.) Because /l/ has no competitor, it will not be inhibited. If it is sufficiently activated during primary activation of *puck,* it may be selected to fill the empty C_2 slot in *puck* yielding *pluck*.

Stemberger uses recent linguistic proposals to suggest that the same kind of account will explain the palatal bias and can predict many other asymmetries in speech errors. These recent linguistic proposals concern *underspecification* in lexical entries for words. We encountered underspecification earlier in regard to the aspiration feature of voiceless syllable-initial stops in English words such as *key*. The proposal there was that predictable features of phonemes are not represented lexically. In a more radical approach to underspecification, some nonredundant, nonpredictable feature values are unspecified lexically. This can be done if all other values of the same feature are specified. For example, if voicing is specified lexically, then voicelessness need not be, because the lack of any voicing specification at all will signify voicelessness. Language-internal evidence, with which we do not concern ourselves here, determines which feature values are identified as underspecified.

In the case of consonantal place of articulation, the underspecified feature value is [coronal], characteristic of /s/ and /t/ among other consonants. Stemberger explains the palatal bias in abstractly the same way as he explained the tendency for errors to create consonant clusters. When /š/ or /č/, which have a place specification, compete with /s/ or /t/, which lack one, the unspecified place feature of /s/ and /t/ is vulnerable to substitution by the specified feature because the specified feature has no competitor to inhibit it.

A number of predictions can be made to test this account. The general prediction is that unspecified feature values should be subject to substitution *by* specified values more than they substitute *for* specified values, given equal opportunity. Both in spontaneous speech errors and in experimentally induced errors, Stemberger (1991a, 1991b) obtained error patterns consistent with underspecification theory and his account of asymmetrical substitution patterns. If Stemberger's account of these error patterns is correct, then phonological segments as planned (and also presumably as specified in the lexicon) are represented abstractly and in ways inconsistent with proposals of Browman and Goldstein. It remains to be seen whether an alternative account of the findings will be offered from the perspective of articulatory phonology.

C. Mowrey and MacKay: Muscular Evidence of Speech Errors

The evidence interpreted as suggesting that errors reveal wholly unabstract planning units is provided by Mowrey and MacKay (1990). These investigators collected productions of such tongue twisters as *Bob flew by Bligh Bay* and *She sells seashells by the seashore*. A novel aspect of their procedure was that they recorded muscle (electromyographic or EMG) activity during the utterances, in particular, that of a muscle of the tongue involved in /l/ production in the first tongue twister and a muscle of the lower lip in the second tongue twister.

Across many productions, they found utterances that sounded correct and were correct as assessed by the EMG data; likewise, they heard such slips as *Bob flew bly Bligh Bay* and saw evidence of the slip in the form of tongue muscle activity during *by*. Remarkably, however, they saw errors that graded evenly between these extremes. There were utterances in which no /l/ could be heard in /b/-V words, but in which some tongue muscle activity was apparent. There were instances in which listeners disagreed about the presence or absence of an intruded /l/ and in which tongue muscle activity was clearly visible. One indisputable conclusion from their findings is that insertions and deletions are not all-or-none. However, the investigators drew stronger conclusions from their findings (Mowrey & MacKay, 1990, p. 1311). They consider the findings to show that errors can be subphonemic and even subfeatural; indeed, they can be errors involving individual muscle actions. One finding they report in support of that conclusion is the occurrence of significant labial activity during a normal sounding [s] in the second tongue twister above. Because substantial lip activity was evident during [š], they identified that activity as the likely trigger for the inappropriate activity accompanying [s]. Because the [s] sounded normal, they infer no intrusion of the alveopalatal feature of [š] on the [s]. They identify the error as subphonemic because the affected [s] is affected in just one respect, not in every respect in which it could be changed by an [š]. They identify it, further, as subfeatural, because [š] is not usually identified as having a rounding or labiality feature. In their view, the intrusion is at the motor output level. They conclude that earlier error collectors may have been misled in their interpretation of speech errors, because they only collected slips that they heard, and because they had no information on the articulatory sources of their perceptions. In their view, there is no compelling evidence yet for phonemes or features as planning units in speech production. Possibly all errors will turn out to be errors at the motor output level.

Mowrey and MacKay's conclusions are not yet compelling, however. First, there must be some organization among the muscle actions that realize a speech utterance. Research on action generally (see, e.g., Bernstein, 1967; Turvey, 1977, 1990) shows that there is no motor output level of the sort Mowrey and MacKay appear to envisage in which independent commands to muscles are issued. To explain the on-line adaptability of the motor system, including the speech system (see Section III), to variation in the context in which actions occur requires invoking the presence of low-level linkages among parts of the motor system responsible for the action. Mowrey and MacKay only recorded from one or two muscle sites at a time, and this would prevent them from seeing evidence of any organization among muscles of the vocal tract. In their example of a subfeatural error described above, they infer that only the labial activity associated with [š] intruded on [s] production, but they base that conclusion on the fact that the [s] sounded normal, a criterion that elsewhere they reject as misleading.

Mowrey and MacKay suggest that: "Units such as features, segments and phonemes may well exist; if it is found at some later time that blocks of motor commands behave as single entities, we should have good evidence of a higher level of organization" (p. 1311). There are at least two reasons for guessing that such evidence will be forthcoming. First is the evidence just alluded to that the motor system is organized in the production of intentional action, including speech. The second is evidence from the errors literature itself. There must be some explanation for the reason why the big speech errors, that is, those that error collectors have heard and recorded, pattern as they do. There are many conceivable big errors (errors in a phoneme and a half, whole syllable errors, movement errors involving single features that do not preserve the identity of the originally planned phonemes) that either do not occur or occur rarely. Others are commonly reported. This suggests that a superordinate organization of motor commands will be found, if one is sought, using Mowrey and MacKay's procedures.

III. ARTICULATORY UNITS

The kinematics of the articulators during production of an utterance do not transparently reflect the units described by classic linguistic theories, such as that of Chomsky and Halle (1968). Naïve expectation would suggest that any articulators involved in the production of a phoneme should initiate their movements synchronously and end them synchronously. Movements for a next phoneme should then begin together and end together. That is not what we see in speech production. Figure 3 reveals just some of the failures of real speech utterance to satisfy those expectations. The figure displays two tokens of the utterance *perfect memory,* the first produced slowly (and represented only through the first syllable of *memory*) and the second produced more quickly. The latter utterance is transcribed phonetically as if the final /t/ in *perfect* had been omitted by the talker. Under the phonetic transcription and acoustic waveform of each utterance are the traces of pellets placed on various articulators and tracked by X ray. Symbols, κ, τ, and β mark constrictions for the /k/ and /t/ in *perfect* and for the /m/ in *memory*. Regarding the expectation that movements of different articulators for a common phoneme should begin and end together, notice that the velum-lowering gesture for /m/ begins well before raising of the lower lip for the same segment. It appears to reach its lowest point around the time that the labial closing gesture *begins*. As for the discreteness of successive phonemes, notice that, in both productions of the phrase, constriction gestures for /k/ and /t/ overlap, and, in the fast production, the labial gesture

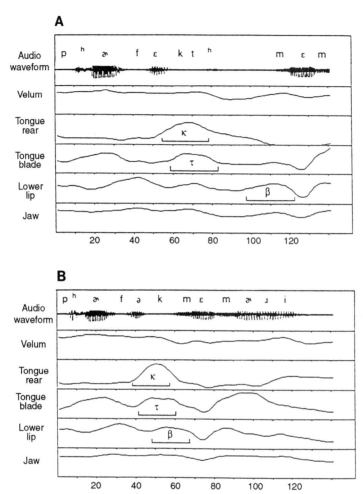

FIGURE 3   Acoustic signal and X-ray pellet trajectories from two utterances of the phrase *perfect memory*. The first utterance (A), produced more slowly than the second (B), is represented only through the first syllable of *memory*. (From Browman & Goldstein, 1990c.)

for /m/ overlaps with that for /t/ to an extent that, although the /t/ constriction is made, it has no apparent acoustic consequences, and was not heard by the transcriber. Gestures for different phonemes overlap, even different phonemes in different words.

At least some reasons why the articulators do not reveal ostensible linguistic or planning units transparently are known. Even if the articulators were stationary when the activation of articulators for a phoneme began, articulators would not begin to move synchronously, because they have different inertias; further, the muscular support for the different articulatory movements may be differentially effective. Of course, the articulators are unlikely to be stationary in fluent speech, and different requirements to change the direction of movement may further introduce asynchronies between movement onsets. However, even factoring out such peripheral sources of asynchrony, articulatory movements would not partition temporally into discrete phonemes. Rather, movements for different consonants and vowels in an utterance overlap in time. This coarticulation means that there can be no boundaries between articulatory movements for consonants and vowels in sequence, that is, no single point in time when movements for one segment cease and those for another begin.

The apparent absence of linguistic units in articulation, of course, does not mean either that linguistic units are absent or that units of any sort are absent. Perhaps the level of description of movement in the vocal tract has been inappropriate for finding units; perhaps we should not attempt to impose on the vocal tract our preconceived ideas of what the units should be (e.g., Kelso, Saltzman, & Tuller, 1986; Moll, Zimmermann, & Smith, 1976). Rather, we first should attempt to discover the natural order in vocal-tract actions, if any, and then worry later about their relation to linguistic units.

A more distanced, less detailed, perspective on the vocal tract does suggest more organization than the one adopted above in which individual movements of individual articulators were tracked. One can describe much of what goes on in the vocal tract during speech as the overlapped, but still serially ordered, achievement and release of constrictions. Frequently, several articulators cooperate in a constriction action, and, at least in this sense, there appears to be a superordinate organization of the vocal tract into systems. If the achievement and release of a constriction can be construed as a unit of action, then perhaps there may be said to be units in articulatory behavior.

Perhaps the earliest kind of evidence suggestive of articulatory systems was provided in the literature on so-called bite-block speech. In this literature (e.g., Lindblom, Lubker, & Gay, 1979; Lindblom & Sundberg, 1971), speakers produce speech, frequently vowels, with bite blocks clenched between their upper and lower teeth so that the jaw cannot move and generally is forced to adopt either a more open position than is typical for a high vowel or a more closed position than is typical for a low vowel. The striking finding is that, with little or no practice, vowels are acoustically normal (or near normal; Fowler & Turvey, 1980) from the first pitch pulse of the vowel. This implies an equifinality in vowel production such that a given configurational target can be reached in a variety of ways. The limited need for practice suggests, too, that this flexibility is somehow already in place in the speaker; it is not learned during the course of the experimental session.

More information about sources of equifinality is obtained using a procedure pioneered by Abbs and his colleagues (e.g., Abbs & Gracco, 1984;

Folkins & Abbs, 1975). In this procedure, speakers produce target utterances repeatedly; on a low proportion of trials, and unexpected by subjects, an articulator is perturbed during production of a consonant. For example, in research by Kelso, Tuller, Vatikiotis-Bateson, and Fowler (1984), the jaw was unexpectedly tugged down during production of the final consonants of target words /bæb/ and /bæz/, produced in a carrier sentence. Within 20–30 ms of the onset of the perturbation, other articulators (the upper lip in /bæb/ and the tongue in /bæz/ began to compensate for the unusually low jaw position, such that consonantal constrictions were achieved, and consonants sounded normal. Findings are generally that the responses to perturbation are, for the most part, functionally specific. That is, articulators that would not compensate for the perturbation are not activated (but see Kelso et al., 1984, for a possible qualification); and, when articulators are perturbed that are not involved in the consonant being produced, the consonant is produced as it is on unperturbed trials (Shaiman, 1989). The short latency onset of the compensatory response implies an existing linkage among articulators, the jaw and lips during /b/ and the jaw and tongue during /z/ in the research by Kelso et al. (1984). Because the linkages are different for different consonants, they must be transiently established during speech production. Researchers in the motor skills literature refer to these linkages as "synergies" or "coordinative structures" (Easton, 1972).

The work on synergies in speech production is limited; accordingly, no catalog of them can be compiled. However, evidence for a synergy to achieve bilabial closure is well established (Abbs & Gracco, 1984; Kelso et al., 1984); some evidence supports synergies for achievement of an alveolar constriction (Kelso et al., 1984) and a labiodental constriction (for /f/; Shaiman, 1989). The partial list invites an inference that synergies exist that achieve consonantal places and manners of articulation. If the research on bite-block speech is interpreted as also revealing synergies of speech production, then the generalization can be extended to establishment of the more open constrictions characteristic of vowels.

This section began with the information that individual articulator movements do not segment temporally into familiar linguistic units. Having moved to a different level of description of vocal-tract actions, we do see unitlike systems, namely synergies, but still, these are not the discrete phonemes of classic linguistic theories. Synergies do appear to map almost transparently onto the phonetic gestures of Browman and Goldstein's articulatory phonology, however, a point we address in Section V.

IV. COMPATIBILITY OF UNITS ACROSS DESCRIPTIVE LEVELS

To what extent are units compatible across the three domains of phonological competence, planning, and articulation? Theorists and researchers have recognized two major barriers to a view that linguistic units can be commensurate with units if there are any behavioral units at all. One barrier is a view that phonological segments as known are different in kind from units as uttered because one is cognitive in nature and the other is physical:

> [P]honological representation is concerned with speakers' implicit knowledge, that is, with information in the mind . . . The hallmarks of phonetic representation follow from the fact that sounds, as well as articulatory gestures and events in peripheral auditory-system processing are observables in the physical world. Representation at this level is not cognitive, because it concerns events in the world rather than events in the mind. (Pierrehumbert, 1990, pp. 376–377)
>
> [Segments] are abstractions. They are the end result of complex perceptual and cognitive processes in the listener's brain. (Repp, 1981, p. 1462)

That problem aside, there is another barrier that, in the phonologies best known to speech researchers, phonological segments have characteristics (such as being static) that are impossible for vocal tracts to implement transparently. This has led to a view already mentioned that research should not seek, in articulatory behavior, units of linguistic description supplied by phonological theories. Rather, it should be designed, in an unbiased way, to discover natural organizational structure in vocal-tract activity (Kelso et al., 1986; Moll, et al., 1976).

For the most part, in the field of psychology, the apparent incommensurability of linguistic units and the articulatory implementation of a speech plan has been accepted, and theorists generally pick a domain in which to work: language planning and sequencing or articulation, without addressing the problem of the interface. There is some motivation for taking another look, however. Certainly, communicative efficacy would be on a more secure basis were the units in vocal-tract actions transparent implementations of units as known and planned. This is because it is only units as produced that immediately structure the acoustic signal for a perceiver.

To motivated theorists, moreover, the barriers above are not insurmountable. Regarding the first, one can challenge the ideas (following Ryle, 1949) both that cognitive things can be only in the mind and that physical things and cognitive things are mutually exclusive sets. Under an alternative conceptualization, vocal-tract action can be linguistic (and therefore cognitive) action. Regarding the second barrier, we have seen that some phonologies do offer units that are compatible with vocal-tract capabilities. It may not be necessary or even desirable for production researchers to design their research wholly unbiased by expectations derived from these new phonologies.

There is one, incomplete, model of speech production that implements phonological units of the language as vocal-tract activity. The model is incomplete in not attempting to handle all the data that a complete model will have to handle, for example, the occurrence of spontaneous speech errors. However, it is unique both in its explicit choice of a phonological theory (articulatory phonology) that eliminates incompatibilities across levels of description and in its handling the evidence described earlier that reveals the role of synergies in speech production. That model is Saltzman's "task dynamic model" (Kelso et al., 1986; Saltzman, 1986; Saltzman & Kelso, 1987; Saltzman & Munhall, 1989).

V. TASK DYNAMICS

The task dynamic model represents a new approach to understanding intentional, goal-directed action (see Turvey, 1990, for a review of this approach). Its novelty is in its recognition that living systems are complex physical systems that behave in some respects like other, even inanimate, complex physical systems. Those aspects may be best explained by invoking relevant physical principles and laws.

Many actions produced by synergies have characteristics in common with various kinds of oscillatory systems, and the approach that Saltzman and others take (Kelso et al., 1986; Kugler, Kelso, & Turvey, 1980; Saltzman, 1986; Saltzman & Kelso, 1987; Saltzman & Munhall, 1989; Turvey, 1990) is to model flexible, goal-directed action as produced by one or more oscillatory subsystems. Saltzman named his model task dynamics to highlight its two salient features. In the model, actions are defined initially in functional terms, that is, in terms of the tasks they are to achieve. That is how the actions acquire and maintain their goal-directed character. In addition, tasks are defined in terms of the dynamics that underlie the actions' surface forms or kinematics.

Actions as diverse as a discrete reach to a location and bilabial closure are described in the same way in their first description, in *task space*. That is because the dynamical control regime that will implement the action is first described functionally, and both discrete reaching and bilabial closure are characterized functionally by *point attractor* dynamics. A point attractor system has point stability, that is, trajectories of the system are attracted to a point at which the system is in equilibrium. An example is a pendulum. Set in motion by a push, it comes to rest hanging parallel to the pull of gravity. In a bilabial closing gesture, a lip aperture system is attracted to a point at which the lips meet.

In the model, equations of motion that represent task achievement in task space undergo two transformations as the model "speaks," first into "body space" (with the jaw as the spatial point of origin) and next into "articulator space," where each articulator is assigned one or more directions of possible movement. In the latter transformation, a small number of dimensions in body space are rewritten as more articulatory dimensions. The redundancy of this transformation permits flexible achievement of task goals. Accordingly, the model, like subjects in the perturbation experiments of Kelso et al. (1984) and others, compensates for perturbations to an articulator. In particular, fixing the model's jaw at an unusually low position during production of bilabial closure leads to compensation, on-line, by the model's upper and lower lips.

Task dynamics has four notable features for our purposes. First, it uses the gestural scores provided by Browman and Goldstein's articulatory phonology as scripts that provide the tract variables and their dynamic parameters to be achieved in production of a word. Second, it *achieves* the task goals specified in gestural scores as vocal-tract activity. Third, the synergies in task dynamics show the equifinality characteristic exhibited by the speech system under perturbation. Fourth, synergies achieve equifinality, because they are treated as complex physical systems, sharing their dynamical characteristics with other physical systems, an approach that many investigators of action generally consider realistic. To my knowledge, this model in which the primitives of a phonological theory are realized nondestructively and in a natural way as vocal-tract action, is unique in the field of speech production.

VI. SEQUENCING

In Section V, attention was focused on the nature of language units as known, planned, and produced. The present topic is the sequencing of these units in speech production.

A. Coarticulation

There is no theory-neutral definition of the term *coarticulation,* and the literature reflects considerable disagreement to its referent. Accordingly, rather than attempt to offer a generic definition, I will offer three in the context of a discussion of findings that each characterization handles well or badly. The characterizations differ in the level of speech production planning or execution at which they propose that coarticulation arises and on the issue of whether coarticulation assimilates a segment to its context or, instead, is overlap of two or more essentially context-free segments.

1. Coarticulation as Feature Spreading

Daniloff and Hammarberg (1973) proposed that the coarticulatory rounding of /š/ in English *shoe* (phonologically /šu/) might be viewed as the consequence of a rule that spreads /u/'s rounding feature. Such spreading of features would serve to assimilate a segment to its context and thereby to smooth articulatory transitions between segments. In the particular feature-spreading theory, known as *look-ahead* theory, ascribed to Henke (1966), in fact a feature such as rounding can spread farther than just to an immediately preceding segment. Generally, a feature will spread anticipatorily to any preceding segment (anticipatory or right-to-left coarticulation) that is unspecified for that feature. Segments are unspecified for a feature if changing the feature value does not change the segment's identity. (Recall the featural representation of *bag* in Section I.) In English, consonants are unspecified for rounding, because rounding them does not change their identity. If features spread in an anticipatory direction to any number of preceding segments that are unspecified for them, then rounding should anticipate a rounded vowel through any number of consonants that precede it up to the first occurrence of an unrounded vowel. [Carryover (left-to-right, perseveratory) coarticulation here is seen as partly due to inertia of the articulators and therefore of somewhat less interest than anticipatory coarticulation.] Supportive evidence for the look-ahead model's account of spreading of rounding was provided by Daniloff and Moll, (1968) for English and by Benguerel and Cowan (1974) for French.

Nasalization in English is complementary to rounding in being specified among consonants but not vowels. According to a look-ahead version of a feature-spreading model, the nasal feature of a nasalized consonant should spread in an anticipatory direction through any number of preceding vowels up to the first oral (i.e., nonnasal) consonant. Supportive evidence on nasality was reported by Moll and Daniloff (1971).

Because, in this theory, coarticulation is spreading of a feature, it makes the strong prediction that coarticulation will be categorial, not gradient both in space and in time. To a first approximation (but see Kent, Carney, & Severeid, 1974, for a qualification), a rounded /š/ should be as rounded as an /u/, and the rounding should always begin at the beginning of a segment to which it has spread, never in the middle. Feature-spreading theories are now generally agreed to have been disconfirmed in part because close examination of the data shows that coarticulation is clearly gradient in character and in part because experiments with improved designs have shown that spreading is less extensive than earlier research had reported. Keating's *window model* of coarticulation (Keating, 1990) and the theory of coarticulation as coproduction both address each source of disconfirmation.

2. The Window Model of Coarticulation

At least some of coarticulation is gradient in nature and does not respect segment boundaries. For example, Benguerrel and Cowan's (1974) frequently cited findings of anticipation of rounding from the first, rounded, vowel in *structure* in the French noun phrase *ministre structure* in fact showed gradience in time. They found anticipatory rounding during the word-initial [str] of *structure* and the word-final [str] of *ministre* as expected because the consonants are unspecified for rounding. However, they also report rounding part way through the second, unrounded, vowel of *ministre*. In a feature-spreading account, this segment should not have been rounded at all, but of central relevance here, there is no provision in the theory for a feature to be spread to part of a segment. Keating (1990) cites other examples from Arabic (Card, 1979; Ghazeli, 1977) in which effects of tongue backing (emphasis) are gradient not only in time, but also in spatial extent.

Keating's proposal retains the idea that coarticulation is assimilation of a segment to its context, and she concurs with Daniloff and Hammarberg (1973) and others that some of coarticulation is categorial and characterizable as feature spreading. However, she suggests that, in cases where coarticulation is gradient, it can be seen as a later, lower-level process rather than as one of feature spreading. Her proposal is to replace the dichotomous concept that segments can be either specified or unspecified for a feature with a graded concept that each segment is associated with target windows of some width on each articulatory dimension involved in realizing its feature values. A maximally wide window corresponds with the earlier unspecified and a minimum window width with specified. However, all window widths between the extremes are possible, as well. Coarticulation is the consequence of the speaker choosing the smoothest or most economical path through a sequence of discrete windows. The theory improves on feature-spreading theory in offering an account of gradience in coarticulatory influences.

There are findings, however, indicating that at least some coarticulatory influences cannot be captured in a theory in which segments (or their windows) do not overlap. Öhman (1966) noticed acoustic influences of V_2 on closing transitions from V_1 to C in V_1CV_2 utterances. X-ray tracings in Öhman (1967) confirmed that the tongue body shape during C was different in the context of different vowels. He proposed that smooth vowel-to-vowel gestures of the tongue body occurred during speech production with consonant articulations superimposed on the diphthongal vocalic gestures (see also Barry & Kuenzel, 1975; Butcher & Weiher, 1976; Carney & Moll, 1971). Vowel-to-vowel gestures can even occur during production of consonants that themselves make demands on the vowels' primary articulator, the tongue body. Perkell (1969) found that the /k/ constriction gesture during production of /həkɛ/ consisted of a sliding tongue movement along the palate from the central location for schwa toward the more front location for /ɛ/. Although the vowel-to-vowel gestures might be seen as windows for each vowel with transitional regions between them, there appears to be no alternative to the conclusion that there is overlap between these windows and those for intervening consonants.

A third view of coarticulation holds that all of coarticulation is gradient in nature, and all of it is overlap in the production of sequences of consonants and vowels.

3. Coarticulation as Coproduction

In one version of this theory (Fowler, 1977; Fowler & Saltzman, 1993), coarticulation is the overlapping implementation of (to a first approximation) context-invariant synergies that realize gestures for consonants and vowels. The context sensitivity apparent in articulation (as when, e.g., lip closure for /b/ is achieved with a lower jaw posture in /ba/ than in /bi/) is seen as a peripheral blending of overlapping movements, not a revision in the plan for achieving a consonant or vowel.

Bell-Berti and Harris's (1981) *frame theory* adds to this characterization a claim that the temporally staggered onsets of the gestures for a consonant or vowel are sequenced in a temporally invariant fashion. This version of the theory appears to be in conflict with data cited earlier in favor of feature-spreading theories, findings that lip rounding and nasalization have extensive anticipatory fields that are linked to the onset of the first segment in a string that is unspecified for the feature. However, research by Bell-Berti and collaborators has shown that a missing control in those earlier investigations led to a considerable overestimation of the extent of coarticulation of lip rounding and nasalization.

Utterances in studies of anticipation of lip rounding have generally been of the form VC_nu, where V is an unrounded vowel and C_n is a consonant string of variable length. The missing control is an utterance type, such as VC_ni in which the ostensible source of any rounding during the consonant string has been eliminated. In the consonant strings of such control utterances, Bell-Berti and colleagues have found lip rounding movement or muscle activity that can be ascribed only to the consonants themselves. Using the control utterances to eliminate such spurious rounding from test utterances reveals an invariant, short-duration anticipation of rounding due to a rounded vowel, consistent with expectations from frame theory (e.g., Boyce, 1990; Gelfer, Bell-Berti, & Harris, 1989; see also Perkell & Matthies, 1992). An interpretation of the earlier findings of more extensive anticipation of rounding is that the earlier evidence was contaminated by lip movements associated with the consonants preceding the rounded vowel.

Research on anticipation of nasalization has the same history. When control utterances of the form V_nC are used to eliminate vowel-related velum lowering the V_nN utterances (where N is a nasal consonant), anticipation of velum lowering for N is found to be short in duration and to precede onset of oral constriction for the nasal by an invariant interval (e.g., Bell-Berti, 1980; Bell-Berti & Krakow, 1991).

Although frame theory appears to provide an account that is compatible with the available data, it is likely that some aspects of the theory will undergo modification. Bell–Berti and colleagues reported that lip rounding anticipates the acoustically defined onset of a rounded vowel by an invariant interval. However, it is unlikely that talkers time lip rounding relative to an acoustically defined landmark. It is more likely that timing or phasing is relative to the gesture achieving the oral configuration for the vowel. Second, as Bell–Berti and Harris (1981) note, it is not likely, in fact, that any real anticipation will be invariant over rate variation. Finally, Krakow's (1989) findings on anticipation of velum lowering for a nasal consonant suggest different phasing rules for pre and post vocalic consonants.

4. Lingual Coarticulation and Coarticulation Resistance: Another Role for Synergies?

In 1976, Bladon and Al-Bamerni introduced the term *coarticulation resistance* to describe the observation that different segments appear to resist coarticulatory influences to greater and lesser degrees. Recasens (1984a, 1984b, 1985, 1987, 1989, 1991) has done much of the work to develop the concept of coarticulation resistance. In a sequence of Catalan consonants that vary in amount of tongue dorsum contact with the palate, he found that consonants with more palatal contact show less coarticulatory influence from neighboring vowels than do consonants with less contact (Recasens, 1984a, 1987). Since vowels also use the tongue dorsum and would tend to lower the tongue away from the palate, the resistance may be seen as an act of "self-preservation" on the part of these consonants. It is interesting that consonants and vowels that strongly resist coarticulatory influences in their own domains in turn exert relatively strong influences on neighbors (see Tables II–VI in Recasens, 1987; see also Butcher & Weiher, 1976; Farnetani, 1990; Farnetani, Vagges, & Magno-Caldognetto, 1985).

A consequence of the different degrees of coarticulation resistance among the gestures of segments in their own domains and a consequence of their correspondingly different degrees of aggression outside of their domains are that production of a given consonant or vowel can appear to differ in different contexts, in particular, its coarticulatory extent will vary. A question is whether this apparent context sensitivity is "deep," that is, whether it reflects changes in a talker's articulatory plan or whether it arises in peripherally established influences on a plan's implementation.

In both Keating's windows theory and the theory of coproduction, the variation arises below the level of a speech plan. For Keating, it arises in the computation of transitions between windows for neighboring segments. A narrow window will exert a stronger influence on the transitional movement than will a wider window. In the theory of coarticulation as coproduction, there are no transitions between segments; there is only overlap. The context sensitivity is hypothesized to arise in the peripheral blending of influences on common articulators of the gestures for different consonants and vowels (Fowler & Saltzman, 1993; also see Saltzman & Munhall, 1989). In the theory, synergies are responsible for flexible achievement of invariant goals of a phonetic gesture as described earlier. They achieve these goals by establishing physiological linkages among articulators that instantiate the appropriate attractor dynamics. But the linkages can be looked at in another way from the perspective of other gestures whose influences on the vocal tract overlap with the target gestures in time. From that perspective, the linkages constitute barriers of variable strengths or resistances to the influences of those overlapping gestures. For a segment such as Catalan /j/ that requires considerable tongue dorsum contact with the palate, the linkages between jaw and tongue that bring about the contact also serve to resist influences from other gestures that would reduce the required contact. In short, in this theory, the constraints that implement synergies are at once the means by which gestural goals are achieved and the sources of resistance to coarticulatory influences that would prevent or hamper goal achievement. The same linkages that make a gesture more or less resistant to coarticulation from neighbors are sources of stronger or weaker coarticulatory influence outside their domain.

B. Models of Sequencing in Speech Production

In a recent discussion of the task dynamic model of speech production, Saltzman and Munhall (1989) point out that, currently, the model offers an intrinsic dynamical account of the implementation of gestures in the vocal tract, but not of sequencing or phasing of gestures themselves. Rather, to generate gestural sequencing, the model uses a gestural score (see Figure 2) in which appropriate sequencing is represented explicitly. Saltzman and Munhall suggest that an approach more compatible with their general theoretical framework would incorporate an adaptation of Jordan's (1986) network model of sequence control into the task dynamic model. Jordan (1986) makes a similar suggestion.

Jordan developed his model to address the problem of serial order in action and, in particular, in speech production. This is the problem, apart from concerns about details of timing or phasing of components of a complex action, of executing the components in the required order. Jordan proposed a model, the structure of which is shown in Figure 4. In the model, a sequence consists of a succession of patterns of activation over the output units of the model. The model learns to produce sequences, by associating each with a unique pattern of activation over the plan units.

Activation at the plan and state level, and again at the level of hidden

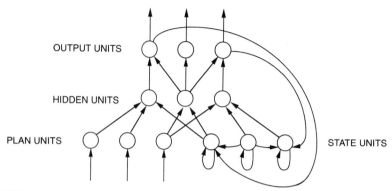

FIGURE 4   A simple example of Jordan's (1986) network model of sequence production. (Adapted from Jordan, 1986, Figure 3.)

units, propagates along links to the next level. Activation at a level is multiplied by the weights on linkages to the next level; products converging on a node are summed and added to a bias value associated with the node. In Jordan's implementation, hidden units and output units follow a rule that, if the activation quantity is positive, a 1 is output; otherwise the output is 0. The pattern of 1s and 0s over the output at a given time represents a set of feature values for one element of the sequence.

A crucial feature of the model that allows sequences with arbitrary numbers of repeated phonemes to be produced is that output units feed back to state units, which themselves are recurrent. This means that outputs, which are functions of activation from both plan and state units, are influenced by their temporal context. (Previous outputs are exponentially weighted so that more recent outputs are represented most strongly.) Because the state reflects the history of the sequence, the first and second /l/s in *lily,* for example, are distinguished by their contexts, and the sequence can be produced without error. Aside from offering a viable solution to the problem of serial order, Jordan's network has two other interesting properties. First, learned sequences (learned trajectories through state space) can serve as limit-cycle attractors, so that compensation for errors is possible. A second interesting feature of the model is that, over learning, generalization occurs so that outputs and states that are temporally close are similar. Therefore, the model's outputs exhibit coarticulatory overlap.

In Saltzman and Munhall's projected incorporation of Jordan's model into task dynamics (described in Saltzman & Munhall, 1989), output units would produce activations for gestures, not the feature values output in Jordan's implementation. Browman and Goldstein's gestural scores would, then, be replaced by plan units that, when inserted into the network, would generate appropriately sequenced gestural activations.

Saltzman and Munhall's proposal may have an unanticipated benefit. As noted, generally, the literature bifurcates into studies of speech production (i.e., studies of articulation) and studies of language production that address plans for producing linguistic units of various grain sizes. Recently, in the literature on language production, Dell, Juliano, and Govindjee (1992) have proposed a model at the level of phoneme production in which a Jordan-like network generates the sequencing of phonemes. This convergence on a single model type from these two directions may offer some hope for the eventual development of a unified model of production.

To put the proposal of Dell et al. in context, I first briefly characterize earlier accounts of phoneme production, based, as the proposal of Dell et al. is, on spontaneous errors of speech production. Some typical single-segment speech errors were listed above in Section II. A striking characteristic of these big errors (i.e., errors audible to an error collector) is their systematicness. In substitution errors, sequences rarely violate the phonotactic constraints of a language; consonants substitute only for consonants and vowels only for vowels; VCs, a constituent of a syllable called the *rime*, are more likely to participate in a substitution than are (nonconstituent) CVs; initial consonants of a word are more likely to participate in a substitution than are postvocalic consonants. Dell et al. called these systematicities *phonological frame constraints,* because they have been interpreted as requiring an explanation in which, during production planning, abstract structural frames for an utterance are distinguished from the phonological contents that fill them.

To explain phonological frame constraints, researchers (e.g., Dell, 1986; Shattuck-Hufnagel, 1983) proposed *slot and filler* or *structure versus content* models in which building a speech plan involves creating abstract structural frames for components of an utterance and then inserting words, morphemes, and phonological segments into the frames. In Dell's (1986) model, sequencing is the consequence of gradient activation in a tiered lexical network and of successive insertion of the most highly activated lexical units of a specified type into appropriate slots in structural frames built for the planned utterance. Errors occur when the most highly activated item in the lexical network that fits the frame's requirements is not the intended item. This can happen because of the spread of activation in the network and because of the presence of some activation noise. Because of the structural frames, however, errors will be systematic. At the phonological level, in particular, most phonological frame constraints (all except the finding that initial consonants are particularly error prone) will be respected. Errors will create phonotactically acceptable sequences because generally if, for example, a vowel is required by the frame, any vowel that is selected will yield an acceptable sequence. Further, because the frame distinguishes initial (onset) consonants, vowels, and final (coda) consonants in a syllable, onset consonants will substitute only for other onset consonants, vowels for vowels, and coda consonants for coda consonants. VCs participate jointly in errors, whereas CVs do not, because VCs (syllable rimes) are units in the lexicon that spread activation to (and receive reinforcing activation from) their component phonological segments.

The model provides a successful account of sequencing in speech production in which most natural error types occur in natural relative proportions. Additionally, the model has been a source of counterintuitive or unexpected error patterns that experimental tests with human subjects have confirmed. It has some unappealing features, however, one of which is its invocation of abstract structural frames. When a lexical item, say, *bag* has been selected at its level, a syllabic frame is created at the next level down that knows that the phonological sequence will consist of a C followed by a V and then a C. But why, if that much is known, is it not already known that the sequence is /b/, /æ/, /g/? And if that is known, why must activation spread in order for selection to occur? The answer is that, as it is, the model generates errors in the proper patterns; without the frame–content distinction it would not.

Dell et al. (1992) suggest an alternative model that almost dispenses with the structural frames; they propose that the frame constraints, the very findings that led Dell (1986) and others to distinguish frames from contents in their models, can arise in the absence of explicit frames. The new model has, in general, the structure of Jordan's model described above. As in Jordan's simulation, words were assigned plans consisting of a unique pattern of 1 and 0 activations on the plan units of the model. There were 18 output units, one for each of Chomsky and Halle's (1968) phonological features. Dell et al. trained the network to generate the appropriate succession of feature values for words in several lexicons consisting of CVCs. Errors occurred in some simulations because sequence learning was incomplete and in other simulations because noise was added to linkage weights. In either case, frame constraints were evident in errors in approximately the same proportions as those in natural error corpora.

As Dell et al. explain, one reason why errors adhere to frame constraints in the absence of explicit frames is that the network is disposed to adhere to well-worn paths (i.e., well-learned sequences serve as attractors; cf. Jordan, 1986). Dell et al. refer to this as the "sequential bias." A second reason is that errors on the output units will be small and therefore will differ by just one or two features from the intended segment (the "similarity bias"). Both biases foster errors in which the output sequence is phonotactically legal. That is, the sequential bias will foster use of a learned, even if not the intended, sequence; the similarity bias will lead to selection of a segment similar to the intended one, and similar segments tend to be phonotactically permissible in similar contexts. The similarity bias will tend to ensure that consonants substitute for consonants and vowels for vowels. The sequential bias fosters a finding that VCs participate in errors more than CVs, in that, in English, VCs are more redundant that are CVs. (That is, given V, the identity of the next C is more constrained than that of the prior C.) Likewise, initial Cs are preceded in Dell et al.'s sequential coding only by a null element signifying a word edge. Consequently, they are less determinate than Cs following vowels and are relatively error prone.

This new model of Dell et al. is an exciting development in part because it eliminates the inelegance of structural frames that are abstracted from, yet tailored to, their contents. It is also exciting in the present context, because, in conjunction with Jordan's sequencing model that coarticulates, and with the possible interfacing of such a model with Saltzman's task dynamic model that generates synergistic actions to a model vocal tract, there is hope for a unified model of production that exhibits many of the central characteristics of natural speech.

The model currently has a major limitation as Dell et al. point out. It generates substitution errors [such as (4) above in Section II] but not the more common movement errors [(1)–(3) in Section II] in which segments in a planned sequence themselves interact. The authors speculate that some characteristics of movement errors may be attained if more than one plan unit (one for a planned first word at, say, 80% activation, and one for a planned next word at 20% activation) is input to the network at the same time. Even so, this would not naturally generate the spectacular exchange errors (e.g., *heft lemisphere*). Consequently, Dell et al. are not able to conclude that frames can be dispensed with. Their more moderate conclusion is that:

> The . . . model can be taken as a demonstration that sequential biases and similarity are powerful principles in explaining error patterns. In fact, we . . . argue that the general frame constraints may simply reflect similarity and sequential effects and not phonological frames, at least not directly. Moreover, we interpret the model's success in its domain as evidence that there is something right about it, [and] that phonological speech errors result from the simultaneous influence of all the words stored in the system, in addition to the rest of words in the intended utterance. (1992, p. 33)

VII. OMISSIONS FROM THE CHAPTER: NEAR OMISSIONS IN THE FIELD

Just as theories of language production have been devised apart from theories of speech production, studies of prosody have been conducted almost independently of research on segmental production of speech (but see Beckman & Edwards, 1992, for a recent exception). Accordingly, theories of speech production have not, typically, explained the macroscopic structure in speaking that metrical or intonational patterning provides (but see Levelt,

1989, for an ambitious attempt). Perhaps a fully integrated account of speech production must await further descriptive studies of the prosodic patternings themselves that are increasingly common.

Eventually, theories of speech production must also provide an account of ordinary variability in speech. Variability in the pronunciation of a word occurs over different speaking styles from formal to casual and more generally over different communicative settings. Words may be produced with ordinary clarity, they may be "hyperarticulated" (e.g., Lindblom, 1990), as when we speak to a deaf person who must lip read, or they may be considerably reduced ("hypoarticulated") when they are redundant for one reason or another (e.g., Browman & Goldstein, 1986a; Fowler & Housum, 1987). No model of production as yet generates this gradience in production that is so natural to, and characteristic of, human speech outside the laboratory.

Acknowledgments

Preparation of this manuscript was supported by NICHD Grant HD-01994 to Haskins Laboratories. I thank Catherine Browman and Gary Dell for comments on parts of the manuscript.

References

Abbs, J., & Gracco, V. (1984). Control of complex gestures: Orofacial muscle responses to load perturbations of the lip during speech. *Journal of Neurophysiology, 51,* 705–723.

Barry, W., & Kuenzel, H. (1975). Co-articulatory airflow characteristics of intervocalic voiceless plosives. *Journal of Phonetics, 3,* 263–282.

Beckman, M., & Edwards, J. (1992). Intonational categories and the articulatory control of duration. In Y. Tohkura, E. Vatikiotis-Bateson, & Y. Sagisaka (Eds.), *Speech perception, production and linguistic structure* (pp. 359–376). Tokyo: IOS Press.

Bell-Berti, F. (1980). Velopharyngeal function: A spatio-temporal model. In N. Lass (Ed.), *Speech and language: Advances in basic research and practice* (pp. 291–316). New York: Academic Press.

Bell-Berti, F., & Harris, K. (1981). A temporal model of speech production. *Phonetica, 38,* 9–20.

Bell-Berti, F., & Krakow, R. (1991). Anticipatory velar lowering: A coproduction account. *Journal of the Acoustical Society of America, 90,* 112–123.

Bendor-Samuel, J.-T. (1960). Some problems of segmentation in the phonological analysis of Terena. *Word, 16,* 348–355.

Benguerel, A., & Cowan, H. (1974). Coarticulation of upper lip protrusion in French. *Phonetica, 30,* 41–55.

Bernstein, N. (1967). *The coordination and regulation of movement.* London: Pergamon Press.

Bladon, A., & Al-Bamerni, A. (1976). Coarticulation resistance in English /l/. *Journal of Phonetics, 4,* 137–150.

Boyce, S. (1990). Coarticulatory organization for lip rounding in Turkish and English. *Journal of the Acoustical Society of America, 88,* 2584–2595.

Browman, C., & Goldstein, L. (1986a). Dynamic processes in linguistics: Casual speech and sound change. *Perceiving Acting Workshop Review (Working Papers of the Center for the Ecological Study of Perception and Action), 1,* 17–18.

Browman, C., & Goldstein, L. (1986b). Towards an articulatory phonology. *Phonology Yearbook, 3,* 219–252.

Browman, C., & Goldstein, L. (1989). Articulatory gestures as phonological units. *Phonology, 6,* 201–252.

Browman, C., & Goldstein, L. (1990a). Gestural specification using dynamically-defined articulatory structures. *Journal of Phonetics, 18,* 299–320.

Browman, C., & Goldstein, L. (1990b). Representation and reality: Physical systems and phonological structure. *Journal of Phonetics, 18,* 411–425.

Browman, C., & Goldstein, L. (1990c). Tiers in articulatory phonology, with some implications for casual speech. In J. Kingston & M. Beckman (Eds.), *Papers in laboratory phonology: I. Between the grammar and the physics of speech* (pp. 341–376). Cambridge, UK: Cambridge University Press.

Browman, C., & Goldstein, L. (1992). Articulatory phonology: An overview. *Phonetica, 49,* 222–234.

Butcher, A., & Weiher, E. (1976). An electropalatographic investigation of coarticulation in VCV sequences. *Journal of Phonetics, 4,* 59–74.

Card, E. (1979). *A phonetic and phonological study of Arabic emphasis.* Doctoral dissertation, Cornell University, Ithaca, NY.

Carney, P., & Moll, K. (1971). A cinefluorographic investigation of fricative consonant-vowel coarticulation. *Phonetica, 23,* 193–202.

Chomsky, N., & Halle, M. (1968). *The sound pattern of English.* New York: Harper & Row.

Clements, G. N. (1985). The geometry of phonological features. *Phonology Yearbook, 2,* 225–252.

Daniloff, R., & Hammarberg, R. (1973). On defining coarticulation. *Journal of Phonetics, 1,* 239–248.

Daniloff, R., & Moll, K. (1968). Coarticulation of lip rounding. *Journal of Speech and Hearing Research, 11,* 707–721.

Dell, G. (1986). A spreading-activation theory of retrieval in speech production. *Psychological Review, 93,* 283–321.

Dell, G., Juliano, C., & Govindjee, A. (1992). *Structure and content in language production: A theory of frame constraints in phonological speech errors* (Cognitive Science Technical Report No. UIUC-BI-CS-91-16). Urbana-Champaign: University of Illinois.

Easton, T. (1972). On the normal use of reflexes. *American Scientist, 60,* 591–599.

Elimelech, B. (1976). A tonal grammar of Etsakǫ. *UCLA Working Papers in Phonetics, 35.*

Farnetani, E. (1990). V-C-V lingual coarticulation and its spatiotemporal domain. In W. Hardcastle & A. Marchal (Eds.), *Speech production and speech modeling* (pp. 93–130). Dordrecht: Kluwer.

Farnetani, E., Vagges, K., & Magno-Caldognetto, E. (1985). Coarticulation in Italian /VtV/ sequences: A palatographic study. *Phonetica, 42,* 78–99.

Folkins, J., & Abbs, J. (1975). Lip and jaw motor control during speech. *Journal of Speech and Hearing Research, 18,* 207–220.

Fowler, C. A. (1977). *Timing control in speech production.* Bloomington: Indiana University Linguistics Club.

Fowler, C. A., & Housum, J. (1987). Talkers' signalling of "new" and "old" words in speech and listeners' perception and use of the distinction. *Journal of Memory and Language, 26,* 489–504.

Fowler, C. A., & Saltzman, E. (1993). Coordination and coarticulation in speech production. *Language and Speech, 36,* 171–195.

Fowler, C. A., & Turvey, M. T. (1980). Immediate compensation for bite block speech. *Phonetica, 37,* 307–326.

Fromkin, V. (1971). The nonamalous nature of anomalous utterances. *Language, 47,* 27–52.

Fromkin, V. (1973). *Speech errors as linguistic evidence.* The Hague: Mouton.

Gelfer, C., Bell-Berti, F., & Harris, K. (1989). Determining the extent of coarticulation: Effects of experimental design. *Journal of the Acoustical Society of America, 86,* 2443–2445.

Ghazeli, S. (1977). *Back consonants and backing coarticulation in Arabic.* Doctoral dissertation, University of Texas, Austin.

Goldsmith, J. (1976). *Autosegmental phonology.* Bloomington: Indiana University Linguistics Club.

Goldsmith, J. (1990). *Autosegmental and metrical phonology.* Oxford: Basil Blackwell.

Henke, W. (1966). *Dynamic articulatory models of speech production using computer simulation.* Doctoral dissertation, MIT, Cambridge, MA.

Jordan, M. (1986). *Serial order: A parallel distributed process.* (ICS Report 8604). San Diego: University of California, Institute for Cognitive Science.

Keating, P. (1990). The window model of coarticulation: Articulatory evidence. In J. Kingston & M. Beckman (Eds.), *Papers in laboratory phonology: Between the grammar and the physics of speech* (pp. 451–470). Cambridge, UK: Cambridge University Press.

Kelso, J. A. S., Saltzman, E., & Tuller, B. (1986). The dynamical perspective on speech production: Data and theory. *Journal of Phonetics, 14,* 29–59.

Kelso, J. A. S., Tuller, B., Vatikiotis-Bateson, E., & Fowler, C. A. (1984). Functionally-specific cooperation following jaw perturbation during speech: Evidence for coordinative structures. *Journal of Experimental Psychology: Human Perception and Performance, 10,* 812–832.

Kenstowicz, M., & Kisseberth, C. (1979)). *Generative phonology.* New York: Academic Press.

Kent, R., Carney, P., & Severeid, L. (1974). Velar movement and timing: Evaluation of a model for binary control. *Journal of Speech and Hearing Research, 17,* 470–488.

Krakow, R. (1989). *The articulatory organization of syllables: A kinematic analysis of labial and velar gestures.* Doctoral dissertation, Yale University, New Haven, CT.

Kugler, P., Kelso, J. A. S., & Turvey, M. (1980). On the concept of coordinative structures as dissipative structures. I. Theoretical lines of convergence. In G. Stelmach & J. Requin (Eds.), *Tutorials in motor behavior* (pp. 3–47). Amsterdam: North-Holland.

Levelt, W. (1989). *Speaking: From intention to articulation.* Cambridge, MA: MIT Press.

Lindblom, B. (1990). Explaining phonetic variation: A sketch of the H&H theory. In W. Hardcastle & A. Marchal (Eds.), *Speech production and speech modeling* (pp. 403–439). Dordrecht: Kluwer.

Lindblom, B., Lubker, J., & Gay, T. (1979). Formant frequencies of some fixed mandible vowels and a model of speech motor programming by predictive simulation. *Journal of Phonetics, 7,* 147–161.

Lindblom, B., & Sundberg, J. (1971). Acoustical consequences of lip, tongue, jaw and larynx movement. *Journal of the Acoustical Society of America, 50,* 1166–1179.

Moll, K., & Daniloff, R. (1971). Investigation of the timing of velar movements during speech. *Journal of the Acoustical Society of America, 50,* 678–684.

Moll, K., Zimmermann, G., & Smith, A. (1976). The study of speech production as a human neuromotor system. In M. Sawashima & F. S. Cooper (Eds.), *Dynamic aspects of speech production* (pp. 71–82). Tokyo: University of Tokyo.

Mowrey, R., & MacKay, I. (1990). Phonological primitives: Electromyographic speech error evidence. *Journal of the Acoustical Society of America, 88,* 1299–1312.

Öhman, S. (1966). Coarticulation in VCV utterances: Spectrographic measurements. *Journal of the Acoustical Society of America, 39,* 151–168.

Öhman, S. (1967). Numerical model of coarticulation. *Journal of the Acoustical Society of America, 41,* 310–320.

Perkell, J. (1969). *Physiology of speech production: Results and implications of a quantitative cineradiographic study.* Cambridge, MA: MIT Press.

Perkell, J., & Matthies, M. (1992). Temporal measures of labial coarticulation for the vowel /u/. *Journal of the Acoustical Society of America, 91,* 2911–2925.

Pierrehumbert, J. (1990). Phonological and phonetic representations. *Journal of Phonetics, 18,* 375–394.

Recasens, D. (1984a). V-to-C coarticulation in Catalan VCV sequences: An articulatory and acoustical study. *Journal of Phonetics, 12,* 61–73.

Recasens, D. (1984b). Vowel-to-vowel coarticulation in Catalan VCV sequences. *Journal of the Acoustical Society of America, 76,* 1624–1635.

Recasens, D. (1985). Coarticulatory patterns and degrees of coarticulation resistance in Catalan CV sequences. *Language and Speech, 28,* 97–114.

Recasens, D. (1987). An acoustic analysis of V-to-C and V-to-V coarticulatory effects in Catalan and Spanish VCV sequences. *Journal of Phonetics, 15,* 299–312.

Recasens, D. (1989). Long range coarticulatory effect for tongue dorsum contact in VCVCV sequences. *Speech Communication, 8,* 293–307.

Recasens, D. (1991). An electropalatal and acoustic study of consonant-to-vowel coarticulation. *Journal of Phonetics, 19,* 177–196.

Repp, B. (1981). On levels of description is speech research. *Journal of the Acoustical Society of America, 69,* 1462–1464.

Ryle, G. (1949). *The concept of mind.* New York: Barnes and Noble.

Saltzman, E. (1986). Task dynamic coordination of the speech articulators. In H. Heuer & C. Fromm (Eds.), *Generation and modeling of action patterns* (pp. 129–144). New York: Springer-Verlag.

Saltzman, E., & Kelso, J. A. S. (1987). Skilled action: A task-dynamic approach. *Psychological Review, 94,* 84–106.

Saltzman, E., & Munhall, K. (1989). A dynamical approach to gestural patterning in speech production. *Ecological Psychology, 1,* 333–382.

Shaiman, S. (1989). Kinematic and electromyographic respones to perturbation of the jaw. *Journal of the Acoustical Society of America, 86,* 78–88.

Shattuck-Hufnagel, S. (1983). Sublexical units and suprasegmental structure in speech production parsing. In P. F. MacNeilage (Ed.), *The Production of speech* (pp. 109–135). New York: Springer-Verlag.

Shattuck-Hufnagel, S., & Klatt, D. (1979). Minimal uses of features and markedness in speech production: Evidence from speech errors. *Journal of Verbal Learning and Verbal Behavior, 18,* 41–55.

Stemberger, J. P. (1983). *Speech errors and theoretical phonology: A review.* Bloomington: Indiana University Linguistics Club.

Stemberger, J. P. (1991a). Apparent anti-frequency effects in language production: The addition bias and phonological underspecification. *Journal of Memory and Language, 30,* 161–185.

Stemberger, J. P. (1991b). Radical underspecification in language production. *Phonology, 8,* 73–112.

Turvey, M. T. (1977). Preliminaries to a theory of action with reference to vision. In R. Shaw & J. Bransford (Eds.), *Perceiving, acting, and knowing: Toward an ecological psychology* (pp. 211–266). Hillsdale, NJ: Erlbaum.

Turvey, M. T. (1990). Coordination. *American Psychologist, 45,* 938–953.

van der Hulst, H., & Smith, N. (1982). An overview of autosegmental and metrical phonology. In H. van der Hulst & N. Smith (Eds.), *The structure of phonological representations.* Part 1 (pp. 1–46). Dordrecht: Foris.

CHAPTER 3

Speech Perception: New Directions in Research and Theory

Lynne C. Nygaard
David B. Pisoni

I. INTRODUCTION

The fundamental problem in the study of speech perception is how to characterize the process by which listeners derive meaning from the acoustic waveform. At first glance, the solution to the problem of how we perceive speech seems deceptively simple. If one could identify stretches of the acoustic waveform that correspond to units of perception, then the path from sound to meaning would be clear. However, this correspondence or mapping has proven extremely difficult to find, even after some forty-five years of research on the problem.

One of the earliest and most basic findings in the study of speech perception was the observation that speech sounds are not organized in the signal like beads on a string (Liberman, 1957; Liberman, Cooper, Shankweiler, & Studdert-Kennedy, 1967) to be picked out of the acoustic signal one at a time by the perceiver for further processing. Rather, the ability to perceive speech is a complex process that involves converting a highly encoded physical stimulus into some kind of abstract neural representation. The ultimate goal of research on speech perception is to explain the structure and function of the perceptual system at each level of description, from signal to percept.

Typically, over the last twenty years, the study of speech has been pur-

Speech, Language, and Communication

sued from an information processing approach (Studdert-Kennedy, 1976). The acoustic waveform was assumed to be analyzed into a set of discrete, symbolic units, which are then compared with stored representations in memory. From this point of view, the end product of perception in speech is a string of abstract, timeless, canonical linguistic units such as distinctive features, phonetic segments, or phonemes in the traditional sense. Although generating a rich and informative body of empirical research and phenomena, this approach to speech perception has left many theoretical issues unexplored and many questions unanswered.

The goal of the present chapter is to provide a selective review of some of the fundamental problems encountered in the study of speech perception. Although a complete and exhaustive discussion of the empirical work is beyond the scope of this chapter (for other reviews, see Cutting & Pisoni, 1978; Darwin, 1976; Goldinger, Pisoni, & Luce, in press; Jusczyk, 1986; Luce & Pisoni, 1987; J. L. Miller, 1990; Pisoni, 1978; Pisoni & Luce, 1986; Studdert-Kennedy, 1974, 1976), we hope to address some key issues in the field and suggest some promising alternative approaches to the old problems that have confronted speech researchers. Our aim is to demonstrate how the accumulated knowledge in the field leads to a rethinking of the nature of linguistic units, how they are represented and how they are processed by the nervous system. Our goal is a reinterpretation of the canonical abstract linguistic unit as the type of representation that underlies the perception of speech. Rather, we emphasize the richness and detail of the neural representations used in speech perception as well as the flexible, context-dependent nature of the processes that act on and use the informationally rich speech representations. In doing so, our discussion focuses primarily on phonetic perception. We maintain a somewhat arbitrary distinction between phonetic perception and spoken word recognition only for convenience and brevity. However, we acknowledge that any complete account of speech perception necessarily must take into consideration all levels of perceptual processing (see Cutler, Chapter 4, this volume) and must also ultimately confront the complex issues in spoken language comprehension.

II. BASIC ISSUES IN SPEECH PERCEPTION

A. Linearity, Segmentation, and Lack of Invariance

One of the most prominent characteristics of speech is that it is a time-varying continuous signal; yet, the impression of the listener is that of a series of discrete linguistic units, the phonemes, syllables, and words that carry meaning. The problem for the theorist working in speech perception is to account for how listeners might carve up the continuous signal of speech into the appropriate units of analysis and recover the linguistic intent of the talker.

Although linguistic units such as phonemes, syllables, and words perceptually appear to follow one after another in time, the same linearity is not found in the physical signal (Chomsky & Miller, 1963). Thus, it is often stated that the speech signal fails to meet the *linearity* condition, which assumes that for each phoneme there must be a particular stretch of sound in the utterance. In natural speech, properties of the acoustic signal associated with one phoneme often overlap or co-occur with the properties of adjacent segments (Delattre, Liberman, & Cooper, 1955; Liberman, Delattre, Cooper, & Gerstman, 1954).

Because of this overlap in the acoustic signal, it is unclear how listeners are able to separate information about one linguistic unit from another. This difficulty in the parsing of the acoustic waveform into discrete linguistic units has been termed the *segmentation problem*. Figure 1 shows a speech spectrogram of an utterance that illustrates this problem. Although a native speaker of English has no problem identifying the phonemes, syllables, and words in the phrase, *I owe you a yo-yo,* there appear to be no obvious acoustic junctures that correspond with perceptual units. The influence of adjacent segments can be seen not only between phonemes, but also across syllable and word boundaries, and although it is possible to identify acoustic segments in the stream of speech reliably (Fant, 1962), these acoustic segments do not always correspond to linguistic units resulting from perceptual analysis.

In addition to the lack of linearity and segmentation in the mapping of acoustic segments onto phonetic percepts, there also exists a lack of

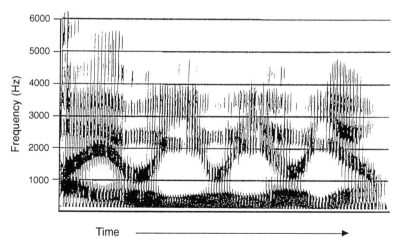

FIGURE 1   Spectrogram of the utterance, *I owe you a yo-yo,* demonstrating that perceptual segmentation is not clearly related to acoustic segmentation.

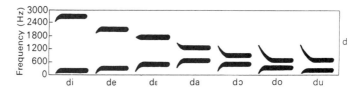

FIGURE 2 Synthetic tokens of syllables beginning with /d/ in which the second formant transitions specify the consonant. (Adapted from Liberman, 1957, with permission of author and publisher.)

acoustic–phonetic invariance in speech perception. Researchers have been unable to find invariant sets of acoustic features or properties that correspond uniquely to individual linguistic units. Instead, because adjacent phonetic segments exert a considerable influence on the acoustic realization of a given phoneme, the acoustic properties that specify a particular phoneme can vary drastically as a function of phonetic context, speaking rate, and syntactic environment. Figure 2 illustrates a classic example of the role of context variability in speech perception (see Liberman, 1957). The first two formants (energy maxima in the acoustic signal resulting from natural resonances of the vocal tract) are shown for a variety of syllables containing the phoneme /d/. The formant transitions that begin each syllable provide information for the /d/ in each syllable context. However, depending on vowel environment, the formant transitions are quite different acoustically and, consequently, the physical realization of the phoneme /d/ is quite different. The paradox for the study of speech perception is that listeners perceive each of these syllables as beginning with a /d/ sound even though the formant transitions for place of articulation in these patterns are anything but invariant acoustically (see Liberman et al., 1967).

The complex relations between acoustic properties of the speech signal and the linguistic units that listeners perceive stem from the way in which speech is produced. The sounds of speech are largely coarticulated, that is, the articulatory gestures associated with adjacent phonetic segments overlap in time. This process of coarticulation results in the smearing together of information in the acoustic signal about individual phonemes. Therefore, as gestures overlap in time, so do the corresponding acoustic properties. The consequence of intended phonetic segments passing through the "articulatory wringer" (Hockett, 1955) is that the acoustic properties of the speech signal do not relate in any simple, obvious, or invariant way to the sequence of phonetic segments resulting from the listener's perceptual analysis of the signal.

B. Units of Perceptual Analysis: Phoneme, Syllable, Word, or Beyond

The principles of linearity, invariance, and segmentation all presuppose a basic unit of analysis in speech perception and, in fact, a great deal of research has been devoted to uncovering such minimal units. Given the momentary and time-varying nature of the speech signal and constraints on auditory memory, it has been reasonable to assume that information in the acoustic waveform must be recoded quickly into a more permanent symbolic representation for further analysis (Broadbent, 1965; Liberman et al., 1967). The essential problem with the idea of the primacy of one type of representation for processing over another has been that no one unit has been found to be the perceptual building block in every situation. Therefore, given the constraints of a task and the nature of the stimuli used in an experiment, evidence has been marshaled for a wide variety of perceptual units, including features, phonemes, syllables, and words.

Empirical results are mixed with regard to what listeners use (features, phonemes, syllables, words, or even larger units) when they are analyzing speech. Numerous studies have shown that listeners appear to initially analyze the acoustic waveform into phoneme-like units and when called upon to make a response based on this type of segmental representation, they do so readily (Cutler, Mehler, Norris, & Segui, 1986; Norris & Cutler, 1988). Other studies have found that subjects are faster and more reliable when their responses are based on a syllable-sized unit (Mehler, 1981; Segui, 1984).

Larger units than the syllable have been considered as well. Studies showing that units such as phonemes and syllables are contingent perceptually on larger perceptual entities such as words and phrases (Bever, Lackner, & Kirk, 1969; Ganong, 1980; G. A. Miller, 1962; Rubin, Turvey, & van Gelder, 1975) suggest that listeners take into account progressively larger stretches of the acoustic waveform when processing the linguistic content of an utterance. Accordingly, it appears that no one unit can be processed without consideration of the context in which it is embedded. This interdependence of representations argues against a strict hierarchical view of the processing of speech in which the signal is segmented into a set of basic units that provide the foundation in every case for the next level of processing (Remez, 1987). Instead, the primacy of any particular unit may rest to a large extent on processing contingencies, attentional demands of the task, and the information available at any given time (e.g., Eimas, Hornstein, & Payton, 1990; Eimas & Nygaard, 1992).

Finally, no discussion of the basic unit of representation in speech would be complete without mentioning that most of the proposed units in speech perception can trace their inspiration to formal linguistic analysis (see Frazier, Chapter 1, and Fowler, Chapter 2, this volume). In general, the type of representation that has provided the cornerstone of almost all theories of speech perception has been the abstract, canonical linguistic unit, the phonetic segment or phoneme or phoneme-like unit. Although both the size of the representational unit and the exact properties comprising the representation may vary with the listening requirements, the basic assumption is that listeners must extract abstract, invariant properties of the speech signal to be compared with prototypical representations that are hypothesized to be stored in long-term memory (Kuhl, 1991; Oden & Massaro, 1978; Samuel, 1982).

Implicit in this notion of the canonical abstract linguistic unit is the assumption that variation in the signal due to phonetic context is "noise" that must be compensated for in the analysis of speech. However, representations such as context-sensitive allophones (Wickelgren, 1969, 1976), context-sensitive spectra (Klatt, 1979), and demisyllables (Fujimura & Lovins, 1978) have been proposed as alternatives to the types of symbolic representations typically assumed in speech perception research. Most of these proposed processing units stem from an interest in implementing speech recognition algorithms and many attempt to sidestep problems of context sensitivity by precompiling variability into the analytic representation. Although these proposed units are contingent on larger perceptual units just as the more traditional linguistic representations are, the attempt implicit in these approaches is to take into account the enormous context sensitivity in speech, which may well prove a promising approach when dealing with the problem of variability in the acoustic speech signal (Church, 1987; Elman & McClelland, 1986). In Section IIC, we address more fully the issue of variability and its effect on linguistic representation.

C. Variability and Perceptual Constancy in Speech

Variation due to phonetic context is just one of a wide variety of factors that can change the acoustic realization of speech sounds. Although much of the research in speech perception has been devoted to studying how listeners achieve consistent percepts in spite of the surrounding phonetic context, the way in which listeners cope with variability from changes in talker and speaking rate is at least as problematic for theories of speech perception. It has long been recognized that variability in talker characteristics and speaking rate among other factors can have profound effects on the acoustic realization of linguistic units. Substantial differences can be found between even two apparently identical utterances produced by the same speaker at the same rate of speech. The question still remains: how do listeners achieve perceptual constancy given the vast amount of acoustic variability that exists in the speech signal?

As mentioned above, the traditional conceptualization of this problem has been to consider this type of variability in the acoustic signal as noise that must be extracted to achieve constant phonetic percepts (Shankweiler, Strange, & Verbrugge, 1977). Listeners are thought to compensate for changes due to talker and speaking rate through a *perceptual normalization* process in which linguistic units are evaluated relative to the prevailing rate of speech (e.g., J. L. Miller, 1987; J. L. Miller & Liberman, 1979; Summerfield, 1981) and relative to specific characteristics of a talker's vocal tract (e.g., Joos, 1948; Ladefoged & Broadbent, 1957; Summerfield & Haggard, 1973). Variation is assumed to be stripped away to arrive at prototypical representations assumed to underlie further linguistic analysis.[1] Indeed, there has been a considerable amount of recent research exploring the nature of perceptual compensation for variability in the speech signal (for a review on rate effects, see J. L. Miller, 1981, 1987; for talker effects, see J. D. Miller, 1989; Nearey, 1989; Pisoni, 1993).

In this section, we consider the role of acoustic variability due to talker characteristics and speaking rate in speech perception. Although our focus is on these two factors, they do not by any means exhaust the sources of acoustic variability that can affect the acoustic fine structure of speech. Syntactic structure of the utterance (Klatt, 1975, 1976; Oller, 1973), utterance length (Klatt, 1975, 1976; Oller, 1973), semantic content, and even room reverberation (Watkins, 1988), to name but a few, all introduce variation in the way in which speech is produced and/or realized acoustically.

1. Talker Variability

One of the first demonstrations that listeners take into account a talker's voice in perceiving speech sounds was provided by Ladefoged and Broadbent (1957). These researchers presented listeners with synthetic precursor phrases in which the formant values had been shifted up or down to simulate vocal-tract differences between speakers. Following the precursor phrases, four target words (*bit, bet, bat,* and *but*) were presented and subjects' identification responses were evaluated with regard to the type of precursor phrase they received. Ladefoged and Broadbent found that subjects' vowel identification responses depended on the relative formant values contained in the precursor phrase and concluded that listeners calibrate their perceptual systems based on the vowel space of each individual talker (e.g., Joos, 1948; Lieberman, Crelin, & Klatt, 1972).

Numerous studies since Ladefoged and Broadbent (1957) have explored the issue of vocal-tract normalization. Researchers have attempted to determine what type of information in the speech signal may be used to compensate for differences in vocal-tract size and shape (Gerstman, 1968; Johnson, 1990; J. D. Miller, 1989; Nearey, 1989) and they have tried to develop normalization algorithms to account for differences among speakers. It is important to note here that all these algorithms have adopted the standard view of normalization and, as such, are generally based on rescaling procedures meant to reduce variation in the static properties of the speech signal (e.g., vowel formant frequencies) to a standard set of acoustic values that can be used for recognition.

Although this notion of vocal-tract normalization may benefit endeavors such as machine recognition of speech, it remains unclear to what extent perceivers use analogous types of procedures and extract prototypical or idealized representations from the acoustic signal. Studies conducted by Verbrugge, Strange, Shankweiler, and Edman (1976) and Verbrugge and Rakerd (1986) suggest that calibration in terms of evaluating phonetic content with regard to a speaker's vowel space may not necessarily occur. Their research showed not only that vowel identification performance is quite good even with extensive talker variability in the stimulus set, but also that exposure to a subset of a talker's vowels appears to provide little to aid in vowel identification performance. They concluded that when identifying vowels, listeners may use higher-order variables such as patterns of spectral change that are assumed to be independent of a talker's specific vocal-tract characteristics.

A growing body of research, however, suggests that the absence of effects due to talker variability in these studies may be the result of identification and discrimination tasks that minimize attentional and time constraints. When tasks are made more difficult or when processing times are measured in addition to accuracy, variability in the signal due to talker characteristics has been found to have a marked effect on listeners' performance. For example, Summerfield and Haggard (1973) have shown that reaction times are slower to recognize words when they are presented in multiple-talker versus single-talker contexts. Peters (1955), Creelman (1957), and, more recently, Mullennix, Pisoni, and Martin (1989) have shown that recognizing words in noise is more difficult when listeners are presented with words produced by multiple talkers compared to words produced by only a single talker. Finally, using a Garner (1974) speeded classification task, Mullennix and Pisoni (1990) reported that subjects had difficulty ignoring irrelevant variation in a talker's voice when asked to classify words by initial phoneme. These findings suggest that variations due to changes in talker characteristics are time and resource demanding. Furthermore, the processing of talker information appears to be dependent on the perception of the phonetic content of the message. The two sources of information are not perceptually independent.

Additional research has suggested that talker variability can affect memory processes as well. Martin, Mullennix, Pisoni, and Summers (1989) and Goldinger, Pisoni, and Logan (1991) found that at relatively fast presentation rates serial recall of spoken words is better in initial list positions when all the words in the list are produced by a single speaker compared to a condition in which each word is produced by a different speaker. It is interesting that at slower presentation rates, Goldinger et al. (1991) found that recall of words from multiple-talker lists was actually superior to recall of words from single-talker lists. These results suggest that at fast presentation rates, variation because of changes in the talker affects the initial encoding and subsequent rehearsal of items in the to-be-remembered lists. At slower presentation rates, on the other hand, listeners are able to fully process, rehearse, and encode each word along with the concomitant talker information. Consequently, listeners are able to use the additional talker information to aid in their recall task.

Further evidence that talker information is encoded and retained in memory comes from recent experiments conducted by Palmeri, Goldinger, and Pisoni (1993). Using a continuous recognition memory procedure, voice-specific information was shown to be retained along with lexical information; these attributes were found to aid later recognition. The finding that subjects are able to use talker-specific information suggests that this source of variability may not be discarded or normalized in the process of speech perception, as widely assumed in the literature. Rather, variation in a talker's voice may become part of a rich and highly detailed representation of the speaker's utterance (Geiselman & Bellezza, 1976, 1977).

Indeed, a recent study from our laboratory investigating the effects of talker familiarity on the perception of spoken words suggests that information about a talker's voice and linguistic information may not be processed and represented independently (Nygaard, Sommers, & Pisoni, 1994). In this experiment, subjects were asked to learn to explicitly identify a set of unfamiliar voices over a nine-day period. Half the subjects then identified novel words mixed in noise that were produced by talkers they were previously trained on and half the subjects then identified words mixed in noise produced by new talkers that they had not been exposed to previously. The results provide evidence for transfer of learning from the explicit voice identification task to the word recognition task. Subjects who heard novel words produced by familiar voices were able to recognize words in noise more accurately than subjects who received the same novel words produced by unfamiliar voices. These findings suggest that exposure to a talker's voice facilitates subsequent perceptual processing of novel words produced by that talker. Thus, these findings provide additional support for the view that the internal representation of spoken words encompasses both a phonetic description of the utterance and a structural description of the source characteristics of the specific talker. Although the exact nature of this type of representation remains to be specified, properties of a talker's voice and linguistic properties of the speech signal are apparently closely interrelated and are not necessarily dissociated in the perceptual analysis of speech.

Despite evidence for the interdependence of talker information and linguistic information, the study of speech perception has traditionally been considered separately from the study of the perception of voice (Laver, 1989; Laver & Trudgill, 1979). In addition to the linguistic content of a talker's utterance, the speech signal carries a considerable amount of personal information about the talker into the communicative setting. The human voice conveys information about a speaker's physical, social, and psychological characteristics (Laver, 1989; Laver & Trudgill, 1979) and these aspects, referred to as *indexical information* (Abercrombie, 1967), also appear to play an important role in speech communication.

In everyday conversation, the indexical properties of the speech signal become quite important as perceivers use this information to govern their own speaking styles and responses. From more permanent characteristics of a speaker's voice that provide information about identity to the short-term vocal changes related to emotion or tone of voice, indexical information contributes to the overall interpretation of a speaker's utterance. That listeners are able to exploit this variation in the signal to apprehend characteristics of a talker and use these characteristics to recover linguistic content suggests a possible reason for a detailed representation of the speech signal. Listeners may retain and use properties of a talker's voice because these properties provide a rich source of information for the listeners. Consequently, it seems that any explanation of perceptual normalization for talker will necessarily need to include an account of the processing and representation of both the information about a talker's voice and the linguistic information that is carried in the speech signal.

2. Variability in Speaking Rate

Changes in speaking rate or the tempo of a talker's speech is another source of variability that can alter the acoustic structure of phonetic segments. In a normal conversation, speakers can vary considerably the speed at which they produce speech. Not only do speakers increase and decrease the number and length of pauses, but they also lengthen or shorten the acoustic underpinnings of linguistic units in the utterance (J. L. Miller, Grosjean, & Lomanto, 1984). This alteration due to speaking rate is particularly profound for phonetic distinctions that are temporal or durational in nature. For example, the timing of voicing onset in voiced versus voiceless stop consonants (J. L. Miller, Green, & Reeves, 1986; Summerfield, 1975), as well as the relative duration and extent of stop–glide contrasts (J. L. Miller & Baer,

1983), may change dramatically with changes in the prevailing rate of speech. Consequently, the theoretical issue concerning rate variability is similar to the one concerning talker variability: how do listeners maintain perceptual constancy given the changes in the temporal properties of phonetic contrasts due to speaking rate? Here again, the notion of perceptual compensation arises. Listeners are thought to utilize some kind of rate normalization process in which articulation rate is taken into consideration when evaluating the linguistic content of an utterance.

A considerable amount of research has been devoted to the effects of speaking rate on the processing of phonetic contrasts that depend on temporal or duration information. By and large, listeners appear to be sensitive to changes in the speech signal due to rate. One of the first studies investigating effects of speaking rate on phonetic identification was conducted by J. L. Miller and Liberman (1979). They presented listeners with synthetic /ba/-/wa/ continua in which the stop–glide distinction was cued primarily by the duration of the formant transitions. Five /ba/-/wa/ continua were synthesized in which overall syllable duration was varied from 80 to 296 ms by changing the duration of the vowel segment. The results showed that listeners required a longer transition duration to hear the glide /w/ as the overall duration of the syllable increased. Thus, a shift was observed in the identification boundaries toward longer values of transition duration as the overall duration of the syllable became longer. According to the authors, the longer syllable duration specified a slower speaking rate and listeners adjusted their perceptual judgments accordingly.

Further research has shown that information about speaking rate *preceding* a phonetic contrast can affect perceptual judgments of phonetic identity as well. Summerfield (1981) conducted a series of experiments to evaluate the effect of a precursor phrase varying in rate of articulation on the identification of voiced versus voiceless stop consonants. His results showed that phoneme identification boundaries shifted to shorter values of voice onset time as the articulation rate of the precursor phrase increased. Thus, listeners were apparently basing their classification of the initial stop consonants on information about the prevailing rate of speech in the precursor phrase.

Although it appears clear that listeners are sensitive to changes in rate of articulation, less attention has been paid to the processing consequences, in terms of attention and resources, of this type of variability. At issue here is whether the observed changes in perceptual judgments are due to compensatory processes that require time and attention or whether adjustments to differences in rate are automatic and cost free in terms of processing. This question has been investigated recently in our laboratory in a series of experiments conducted by Sommers, Nygaard, and Pisoni (1994). They presented subjects with lists of words mixed in noise under two conditions, one in which all the words in the list were presented at a single speaking rate and one in which words in the list were presented at multiple speaking rates. The results mirrored those found earlier for talker variability (Mullennix et al., 1989). Subjects were better able to identify words mixed in noise if all the words were produced at a single speaking rate. Changes in speaking rate from word to word in a list apparently incurred some kind of processing cost that made identifying words more difficult. Again, the conclusion is that if a compensatory process exists, it must demand the attention and processing resources of the listener.

These studies and numerous others demonstrating the effects of speaking rate on perceptual judgments (see J. L. Miller, 1981, 1987, for a comprehensive review of the research on effects of speaking rate) all indicate that changes in speaking rate, both internal and external to the target segment, produce shifts in category boundaries. Recently, Miller and her colleagues (J. L. Miller & Volaitis, 1989; Volaitis & Miller, 1992) have shown that internal phonetic category *structures* that rely on temporal information are also sensitive to relative changes in rate of articulation. Their results indicate that changes in speaking rate affect the mapping of acoustic information onto the organization of phonetic category structures. Thus, listeners seem to compensate for changes in speaking rate not only by shifting or readjusting category boundaries, but also by reorganizing the entire structure of their phonetic categories. The implication of this finding is that any type of normalization or compensation process for speaking rate may be much more complex than just stripping away or normalizing rate information to arrive at idealized, time-invariant linguistic units. Instead, it seems that a great deal of temporal information, enough to specify category structure, is preserved in the initial encoding of the speech signal and is represented in memory.

One potential reason for a rich representation of variability in the speech signal due to speaking rate may be found in research on the contributions of prosodic information to the perception of speech. Just as indexical properties constitute a rich source of information for perceivers of speech, so do the prosodic or suprasegmental attributes of the speech signal. Similarly, as in the case of indexical information, the role of these attributes in speech perception has received relatively little attention. Prosody refers to the melody of speech or, more precisely, to differences in pitch, intensity, duration, and the timing of segments and words in sentences. Since most research in speech perception has concentrated on the segmental analysis of phonemes, there has always been a wide gap between research conducted on the perception of isolated segments and the role of prosodic factors in the processing of connected speech (see Cohen & Nooteboom, 1975). Nevertheless, it is apparent that prosody provides a crucial connection between phonetic segments, features, and words and higher-level grammatical processes (see

Darwin, 1975; Huggins, 1972; Nooteboom, Brokx, & de Rooij, 1978, for reviews). In addition, prosody provides useful information regarding lexical identity, syntactic structure, and the semantic content of a talker's utterance.

In the preceding sections, we have reviewed two sources of variability that can affect the processing of the linguistic content of a speaker's utterance. In addition, we have outlined the types of information, indexical and prosodic, that variations in talker and rate provide to the listener in everyday communication. Taken together, the research on these factors suggests that traditional explanations of speech perception may need to reconsider their long-standing emphasis on the search for abstract, canonical linguistic units as the end point of perception. It appears that a great deal of information is conveyed by the same factors that also exacerbate the problem of acoustic–phonetic invariance. Therefore, any account of speech perception will necessarily need to consider the apparently contradictory nature of these different sources of variability in the speech signal. In traditional accounts of speech perception, variability was considered to be noise, something to be eliminated so that the idealized symbolic representations of speech as a sequence of segments could emerge from the highly variable acoustic signal. Current thinking on these problems suggests a different view. Variation in speech should be considered as a rich source of information that is encoded and stored in memory along with the linguistic content of the talker's utterance. By this account, speech perception does not involve a mapping of invariant attributes or features onto idealized symbolic representations, but rather a highly detailed and specific encoding of the acoustic speech signal.

D. Perceptual Organization of Speech

Another area in speech perception that has been neglected relative to the emphasis on the search for idealized linguistic representations is the issue of perceptual organization of speech. In normal conversation, speech communication occurs in a rich acoustic environment consisting of a mixture of other speakers' conversations and competing environmental sounds. The classic example of this problem is the situation a listener encounters at a cocktail party (Cherry, 1953). Upon arriving at the party, to strike up and maintain a conversation listeners must be able to perceptually isolate the speech signal produced by their conversational partners from background noise consisting of music, voices, and other party noise. Thus, a listener attempting to follow a particular talker's message must somehow separate the acoustic energy attributable to that talker's utterance from acoustic energy attributable to other sounds occurring simultaneously. The success of this perceptual feat depends not only on the listener's ability to separate sources of sound but, more important perhaps, on the listener's ability to integrate the acoustic components that comprise the particular speech signal to which the listener is attending. The acoustic elements that constitute a particular utterance must somehow cohere into an identifiable perceptual object.

To date, theories of speech perception have typically taken as their starting point a coherent perceptual object, implicitly assuming that perceptual organization has already taken place. Indeed, the study of speech has concentrated almost exclusively on laboratory experiments designed to evaluate the perception of speech produced by a single speaker in an acoustically sterile environment. The consequence of this approach has been the neglect of issues relating to perceptual organization. Recently, however, a growing body of theoretical and empirical work has been conducted that significantly narrows this gap. This research concentrates on the issue of perceptual coherence, how the perceptual system integrates different components of the speech signal while at the same time segregating competing acoustic input.

1. Gestalt Principles of Perceptual Grouping

In general, two types of explanations have been proposed to account for the listener's ability to organize acoustic energy into coherent perceptual objects. The first is based on Gestalt principles of organization as applied to auditory perception (Julesz & Hirsch, 1972; Wertheimer, 1923). In particular, Bregman (1990) has proposed that general auditory grouping mechanisms underlie the perceptual segregation of frequencies from separate sound sources and the perceptual integration of acoustic energy from the same sound source. Principles such as proximity, common fate, symmetry, and closure are hypothesized to be the basis for perceptual coherence in speech. There is considerable evidence that these grouping tendencies might describe the organization of nonspeech auditory stimuli consisting of tone and noise patterns (Bregman & Campbell, 1971; Bregman & Doehring, 1984; Dannenbring & Bregman, 1978). It is less clear, however, if these principles can explain the organization of the complex acoustic properties found in speech.

Evidence that this type of explanation may account for perceptual organization in speech comes from experiments suggesting that perceptual organization based on properties such as those proposed by Bregman (1990) can have a marked effect on phonetic coherence. For example, Ciocca and Bregman (1989) studied the effects of auditory streaming on the integration of syllable components in a dichotic listening task. Using the standard "duplex" paradigm (see Rand, 1974), they presented listeners with a three-formant synthetic syllable split so that the third-formant transition was presented to one ear and the rest of the syllable was presented to the other ear. In addition, Ciocca and Bregman embedded the isolated third-formant transition into a series of capturing tones (repetitions of third-formant transitions that preceded or followed the duplex transitions). Their results showed that the capturing tones successfully created a perceptual stream with the isolated third-formant transition that reduced its phonetic contribution to the syllable percept. Thus, it appears that presence of capturing tones similar in frequency and spatial location created the basis for perceptual coherence of the components within the syllable.

Similarly, Darwin and his colleagues (Darwin, 1981; Darwin & Gardner, 1986; Darwin & Sutherland, 1984; Gardner, Gaskill, & Darwin, 1989) have shown that onset time and fundamental frequency differences can also serve to segregate acoustic/phonetic components within the speech signal. For example, Darwin (1981) presented listeners with four formant composite syllables. When all four formants are excited at the same fundamental frequency and start and stop simultaneously, the predominant percept is that of the syllable /ru/. However, when the composite's second formant is perceptually segregated, the predominant percept becomes /li/. Darwin found that onset asynchronies between the second formant and the rest of the composite accomplished this perceptual segregation. Likewise, sufficient differences in the fundamental frequency of the second formant caused a shift in phonetic quality.

Although these experiments demonstrate the influence of principles of segregation/grouping based on low-level acoustic dimensions on perceptual organization, it should be noted that the results also suggest that factors associated with the phonetic integrity of the stimuli are influential as well. In both examples, residual phonetic coherence persists even when Gestalt principles of organization are violated. Often, relatively extreme differences along an acoustic dimension or even combinations of differences must exist before components of a speech sound will segregate perceptually.

2. Phonetic Organization

Alternative accounts of perceptual organization in speech (Best, Studdert-Kennedy, Manuel, & Rubin-Spitz, 1989; Fowler, 1986; Remez, Rubin, Berns, Nutter, & Lang, 1994; Remez, Rubin, Pisoni, & Carrell, 1981) have proposed that the perceptual coherence found in speech is based on complex principles of organization that are highly specific to the vocal source of the speech signal. Perceivers are assumed to be sensitive to patterns of spectral-temporal change that provide information about the acoustic event that has occurred. In short, these accounts claim that perceptual organization of speech is not dependent on low-level auditory grouping principles. Rather, perceivers are thought to use higher-order organizational principles that are based on "perceptual sensitivity to properties of vocally produced sound" (Remez et al., 1994).[2]

Evidence for the second approach stems in a large part from experiments

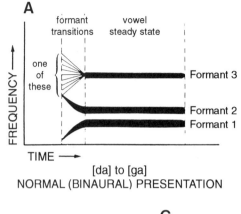

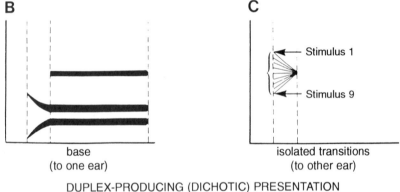

FIGURE 3   Stimuli used in a duplex perception experiment. (A) shows a synthetic speech syllable with a continuum of third-formant transitions ranging from /da/ to /ga/; (B) shows the constant syllable base; and (C) shows the /da/ to /ga/ continuum of third-formant transitions. (From Mann & Liberman, 1983, with permission of authors and publisher.)

that demonstrate phonetic coherence in spite of severe violations of general auditory grouping principles. One such demonstration comes from experiments on duplex perception (Liberman, Isenberg, & Rakerd, 1981; Mann & Liberman, 1983; Rand, 1974). As mentioned earlier, duplex perception occurs when a synthetic consonant–vowel (CV) syllable is split so that the third-formant transition is presented to one ear and the rest of the syllable (or base) is presented to the other ear. Figure 3 shows an example of these types of stimuli. When presented with these signals, listeners report hearing two distinct percepts, a complete syllable in the ear presented with the base and a nonspeech chirp in the ear presented with the isolated transition. This finding suggests that information from the isolated formant transition integrates with the base to form a unitary percept despite the difference in location of the syllable components. In addition, experiments have shown that discontinuities or differences along additional acoustic dimensions such as onset time, fundamental frequency, and amplitude (Bentin & Mann, 1990; Cutting, 1976; Nygaard & Eimas, 1990) do not necessarily disrupt the integration of the isolated formant transitions with the base component presented to the other ear (also see Nygaard, 1993; Whalen & Liberman, 1987). Furthermore, Eimas and Miller (1992) have shown that 3- and 4-month-old infants are susceptible to the duplex perception phenomenon as well. Not only do infants appear to integrate the disparate syllable components presented to each ear, but they also exhibit a tolerance for additional acoustic discontinuities. These findings suggest that the perceptual coherence of speech relies on some type of perceptual organization other than simple auditory grouping. Listeners seem to be sensitive to higher-order, perhaps phonetic, principles of perceptual organization rather than to principles of grouping based on low-level acoustic dimensions. This underlying phonetic coherence of speech seems to be present quite early in life, suggesting that infants may be born with, or acquire very early, a sensitivity to the unique properties of vocally produced sound.

Further evidence for the tolerance of mechanisms of perceptual organization to violations of general auditory grouping principles comes from a set of studies using sine wave analogs of speech (Remez & Rubin, in press; Remez et al., 1981). In these experiments, time-varying sinusoids were used to reproduce the center frequencies and amplitudes of the first three formants of a naturally spoken utterance. Figure 4 provides an example of a

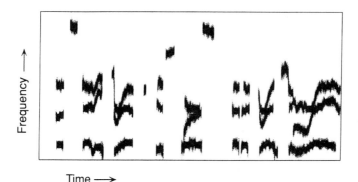

FIGURE 4   A sinusoidal version of the utterance, *The steady drip is worse than a drenching rain.* Time-varying sinusoids are used to replicate the center frequencies of the first three formants of a natural utterance. (Copyright 1994 by the American Psychological Association. Adapted from Remez, Rubin, Berns, Nutter, & Lang, 1994, with permission of authors and publisher.)

sine wave approximation of the utterance, *The steady drip is worse than a drenching rain*. Sinusoidal utterances preserve the time-varying information found in natural speech but have none of the short-time acoustic attributes that are commonly thought to underlie segmental phonetic perception. When asked to attend to the phonetic quality of these types of stimuli, subjects are able to transcribe the sine wave utterances. It is interesting that sine wave speech seems to violate several of the grouping principles that have been proposed; yet these sine wave patterns do cohere phonetically. For example, the three time-varying sinusoids are not related harmonically; the sine wave elements do not have similar trajectories with similar onsets and offsets; and the sinusoids are different in frequency range and change. Yet, the three time-varying sinusoids cohere phonetically.

Additional experiments conducted by Remez and his colleagues (1994) have shown that the phonetic coherence evident in sine wave speech is not a result of cochlear distortion products, on one hand, or cognitive restoration strategies, on the other hand. Rather, it is the highly constrained pattern of spectral–temporal change in these sine wave analogs that provided the basis for phonetic coherence. Thus, these results demonstrate that general auditory grouping principles may be insufficient to account for the perceptual organization of speech. In addition, they also provide evidence for the alternative account; namely, that the perceptual organization of speech is based on characteristic spectral–temporal variation related to the dynamic properties of the vocal source used to produce speech.

In summary, the balance of evidence seems to suggest that Gestalt principles of perceptual organization may not be sufficiently complex to account for the coherence of the speech signal. While these general principles may loosely constrain possible groupings of acoustic–phonetic components and help segregate extraneous acoustic energy, they do not seem to provide the primary basis for the formation of phonetic objects. It seems more likely that the time-varying spectral information related to the vocal source provides the underlying perceptual coherence in the speech signal and that this sensitivity to information from the vocal source may be present early in development.

E. Autonomous versus Interactive Processing in Speech Perception

The nature of the perceptual mechanisms employed in speech perception is obviously highly complex and as such, must involve numerous stages of analysis and representation. As the speech signal arrives at the listener's ear, it must first undergo a peripheral auditory analysis and then be quickly recoded for further processing. Along the way, the information contained in the physical signal must make contact with the listener's linguistic and general knowledge, eventually resulting in the comprehension of the speaker's message. The question for theories of speech perception is not only what kind of representations are constructed and used at each level of linguistic analysis but also how many and what kinds of analyses are involved in the apprehension of linguistic content? Do sources of knowledge interact flexibly with information from the incoming signal, or is perceptual processing carried out in a strict hierarchical manner?

In general, two basic approaches to the nature of perceptual processing have been proposed. The first, inspired by Fodor's (1983) modularity thesis, assumes that analysis of the speech signal proceeds in a strictly bottom-up fashion. That is, discrete stages of processing are assumed (from phonetic, lexical, syntactic, to semantic), in which linguistic information is processed with regard to a limited pool of knowledge specific to that particular stage. The end product of one stage of processing is assumed to provide the input to the next level of processing, and the analysis of speech is presumed to proceed in a uniformly serial manner (see Studdert-Kennedy, 1974, 1976).

Alternative accounts hypothesize that speech perception is highly interactive (Connine, 1990; Elman & McClelland, 1988; Samuel, 1990). That is, the construction of linguistic representations is determined not only by information accrued from the acoustic signal but also from information and knowledge from higher levels of processing. These explanations emphasize the dynamic adaptive nature of speech perception and, in their most extreme formulation, propose that many diverse types of knowledge are brought to bear on linguistic decisions at any level of analysis.

The relative usefulness of each of these approaches has been a hotly debated topic in the field of speech perception for many years and numerous studies have been conducted in an attempt to marshal evidence for each view. Although a comprehensive evaluation of the empirical work relating to this topic is beyond the scope of this chapter, we review two representative experiments. The first is a well-known experiment conducted by Ganong (1980) in which he found that lexical information affected the placement of the perceptual boundary between two phonetic categories. When subjects were asked to identify initial consonants from a voicing continuum, stimuli with ambiguous voice-onset time (VOT) values were more often identified as having the initial consonant that formed a word compared to a nonword. This so-called lexical effect suggested that the status of the stimulus item as a word or nonword influenced phonetic identification (also see McQueen, 1991). Ganong argued that this influence of lexical information on phonetic categorization reflected top-down or interactive processes at work in speech perception and he argued that this finding provided evidence against a strictly bottom-up modular processing system.

In a related experiment, Burton, Baum, & Blumstein (1989) questioned the generality of Ganong's findings. Their experiment consisted of a replication of Ganong's study (1980) with one interesting difference: their voicing continuum used edited natural speech designed to provide a more complete set of voicing cues. The authors argued that Ganong had found lexical effects simply because his stimulus continuum, although edited natural speech as well, provided listeners with impoverished and contradictory voicing information. They reasoned that if the speech signal provided more natural and consistent cues to voicing, perceptual processing would proceed in a strictly bottom–up fashion based entirely on the information contained in the speech signal. In fact, this is exactly what Burton et al. found. Their results showed that lexical effects disappeared when the stimulus set preserved the redundant multiple cues to voicing found in natural speech.

How are the results of these two experiments to be reconciled with regard to the claims about the processing architecture in speech perception? It seems that listeners are able to flexibly alter their processing strategies based on the information available to them in the signal and the information available from their store of linguistic knowledge. On one hand, if the physical signal provides rich, unambiguous information about a phonetic contrast, listeners appear to attend primarily to the physical signal when making their phonetic identifications. On the other hand, if the physical signal is noisy, impoverished, or degraded, as synthetic speech often is, listeners may shift their attention to different levels of processing to assist in phonetic categorization (see Pisoni, Nusbaum, & Greene, 1985). Thus, speech perception appears to be a highly adaptive process in which listeners flexibly adjust to the demands of the task and to the properties of the signal.

III. THEORETICAL APPROACHES TO SPEECH PERCEPTION

In the preceding sections, we have considered several problems and issues that confront researchers in the field of speech perception. In general, the long-standing nature of these problems illustrates the complexity of the speech perceptual system. The numerous processes involved in the analysis of the auditory signal during speech perception draw upon many sources of knowledge and multiple levels of representations. As a consequence of this complexity, the theoretical models and approaches that have been proposed to date to explain speech perception often fall short of being detailed and testable accounts. Rather, most of the theoretical approaches that have been proposed offer possible frameworks in which to place the specific phenomena and paradigms that seem to be the focus of the field.

In this section, we briefly introduce and discuss some of the models and theories that have attempted to account for the complex process of speech perception (also see Massaro, 1987; Massaro & Oden, 1980; Oden & Massaro, 1978; Sussman, 1988, 1989). We focus primarily on a few representative and influential theoretical approaches in the field (but see Klatt, 1989, for a recent comprehensive review). Our aim is to introduce the basic assumptions and unique properties of each approach and to discuss how these accounts deal with the basic problems in speech perception.

A. Invariant Feature or Cue-Based Approaches

Each of the theoretical issues outlined in the preceding sections has to some extent centered on the problem of variability in the speech signal, whether because of phonetic context, changes in speaking rate, talker characteristics, or competing signals. One theoretical approach that has been proposed to account for listeners' success in spite of this vast amount of variation in the speech signal has simply assumed that the lack of invariance in the speech signal is more apparent than real (e.g., Cole & Scott, 1974a, 1974b; Fant, 1967). The assumption here is that invariant acoustic properties corresponding directly to individual features or phonetic segments could be uncovered if the speech signal were examined in the correct way. That is, it is assumed that traditional analyses of the speech signal that relied on highly simplified synthetic speech stimuli may have overlooked the presence of invariant acoustic properties in the signal. Consequently, proponents of this approach have engaged in a careful and systematic search for the invariant properties in the acoustic signal that might correspond uniquely to individual phonetic attributes (Kewley-Port, 1982, 1983; Stevens & Blumstein, 1978, 1981).

Although sharing the basic assumption that acoustic–phonetic invariance can be found, researchers have differed in their assessment of the most likely candidate acoustic features or cues. Stevens and Blumstein (1978; Blumstein & Stevens, 1979, 1980), for example, have focused primarily on gross spectrum shape at the onset of burst release as a possible invariant for place of articulation in stop consonants. Thus, their emphasis has been on *static* properties of the speech signal as the primary acoustic correlates of phonetic segments. In contrast, Kewley-Port (1982, 1983) has emphasized a more dynamic type of invariant representation. Her approach has been to examine both the auditory transformations of the speech signal and the dynamic changes within these transformations. Thus, it is hypothesized that dynamic invariants as opposed to the more static ones proposed by Stevens and Blumstein (1978) may underlie the perception of speech (see Walley & Carrell, 1983). More recently, however, both approaches have acknowledged the possibility of invariant dynamic representations (Mack & Blumstein, 1983).

The assumption of invariant acoustic properties, regardless of their static or dynamic nature, necessarily constrains the types of processing operations that can underlie the perception of speech. Thus, according to this view, speech perception consists of a primarily bottom-up process by which stable invariant acoustic cues are extracted from the speech signal for recognition. Accordingly, this type of approach makes explicit the assumption that the theoretical end point of perception is a series of canonical linguistic units like features, phonemes, syllables, or words; because, in this case, the representation is, by definition, free of any variability or noise.

In summary, the search for invariance advocated by this class of models has yielded a wealth of information regarding the acoustic structure underlying linguistic content and has, in some cases, provided promising candidates for the role of acoustic invariants and for how invariance might be extracted by the auditory system (see Sussman, 1988, 1989). However, it is unfortunate that this approach has not yet discovered a complete set of invariants that are both impervious to phonetic context and are used consistently by perceivers in recognizing the linguistic content of an utterance. Further, these models provide no account of the representation and processing of indexical and prosodic information, for example, and their interaction with the analysis of the linguistic content of an utterance. Variation in the signal, even if it is informative, is discarded by the speech processing system in the extraction of phonetic representations. Thus, although it is appealing to consider the possibilities and advantages of a direct and invariant mapping from acoustic properties to phonetic percepts, it may be unrealistic to assume that these properties alone will be used by perceivers of speech in all listening situations.

B. Motor Theory of Speech Perception

In contrast to models that assume acoustic–phonetic invariance in the signal, an alternative approach has been to explain speech perception by focusing on perceptual processes by which listeners might unravel the complicated articulatory encoding characteristic of speech (Liberman et al., 1967; Liberman & Mattingly, 1989). This view looks to processes *within* the listener that take into account context sensitivity and variability when analyzing the speech signal. Thus, rather than searching for invariant features in the acoustic waveform that uniquely specify particular linguistic units, perceivers are thought to reconstruct or recover the phonetic intent of the talker from incomplete, impoverished, or highly encoded information provided by the speech signal.

The most influential of this class of explanation is the motor theory of speech perception. In Liberman et al.'s (1967; Liberman, Cooper, Harris, & MacNeilage, 1963) original formulation, the complicated articulatory encoding was assumed to be decoded in the perception of speech by the same processes that are involved in production. That is, articulatory movements and their sensory consequences are assumed to play a direct role in the analysis of the acoustic signal. Subsequent versions of the model have abandoned articulatory movements per se as the basis of the perception of speech in favor of neural commands to the articulators (Liberman, 1970; Liberman et al., 1967) or most recently, intended articulatory gestures (Liberman & Mattingly, 1985, 1989).

This view of speech perception was motivated to a large extent by the observation that listeners are also speakers and, as such, a common type of representation must underlie both perceptual and productive activities. Because speech sounds undergo a complex process of encoding during production, it was assumed that the same processes responsible for production would be responsible for decoding the message back to the underlying phonetic segments. The complex overlapping of speech sounds in the speech signal due to coarticulation was assumed to be unraveled in perception by reference to the same rules used in production.

In the original motor theory, the crucial relationship underlying speech perception was the one between articulatory movement and phonetic segment. It was assumed that a direct relationship might exist between these two types of representations. Regrettably, research on articulation provided little evidence for a more invariant relationship between articulatory movement and phonetic segment than that between acoustic signal and phonetic segment (MacNeilage, 1970). Consequently, the revised motor theory has concentrated on the intended articulatory gestures of the talker. Speech perception is proposed to occur with reference to abstract knowledge of a speaker's vocal tract.

In addition to the assumption that the object of perception in speech is the phonetic gesture, the motor theory contends that speech perception is subserved by an innate, special-purpose phonetic module conforming to the specifications for modularity proposed by Fodor (1983). Speech perception is considered to be special because the mechanisms and processes that are used to extract the linguistic content of an utterance are separate from those used to perceive other kinds of auditory events (Mattingly & Liberman, 1988, 1989). In fact, the speech perceptual system is assumed to have evolved for the special purpose of extracting intended articulatory gestures (Liberman, 1982; Mattingly & Liberman, 1988, 1989).

In terms of the nature of the neural representation of speech, the motor theory, though vastly different in other respects, assumes, like models of acoustic–phonetic invariance, that linguistic representations are abstract, canonical, phonetic segments or the gestures that underlie these segments. The speech perceptual module is assumed to be tuned to the phonetic intent of the speaker, but no account is given for how information about voice is integrated with information regarding linguistic intent. It is unclear, assuming this type of conceptualization of the speech perceptual process, when information about talker identity or prosody might be extracted and how it would be used in ongoing processing of the acoustic signal.

The claims about intended articulatory gestures as the objects of perception and about the specialized nature of speech processing have spawned a great deal of controversy in the field and have, as a result, generated a considerably body of research. Support for the revised motor theory has stemmed in a large part from its ability to account for a wide range of phenomena in a principled and consistent manner. However, the theory itself has received little direct unequivocal empirical support, in large part because of the abstract nature of the proposed perceptual mechanisms. Obviously, a more precise specification of how listeners extract the underlying articulatory gestures and how those gestures are decoded into phonetic segments is needed.

C. Direct-Realist Approach to Speech Perception

The direct-realist approach to speech perception outlined by Fowler (1986; Fowler & Rosenblum, 1991) shares with the motor theory the basic assumption that the objects of perception in speech are articulatory gestures. However, despite this shared assumption, many crucial differences exist. Most important, the two theories approach the perception of the signal in fundamentally different ways. Motor theory assumes that the speech signal is highly encoded and, as such, must be subjected to computations to retrieve the underlying gestures. The direct-realist approach, on the other hand, assumes that cognitive mediation is not necessary to support perception. Articulatory gestures are assumed to be readily available to the perceiver in the speech signal and, consequently, are perceived directly. Another important difference between the two types of theories is the assumption of the specialized nature of speech. In contrast to the motor theory, the direct-realist approach assumes that the perception of speech is just like the perception of other events in the world, auditory or otherwise (Fowler & Rosenblum, 1991).

The direct-realist approach derives its inspiration from Gibson's (1966, 1979) ecological approach to visual perception, which views perception in terms of the recognition of events in the world (in the case of speech, natural phonetic events), rather than in terms of recognition of sensory stimulation. Thus, a fundamental distinction is made between the object of perception or the event in the world and the informational medium. For example, consider the perception of a chair. According to this view, the chair constitutes the object that is perceived. The structured reflected light that hits the sensory apparatus is termed the proximal stimulus and provides information about the chair that is the end point of perception. It is important to note that it is not the light, per se, that is perceived according to this view, but rather the object or event in the world. In terms of speech perception, Fowler (1986) has proposed that the acoustic signal provides information about articulatory events. The acoustic signal serves as the proximal stimulus and it is the articulatory gestures that are assumed to be the objects of perception.

In general, the direct-realist approach differs from all other models of speech perception principally in terms of its de-emphasis on the role of representation in the analysis of speech. Because no cognitive mediation is assumed and articulatory gestures are thought to be perceived directly, the focus of this approach is on the rich information in the speech signal that uniquely specifies phonetic events. Consequently, this view may provide one of the more promising accounts of the role that variability may play in the perception of speech. Just as articulatory gestures specific to phonetic events can be perceived directly, it seems reasonable to assume that the acoustic signal provides information regarding talker identity and prosodic structure, for example. The relationship between indexical properties, for instance, and phonetic properties of the speech signal would then be a problem of perceptual organization of the information in the speech signal rather than a problem of perceptual normalization (Fowler, 1990). Thus, according to this approach, the perception of speech is conceptualized as a general process of listener–talker attunement in which listeners perceive "the separation of gestures for different segments or for suprasegmental information, that are layered in articulation and hence in the acoustic speech signal (Fowler, 1990 p. 126)."

Although the direct-realist view is appealing in its ability to account for a wide variety of phenomena in speech perception and in its alternative conceptualization of the analysis of speech, it remains unclear empirically whether articulatory gestures are the essential objects of perception. The choice of the proper perceptual object in speech is problematic (Remez, 1986). Because language is symbolic, the acoustic speech signal may provide information about articulatory gestures; but obviously, these articulations are not the ultimate end point of perception. Rather, articulatory gestures provide information themselves about the intended words, phrases, and even ideas of the talker that constitute the essence of language perception. Nevertheless, the direct-realist approach has provided a viable alternative to the solution of the classic problems in speech perception. As more empirical work is carried out from this theoretical point of view, the role of articulatory gestures in the perception of speech should become clearer.

D. TRACE

In sharp contrast to the accounts or approaches outlined in the preceding sections, the TRACE model (Elman, 1989; Elman & McClelland, 1986; McClelland & Elman, 1986) is an example of an interactive connectionist model applied to the problem of speech perception. As such, TRACE advocates multiple levels of representation and extensive feed-forward and feed-back connections between processing units. These functional units in TRACE are simple, highly interconnected processing units called nodes that are arranged in three different levels of representation. At each level, nodes represent the phonetic features, phonetic segments, and words that are assumed to underlie the processing of speech.

When a speech signal is presented to the network, as information passes upward through each level, nodes collect evidence for the presence of specific information (featural, phonemic, or lexical) in the input representation. Nodes fire when some threshold of activation is reached and activation is then passed along weighted links to connected nodes. In this manner, nodes act as feature detectors, firing when information in the signal is consistent with their specific sensitivity.

In addition to this feed-forward flow of information, excitatory links exist between nodes at different levels and inhibitory links exist between nodes within the same level. This key property of TRACE has important implications for the types of processing operations possible within the model. Inhibitory links between nodes at the same level of representation allow highly activated nodes to inhibit their nearest competitors resulting in a type of "winner take all" form of perceptual decision. In addition, the presence of excitatory feedback allows for the contribution of top-down processing to the perception of phonetic segments. Not only is information accrued from the features present in the physical signal, but information from higher-level lexical information influences phonetic identification as well.

The highly interactive processing and the types of representations that are assumed within the framework of TRACE contrast sharply with the motor theory and traditional accounts emphasizing acoustic–phonetic invariance. In terms of representation, TRACE does not necessarily assume that coarticulatory effects introduce noise onto an idealized string of phonemes. Rather, variability due to phonetic context is considered lawful and can serve as a rich source of information for processing in TRACE (Elman & McClelland, 1986). Less clear, however, is how TRACE might cope with variability due to factors other than phonetic context. As we have argued, variation due to talker and rate, for example, is lawful as well and, as such, provides an additional rich source of information in speech analysis. Yet, within the framework of TRACE, there is no mechanism proposed for extracting these other types of information or for accounting for their effects on phonetic processing. Nevertheless, TRACE is an impressive model of speech perception and spoken word recognition. Its precise description of the speech perceptual process as well as its clearly testable claims make it a significant contribution to the study of speech perception.

IV. SUMMARY AND CONCLUSIONS

This review elucidates several of the fundamental problems confronting research and theory in speech perception. Theoretical and empirical issues such as acoustic–phonetic invariance, perceptual normalization, and perceptual organization have been identified and discussed with regard to the types of representation and analysis that underlie speech perception. In particular, we have attempted to point out the basic assumptions that have motivated and constrained the investigation of these issues.

One of the most important of these assumptions that we have highlighted in this chapter stems from the problem of variability in the signal. Variation and perceptual constancy have emerged as reoccurring themes both in empirical work generated by speech researchers and in the theoretical perspectives that have been endorsed. In general, representations in speech perception have been characterized as highly abstract idealized constructs. However, much of the empirical work outlined points to a different conclusion; namely, that variation in the speech signal is an important source of information that interacts flexibly with processing of the phonetic content of speech. If this revised notion of variability proves to be true, then important changes in the basic assumptions regarding representation and processing will have to occur. Perhaps the traditional idealized phonetic segment may need to be abandoned for a more rich, highly detailed representation. However, in any such account, the evidence for detail in the representation must of course be balanced with the evidence for abstraction. In short, we believe that a more careful assessment of the role of variability in the processing of speech is warranted.

In addition, we believe that speech analysis is a highly flexible adaptive process in which information from a variety of knowledge sources may interact to meet particular processing situations and task demands. The body of research presented in this chapter suggests that listeners encode and utilize any information available to them from the physical signal itself as well as from their own linguistic experience to extract the linguistic intent of a talker's utterance. We have also seen that information above and beyond a strict segmental analysis is derived from the communicative setting and may interact with the on-line processing of the phonemes, words, and phrases that carry linguistic information in speech.

In summary, we believe the theoretical and empirical work presented in this chapter lead to a reassessment of the nature of linguistic units and analysis. In the future, emphasizing informationally rich, detailed representations in speech as well as flexible, adaptive analysis may well provide the key that will unlock the long-standing problems confronting speech perception research.

Acknowledgments

This work was supported by NIH Research Grant DC-000111-16 and NIH Training Grant DC-00012-14 to Indiana University, Bloomington, Indiana. We thank Scott Lively, Joanne Miller, and Peter Eimas for comments on an earlier draft of the chapter.

Endnotes

1. For the purpose of this discussion, we have adopted the standard definition of normalization as a reduction to a normal or standard state. As applied to speech analysis, if listeners normalize a speech sound, then they are bringing it into conformity with a standard, pattern, or model. It should be noted, however, that the term normalization is also used within the field of speech perception to refer in general to a process of perceptual compensation. In this sense, there is not necessarily a reduction of information per se. Nevertheless, most accounts of speech perception have implicitly assumed that the normalization involves some kind of reduction of information and transformation of the signal into some common representational format.

2. It should be noted that speech signals or vocally produced sounds are not arbitrary acoustic signals. Speech is produced by a well-defined sound source with highly constrained parameters for signal space (Stevens, 1972).

References

Abercrombie, D. (1967). *Elements of general phonetics*. Chicago: Aldine.

Bentin, S., & Mann, V. A. (1990). Masking and stimulus intensity effects on duplex perception: A confirmation of the dissociation between speech and nonspeech modes. *Journal of the Acoustical Society of America, 88,* 64–74.

Best, C. T., Studdert-Kennedy, M., Manuel, S., & Rubin-Spitz, J. (1989). Discovering phonetic coherence in acoustic patterns. *Perception & Psychophysics, 45,* 237–250.

Bever, T. G., Lackner, J., & Kirk, R. (1969). The underlying structures of sentences are the primary units of immediate speech processing. *Perception & Psychophysics, 5,* 191–211.

Blumstein, S. E., & Stevens, K. N. (1979). Acoustic invariance in speech production: Evidence from measurements of the spectral characteristics of stop consonants. *Journal of the Acoustical Society of America, 66,* 1001–1017.

Blumstein, S. E., & Stevens, K. N. (1980). Perceptual invariance and onset spectra for stop consonants in different vowel environments. *Journal of the Acoustical Society of America, 67,* 648–662.

Bregman, A. S. (1990). *Auditory scene analysis*. Cambridge, MA: MIT Press.

Bregman, A. S., & Campbell, J. (1971). Primary auditory stream segregation and perception of order in rapid sequences of tones. *Journal of Experimental Psychology, 89,* 244–249.

Bregman, A. S., & Doehring, P. (1984). Fusion of simultaneous tonal glides: The role of parallelness and simple frequency relations. *Perception & Psychophysics, 36,* 251–256.

Broadbent, D. E. (1965). Information processing in the nervous system. *Science, 150,* 457–462.

Burton, M., Baum, S., & Blumstein, S. (1989). Lexical effects on the phonetic categorization of speech: The role of acoustic structure. *Journal of Experimental Psychology: Human Perception and Performance, 15,* 567–575.

Cherry, C. (1953). Some experiments on the recognition of speech with one and with two ears. *Journal of the Acoustical Society of America, 25,* 975–979.

Chomsky, N., & Miller, G. A. (1963). Introduction to the formal analysis of natural language. In R. D. Luce, R. Bush, & E. Galanter (Eds.), *Handbook of mathematical psychology* (Vol. 2, pp. 269–321). New York: Wiley.

Church, K. W. (1987). Phonological parsing and lexical retrieval. In U. H. Frauenfelder & L. K. Tyler (Eds.), *Spoken word recognition* (pp. 53–69). Cambridge, MA: MIT Press.

Ciocca, V., & Bregman, A. S. (1989). The effects of auditory streaming on duplex perception. *Perception & Psychophysics, 46,* 39–48.

Cohen, A., & Nooteboom, S. G. (Eds.). (1975). *Structure and process in speech perception*. Heidelberg: Springer-Verlag.

Cole, R. A., & Scott, B. (1974a). The phantom in the phoneme: Invariant cues for stop consonants. *Perception & Psychophysics, 15,* 101–107.

Cole, R. A., & Scott, B. (1974b). Toward a theory of speech perception. *Psychological Review, 81,* 348–374.

Connine, C. M. (1990). Effects of sentence context and lexical knowledge in speech processing. In G. T. M. Altmann (Ed.), *Cognitive models of speech processing* (pp. 281–294). Cambridge, MA: MIT Press.

Creelman, C. D. (1957). The case of the unknown talker. *Journal of the Acoustical Society of America, 29,* 655.

Cutler, A., Mehler, J., Norris, D., & Segui, J. (1986). The syllable's differing role in the segmentation of French and English. *Journal of Memory and Language, 25,* 385–400.

Cutting, J. E. (1976). Auditory and linguistic processes in speech perception: Inferences from six fusions in dichotic listening. *Psychological Review, 83,* 114–140.

Cutting, J. E., & Pisoni, D. B. (1978). An information-processing approach to speech perception. In J. F. Kavanagh & W. Strange (Eds.), *Speech and language in the laboratory, school, and clinic* (pp. 38–72). Cambridge, MA: MIT Press.

Dannenbring, G. L., & Bregman, A. S. (1978). Streaming vs. fusion of sinusoidal components of complex tones. *Perception & Psychophysics, 24,* 544–555.

Darwin, C. J. (1975). On the dynamic use of prosody in speech perception. In A. Cohen & S. G. Nooteboom (Eds.), *Structure and process in speech perception.* Heidelberg: Springer-Verlag.

Darwin, C. J. (1976). The perception of speech. In E. C. Carterette & M. P. Friedman (Eds.), *Handbook of perception* (pp. 175–216). New York: Academic Press.

Darwin, C. J. (1981). Perceptual grouping of speech components differing in fundamental frequency and onset-time. *Quarterly Journal of Experimental Psychology, 33,* 185–207.

Darwin, C. J., & Gardner, R. B. (1986). Mistuning a harmonic of a vowel: Grouping and phase effects on vowel quality. *Journal of the Acoustical Society of America, 79,* 838–845.

Darwin, C. J., & Sutherland, N. S. (1984). Grouping frequency components of vowels: When is a harmonic not a harmonic? *Quarterly Journal of Experimental Psychology, 36A,* 193–208.

Delattre, P. C., Liberman, A. M., & Cooper, F. S. (1955). Acoustic loci and transitional cues for consonants. *Journal of the Acoustical Society of America, 27,* 769–773.

Eimas, P. D., Hornstein, S. B. M., & Payton, P. (1990). Attention and the role of dual codes in phoneme monitoring. *Journal of Memory and Language, 29,* 160–180.

Eimas, P. D., & Miller, J. L. (1992). Organization in the perception of speech by young infants. *Psychological Science, 3,* 340–345.

Eimas, P. D., & Nygaard, L. C. (1992). Contextual coherence and attention in phoneme monitoring. *Journal of Memory and Language, 31,* 375–395.

Elman, J. L. (1989). Connectionist approaches to acoustic/phonetic processing. In W. D. Marslen-Wilson (Ed.), *Lexical representation and process* (pp. 227–260). Cambridge, MA: MIT Press.

Elman, J. L., & McClelland, J. L. (1986). Exploiting lawful variability in the speech waveform (pp. 360–385). In J. S. Perkell & D. H. Klatt (Eds.), *Invariance and variability in speech processing.* Hillsdale, NJ: Erlbaum.

Elman, J. L., & McClelland, J. L. (1988). Cognitive penetration of the mechanisms of perception: Compensation for coarticulation of lexically restored phonemes. *Journal of Memory and Language, 27,* 143–165.

Fant, G. (1962). Descriptive analysis of the acoustic aspects of speech. *Logos, 5,* 3–17.

Fant, G. (1967). Auditory patterns of speech. In W. Wathen-Dunn (Ed.), *Models for the perception of speech and visual form* (pp. 111–125). Cambridge, MA: MIT Press.

Fodor, J. A. (1983). *The modularity of mind.* Cambridge, MA: MIT Press.

Fowler, C. A. (1986). An event approach to the study of speech perception from a direct-realist perspective. *Journal of Phonetics, 14,* 3–28.

Fowler, C. A. (1990). Listener-talker attunements in speech. *Haskins Laboratories Status Report on Speech Research, SR-101/102,* 110–129.

Fowler, C. A., & Rosenblum, L. D. (1991). The perception of phonetic gestures. In I. G. Mattingly & M. Studdert-Kennedy (Eds.), *Modularity and the motor theory of speech perception* (pp. 33–59). Hillsdale, NJ: Erlbaum.

Fujimura, O., & Lovins, J. B. (1978). Syllables as concatenative phonetic units. In A. Bell & J. B. Hooper (Eds.), *Syllables and segments.* Amsterdam: North-Holland.

Ganong, W. F. (1980). Phonetic categorization in auditory word perception. *Journal of Experimental Psychology: Human Perception and Performance, 6,* 110–125.

Gardner, R. B., Gaskill, S. A., & Darwin, C. J. (1989). Perceptual grouping of formants with static and dynamic differences in fundamental frequency. *Journal of the Acoustical Society of America, 85,* 1329–1337.

Garner, W. (1974). *The processing of information and structure.* Hillsdale, NJ: Erlbaum.

Geiselman, R. E., & Bellezza, F. S. (1976). Long-term memory for speaker's voice and source location. *Memory & Cognition, 4,* 483–489.

Geiselman, R. E., & Bellezza, F. S. (1977). Incidental retention of speaker's voice. *Memory & Cognition, 5,* 658–665.

Gerstman, L. H. (1968). Classification of self-normalized vowels. *IEEE Transactions on Audio and Electroacoustics, AU-16,* 78–80.

Gibson, J. J. (1966). *The senses considered as perceptual systems.* Boston: Houghton Mifflin.

Gibson, J. J. (1979). *The ecological approach to visual perception.* Boston: Houghton Mifflin.

Goldinger, S. D., Pisoni, D. B., & Logan, D. B. (1991). The nature of talker variability effects on recall of spoken word lists. *Journal of Experimental Psychology: Learning, Memory, and Cognition, 17,* 152–162.

Goldinger, S. D., Pisoni, D. B., & Luce, P. A. (in press). Speech perception and spoken work recognition: Research and theory. In N. J. Lass (Ed.), *Principles of experimental phonetics.* Toronto: B. C. Decker.

Hockett, C. (1955). *Manual of phonology* (Publications in Anthropology and Linguistics, No. 11). Bloomington: Indiana University Press.

Huggins, A. W. F. (1972). On the perception of temporal phenomena in speech. In J. Requin (Ed.), *Attention and performance VII* (pp. 279–297). Hillsdale, NJ: Erlbaum.

Johnson, K. (1990). The role of perceived speaker identity in F0 normalization of vowels. *Journal of the Acoustical Society of America, 88,* 642–654.

Joos, M. A. (1948). Acoustic phonetics. *Language, 24*(Suppl. 2), 1–136.

Julesz, B., & Hirsch, I. J. (1972). Visual and auditory perception: An essay of comparison. In E. E. David & P. B. Denes (Eds.), *Human communication: A unified view* (pp. 283–340). New York: McGraw-Hill.

Jusczyk, P. (1986). Speech perception. In K. R. Boff, L. Kaufman, & J. P. Thomas (Eds.), *Handbook of perception and human performance: Vol. 2. Cognitive processes and performance* (pp. 1–57). New York: Wiley.

Kewley-Port, D. (1982). Measurement of formant transitions in naturally produced stop consonant-vowel syllables. *Journal of the Acoustical Society of America, 72,* 379–389.

Kewley-Port, D. (1983). Time-varying features as correlates of place of articulation in stop consonants. *Journal of the Acoustical Society of America, 73,* 322–335.

Klatt, D. H. (1975). Vowel lengthening is syntactically determined in connected discourse. *Journal of Phonetics, 3,* 129–140.

Klatt, D. H. (1976). Linguistic uses of segmental duration in English: Acoustic and perceptual evidence. *Journal of the Acoustic Society of America, 59,* 1208–1221.

Klatt, D. H. (1979). Speech perception: A model of acoustic-phonetic analysis and lexical access. *Journal of Phonetics, 7,* 279–312.

Klatt, D. H. (1989). Review of selected models of speech perception. In W. D. Marslen-Wilson (Ed.), *Lexical representation and process* (pp. 169–226). Cambridge, MA: MIT Press.

Kuhl, P. K. (1991). Human adults and human infants show a "perceptual magnet effect" for the prototypes of speech categories, monkeys do not. *Perception & Psychophysics, 50,* 93–107.

Ladefoged, P., & Broadbent, D. E. (1957). Information conveyed by vowels. *Journal of the Acoustical Society of America, 29,* 948–104.

Laver, J. (1989). Cognitive science and speech: A framework for research. In H. Schnelle & N. O. Bernsen (Eds.), *Logic and linguistics: Research directions in cognitive science: Vol. 2. European perspectives.* (pp. 37–70). Hillsdale, NJ: Erlbaum.

Laver, J., & Trudgill, P. (1979). Phonetic and linguistic markers in speech. In K. R. Scherer & H. Giles (Eds.), *Social markers in speech* (pp. 1–32). Cambridge, UK: Cambridge University Press.

Liberman, A. M. (1957). Some results of research on speech perception. *Journal of the Acoustical Society, 29,* 117–123.

Liberman, A. M. (1970). The grammars of speech and language. *Cognitive Psychology, 1,* 301–323.

Liberman, A. M. (1982). On finding that speech is special. *American Psychologist, 37,* 148–167.

Liberman, A. M., Cooper, F. S., Harris, K. S., & MacNeilage, P. F. (1963). A motor theory of speech perception. In C. G. M. Fant (Ed.), *Proceedings of the Speech Communication Seminar, Stockholm, 1962.* Stockholm: Royal Institute of Technology, Speech Transmission Laboratory.

Liberman, A. M., Cooper, F. S., Shankweiler, D. P., & Studdert-Kennedy, M. (1967). Perception of the speech code. *Psychological Review, 74,* 431–461.

Liberman, A. M,. Delattre, P. C., Cooper, F. S., & Gerstman, L. H. (1954). The role of consonant-vowel transitions in the perception of the stop and nasal consonants. *Psychological Monographs, 68,* 1–13.

Liberman, A. M., Isenberg, D., & Rakerd, B. (1981). Duplex perception of cues for stop consonants: Evidence for a phonetic mode. *Perception & Psychophysics, 30,* 133–143.

Liberman, A. M., & Mattingly, I. G. (1985). The motor theory of speech perception revised. *Cognition, 21,* 1–36.

Liberman, A. M., & Mattingly, I. G. (1989). A specialization for speech perception. *Science, 243,* 489–494.

Lieberman, P., Crelin, E. S., & Klatt, D. H. (1972). Phonetic ability and related anatomy of the newborn, adult human, Neanderthal man, and the chimpanzee. *American Anthropology, 74,* 287–307.

Luce, P. A., & Pisoni, D. B. (1987). Speech perception: New directions in research, theory, and applications. In H. Winitz (Ed.), *Human communication and its disorders* (pp. 1–87). Norwood, NJ: Ablex.

Mack, M., & Blumstein, S. E. (1983). Further evidence of acoustic invariance in speech production: The stop-glide contrast. *Journal of the Acoustical Society of America, 73,* 1739–1750.

MacNeilage, P. F. (1970). Motor control of serial ordering of speech. *Psychological Review, 77,* 182–196.

Mann, V. A,. & Liberman, A. M. (1983). Some differences between phonetic and auditory modes of perception. *Cognition, 14,* 211–235.

Martin, C. S., Mullennix, J. W., Pisoni, D. B., & Summers, W. V. (1989). Effects of talker variability on recall of spoken word lists. *Journal of Experimental Psychology: Learning, Memory, and Cognition, 15,* 676–681.

Massaro, D. W. (1987). *Speech perception by ear and eye: A paradigm for psychological inquiry.* Hillsdale, NJ: Erlbaum.

Massaro, D. W., & Oden, G. C. (1980). Speech perception: A framework for research and theory. In N. J. Lass (Ed.), *Speech and language: Advances in basic research and practice* (Vol. 3, pp. 129–165). New York: Academic Press.

Mattingly, I. G., & Liberman, A. M. (1988). Specialized perceiving systems for speech and other biologically-significant sounds. In G. Edelman, W. Gall, & W. Cohen (Eds.), *Auditory function: The neurobiological bases of hearing* (pp. 775–793). New York: Wiley.

Mattingly, I. G., & Liberman, A. M. (1989). Speech and other auditory modules. *Science, 243,* 489–494.

McClelland, J. L., & Elman, J. L. (1986). The TRACE model of speech perception. *Cognitive Psychology, 18,* 1–86.

McQueen, J. M. (1991). The influence of the lexicon on phonetic categorization: Stimulus quality in word-final ambiguity. *Journal of Experimental Psychology: Human Perception and Performance, 17,* 433–443.

Mehler, J. (1981). The role of syllables in speech processing. *Philosophical Transactions of the Royal Society of London, Series B, 295,* 333–352.

Miller, G. A. (1962). Decision units in the perception of speech. *IRE Transactions on Information Theory, IT-8,* 81-83.

Miller, J. D. (1989). Auditory-perceptual interpretation of the vowel. *Journal of the Acoustical Society of America, 85,* 2114–2134.

Miller, J. L. (1981). Effects of speaking rate on segmental distinctions. In P. D. Eimas & J. L. Miller (Eds.), *Perspectives on the study of speech* (pp. 39–74). Hillsdale, NJ: Erlbaum.

Miller, J. L. (1987). Rate-dependent processing in speech perception. In A. Ellis (Ed.), *Progress in the psychology of language* (pp. 119–157). Hillsdale, NJ: Erlbaum.

Miller, J. L. (1990). Speech perception. In D. N. Osherson & H. Lasmik (Eds.), *An invitation of cognitive science* (Vol. 1, pp. 69–93). Cambridge, MA: MIT Press.

Miller, J. L., & Baer, T. (1983). Some effects of speaking rate on the production of /b/ and /w/. *Journal of the Acoustical Society of America, 73,* 1751–1755.

Miller, J. L., Green, K. P., & Reeves, A. (1986). Speaking rate and segments: A look at the relation between speech production and perception for the voicing contrast. *Phonetica, 43,* 106–115.

Miller, J. L., Grosjean, F., & Lomanto, C. (1984). Articulation rate and its variability in spontaneous speech: A reanalysis and some implications. *Phonetica, 41,* 215–225.

Miller, J. L., & Liberman, A. M. (1979). Some effects of later occurring information on the perception of stop consonant and semivowel. *Perception & Psychophysics, 25,* 457–465.

Miller, J. L., & Volaitis, L. E. (1989). Effects of speaking rate on the perceived internal structure of phonetic categories. *Perception & Psychophysics, 46,* 505–512.

Mullennix, J. W., & Pisoni, D. B. (1990). Stimulus variability and processing dependencies in speech perception. *Perception & Psychophysics, 47,* 379–390.

Mullennix, J. W., Pisoni, D. B., & Martin, C. S. (1989). Some effects of talker variability on spoken word recognition. *Journal of the Acoustical Society of America, 85,* 365–378.

Nearey, T. M. (1989). Static, dynamic, and relational properties in vowel perception. *Journal of the Acoustical Society of America, 85,* 2088–2113.

Nooteboom, S. G., Brokx, J. P. L., & de Rooij, J. J. (1978). Contributions of prosody to speech perception. IN W. J. M. Levelt & G. B. Flores d'Arcais (Eds.), *Studies in the perception of language* (pp. 75–107). New York: Wiley.

Norris, D. G., & Cutler, A. (1988). The relative accessibility of phonemes and syllables. *Perception and Psychophysics, 43,* 541–550.

Nygaard, L. C. (1993). Phonetic coherence in duplex perception: Effects of acoustic differences and lexical status. *Journal of Experimental Psychology: Human Perception and Performance, 19,* 268–286.

Nygaard, L. C., & Eimas, P. D. (1990). A new version of duplex perception: Evidence for phonetic and nonphonetic fusion. *Journal of the Acoustical Society of America, 88,* 75–86.

Nygaard, L. C., Sommers, M. S., & Pisoni, D. B. (1994). Speech perception as a talker-contingent process. *Psychological Science, 5,* 42–46.

Oden, G. C., & Massaro, D. W. (1978). Integration of featural information in speech perception. *Psychological Review, 85,* 172–191.

Oller, D. K. (1973). The effect of position in utterance on speech segment duration in English. *Journal of the Acoustical Society of America, 54*, 1235–1247.

Palmeri, T. J., Goldinger, S. D., & Pisoni, D. B. (1993). Episodic encoding of voice attributes and recognition memory for spoken words. *Journal of Experimental Psychology: Learning, Memory, and Cognition, 19*, 309–328.

Peters, R. W. (1955). *The relative intelligibility of single-voice and multiple-voice messages under various conditions of noise* (Joint Project Report, Vol. 56, pp. 1–9). Pensacola, FL: U.S. Naval School of Aviation Medicine.

Pisoni, D. B. (1978). Speech perception. In W. K. Estes (Ed.), *Handbook of learning and cognitive processes* (Vol. 6, pp. 167–233). Hillsdale, NJ: Erlbaum.

Pisoni, D. B. (1993). Long-term memory in speech perception: Some new findings on talker variability, speaking rate, and perceptual learning. *Speech Communication, 13*, 109–125.

Pisoni, D. B., & Luce, P. A. (1986). Speech perception: Research, theory, and the principal issues. In E. C. Schwab & H. C. Nusbaum (Eds.), *Perception of speech and visual form: Theoretical issues, models, and research* (pp. 1–50). New York: Academic Press.

Pisoni, D. B., Nusbaum, H. C., & Greene, B. (1985). Perception of synthetic speech generated by rule. *Proceedings of the IEEE, 73*, 1665–1676.

Rand, T. C. (1974). Dichotic release from masking for speech. *Journal of the Acoustical Society of America, 55*, 678–680.

Remez, R. E. (1986). Realism, language, and another barrier. *Journal of Phonetics, 14*, 89–97.

Remez, R. E. (1987). Units of organization and analysis in the perception of speech. In M. E. H. Schouten (Ed.), *The psychophysics of speech perception* (pp. 419–432). Dordrecht: Martinus Nijhoff.

Remez, R. E., & Rubin, P. E. (in press). Acoustic shards, perceptual glue. In P. A. Luce & J. Charles-Luce (Eds.), *Proceedings of a workshop on spoken language*. Hillsdale, NJ: Ablex.

Remez, R. E., Rubin, P. E., Berns, S. M., Nutter, J. S., & Lang, J. M. (1994). On the perceptual organization of speech. *Psychological Review, 101*, 129–156.

Remez, R. E., Rubin, P. E., Pisoni, D. B., & Carrell, T. D. (1981). Speech perception without traditional speech cues. *Science, 212*, 947–950.

Rubin, P. E., Turvey, M. T., & van Gelder, P. (1975). Initial phonemes are detected faster in spoken words than in spoken nonwords. *Perception & Psychophysics, 19*, 394–3948.

Samuel, A. G. (1982). Phonetic prototypes. *Perception & Psychophysics, 31*, 307–314.

Samuel, A. G. (1990). Using perceptual-restoration effects to explore the architecture of perception. In G. T. M. Altmann (Ed.), *Cognitive models of speech processing* (pp. 295–314). Cambridge, MA: MIT Press.

Segui, J. (1984). The syllable: A basic perceptual unit in speech processing. In H. Bouma & D. G. Bouwhuis (Eds.), *Attention and performance X: Control of language processes*. Hillsdale, NJ: Erlbaum.

Shankweiler, D. P., Strange, W., & Verbrugge, R. R. (1977). Speech and the problem of perceptual constancy. In R. Shaw & J. Bransford (Eds.), *Perceiving, acting, and knowing: Toward an ecological psychology* (pp. 315–345). Hillsdale, NJ: Erlbaum.

Sommers, M. S., Nygaard, L. C., & Pisoni, D. B. (1994). Stimulus variability and spoken word recognition. I. Effects of variability in speaking rate and overall amplitude. *Journal of the Acoustical Society of America, 96*, 1314–1324.

Stevens, K. N. (1972). The quantal nature of speech: Evidence from articulatory-acoustic data. In E. E. David, Jr., & P. B. Denes (Eds.), *Human communication: A unified view* (pp. 51–66). New York: McGraw-Hill.

Stevens, K. N., & Blumstein, S. E. (1978). Invariant cues for place of articulation in stop consonants. *Journal of the Acoustical Society of America, 64*, 1358–1368.

Stevens, K. N., & Blumstein, S. E. (1981). The search for invariant acoustic correlates of phonetic features. In P. D. Eimas & J. L. Miller (Eds.), *Perspectives on the study of speech* (pp. 1–38). Hillsdale, NJ: Erlbaum.

Studdert-Kennedy, M. (1974). The perception of speech. In T. A. Sebeok (Ed.), *Current trends in linguistics* (Vol. 12, pp. 2349–2385). The Hague: Mouton.

Studdert-Kennedy, M. (1976). Speech perception. In N. J. Lass (Ed.), *Contemporary issues in experimental phonetics* (pp. 213–293). New York: Academic Press.

Summerfield, Q. (1975). *Aerodynamics versus mechanics in the control of voicing onset in consonant-vowel syllables* (Speech perception: Series 2, No. 4, Spring). Belfast: Queen's University, Department of Psychology.

Summerfield, Q. (1981). On articulatory rate and perceptual constancy in phonetic perception. *Journal of Experimental Psychology: Human Perception and Performance, 7,* 1074–1095.

Summerfield, Q., & Haggard, M. P. (1973). Vocal tract normalization as demonstrated by reaction times. In *Report of speech research in progress* (Vol. 2, No. 2, pp. 12–23). Queens University of Belfast.

Sussman, H. M. (1988). The neurogenesis of phonology. In H. A. Whitaker (Ed.), *Phonological processes and brain mechanisms* (pp. 1–23). New York: Springer-Verlag.

Sussman, H. M. (1989). Neural coding of relational invariance in speech: Human language analogs to the barn owl. *Psychological Review, 96,* 631–642.

Verbrugge, R. R., & Rakerd, B. (1986). Evidence of talker-independent information for vowel. *Language and Speech, 29,* 39–57.

Verbrugge, R. R., Strange, W., Shankweiler, D. P., & Edman, T. R. (1976). What information enables a listener to map a talker's vowel space? *Journal of the Acoustical Society of America, 60,* 198–212.

Volaitis, L. E., & Miller, J. L. (1992). Phonetic prototypes: Influences of place of articulation and speaking rate on the internal structure of voicing categories. *Journal of the Acoustical Society of America, 92,* 723–735.

Walley, A. C., & Carrell, T. D. (1983). Onset spectra and formant transitions in the adult's and child's perception of place of articulation in stop consonants. *Journal of the Acoustical Society of America, 73,* 1011–1022.

Watkins, A. J. (1988, July). *Effects of room reverberation on the fricative/affricate distinction.* Paper presented at the Second Franco-British Speech meeting, University of Sussex.

Wertheimer, M. (1923). Untersuchungen zur Lehre von der Gestalt. II. *Psycholigische Forschung, 41,* 301–350. (Reprinted in translation as Laws of organization in perceptual forms. In *A sourcebook of Gestalt psychology,* pp. 71–88, by W. D. Ellis, Ed., London: 1938, Routledge & Kegan Paul).

Whalen, D. H., & Liberman, A. M. (1987). Speech perception takes precedence over non-speech perception. *Science, 237,* 169–171.

Wickelgren, W. A. (1969). Context-sensitive coding, associative memory, and serial order in (speech) behavior. *Psychological Review, 76,* 1–15.

Wickelgren, W. A. (1976). Phonetic coding and serial order. In E. C. Carterette & M. P. Friedman (Eds.), *Handbook of perception* (Vol. 7, pp. 227–264). New York: Academic Press.

CHAPTER 4

Spoken Word Recognition and Production

Anne Cutler

I. INTRODUCTION

Most language behavior consists of speaking and listening. However, the recognition and production of spoken words have not always been central topics in psycholinguistic research. Considering the two fields together in one chapter reveals differences and similarities. Spoken-word recognition studies began in earnest in the 1970s, prompted on one hand by the development of laboratory tasks involving auditory presentation and on the other hand by the realization that the growing body of data on visual word recognition (see Seidenberg, Chapter 5, this volume) did not necessarily apply to listening, because of the temporal nature of speech signals. This recognition research has been, to a great extent, model driven. Spoken-word production research, on the other hand, has a longer history but a less intimate relationship with theory. Laboratory tasks for studying production are difficult to devise, so that much research addressed production *failure,* such as slips of the tongue. An unhappy result of this focus has been models of production that are largely determined by the characteristics of failed rather than successful operation of the processes modeled; moreover, the models have rarely prompted new research. Only in recent years have models and laboratory studies of successful production become widely available. Despite these differences, theoretical questions in recognition and produc-

Speech, Language, and Communication

tion are similar, and central to both has been the question of autonomy versus interaction in levels of processing. As this chapter describes, the balance of evidence indicates a similar answer for both fields.

II. SPOKEN WORD RECOGNITION

A. Methodology

The simplest methods for studying spoken word recognition measure recognizability per se, for example, of words or sentences under noise masks (e.g., Savin, 1963) or of filtered or truncated ("gated"; Ellis, Derbyshire, & Joseph, 1971) speech signals. None of these tasks reflects the time course of recognition.

Among tasks that do attempt to tap processing on-line are those of lexical decision, deciding whether or not a stimulus is a real word (see Seidenberg, Chapter 5, this volume); as this merely requires affirming that recognition has occurred, it has a certain ecological validity. In the auditory form of this task, however, subjects cannot respond before the end of a word in case it becomes a nonword at the last opportunity (*recognitious* rather than *recognition*, for instance); thus response time (RT) varies with word length (Bradley & Forster, 1987). Also, subjects can be reluctant to reject nonwords, perhaps reflecting all listeners' practice in guessing from unclear speech input. Variants of lexical decision are "word-spotting" (Cutler & Norris, 1988), in which a largely nonsense input contains occasional real words and a single positive response to a real word replaces lexical decision's choice response, and "phoneme-triggered lexical decision" (Blank, 1980), in which subjects listen for a specified initial phoneme and then decide whether it begins a word or nonword. Both can be used with continuous speech input. Speeded repetition of words ("auditory naming"; Whalen, 1991) or continuous speech ("shadowing"; Marslen-Wilson, 1985) may also be used to study recognition, but these tasks have the disadvantage of confounding recognition and production processes.

In phonetic categorization, principally used to study segmental perception (see Nygaard and Pisoni, Chapter 3, this volume), the stimuli are *unnatural* tokens, along a continuum formed by some acoustic parameter between one natural speech sound and another. For word recognition studies the tokens may be embedded in words versus nonwords (e.g., Ganong, 1980).

In dual-task experiments, RT to perform the secondary task can reflect momentary changes in difficulty of the primary task. Many such tasks require subjects to monitor incoming speech for a prespecified target, which can be part of the speech stream itself (a word, a syllable, a phoneme), something wrong with the speech (e.g., a mispronunciation; Cole, 1973), or an extraneous signal (e.g., a click; Ladefoged & Broadbent, 1960). In phoneme monitoring (Foss, 1969), subjects detect a target phoneme (usually in word-initial position). The task must be performed at a phonemic rather than an acoustic match level, since the acoustic patterns of phonemes differ with context. Phoneme monitoring has featured in many studies of prelexical processing, as has syllable monitoring (e.g., Mills, 1980b), in which the target is a sequence such as /ba/. Rhyme monitoring (detection of a word rhyming with the target; e.g., Seidenberg & Tanenhaus, 1979) has been used to study phonological characteristics of lexical entries. In word monitoring (e.g., Marslen-Wilson & Tyler, 1980), specification of the target involves recognition of the very word to which a response is later made; responses are therefore subject to repetition priming, that is, facilitation of recognition on a second occurrence (e.g., Slowiaczek, Nusbaum, & Pisoni, 1987).

Another indirect measure is cross-modal priming (Swinney, Onifer, Prather, & Hirschkowitz, 1979), in which listeners perform a lexical decision to a visually presented string while simultaneously listening to words or sentences. Response time to the visual words is measured as a function of their associative relationship to the spoken words. Facilitatory effects, and the time at which they appear relative to presentation of the spoken word, reflect lexical processing of the latter. This task has proved particularly useful for studying patterns of activation in the lexicon during word recognition.

B. Issues

1. The Input to the Lexicon

Lexical access from spectra (LAFS; Klatt, 1979) is the only recognition model in which lexical hypotheses are generated directly from a spectral representation of input. In this model, the lexicon consists of a tree of possible sequences, in which the end of every word is connected to the beginning of every other word, with phonological rules supplying the appropriate allophone; the result is a decoding network for phonetic sequences. Each state transition in this network is a mininetwork of spectral templates. Lexical recognition consists of finding the best match between the input sequence of spectral templates and paths through the network.

LAFS is neither an implemented engineering system nor a psychological model specified in terms that make predictions about human performance. Its main advantage is that it offers a way to preserve useful low-level information that is often lost in the process of making all-or-none phonemic decisions. However, it incorporates some psychologically implausible features, such as the redundancy of having similar word boundary transitions represented for every possible word pair separately. Problems of variability (Nygaard and Pisoni, Chapter 3; this volume) eventually proved insuperable for actual implementation of LAFS (Klatt, 1989). The model requires a spectral distance metric for the computation of matching scores for each input spectrum with the stored spectral templates; but the spectral variability of real speech input defeated efforts to devise such a metric.

Other models of spoken word recognition assume that speech input is translated into a more abstract representation for contact with the lexicon. Obvious candidates for such representations have been the units of linguistic analysis, and of these, the phoneme, by definition the smallest unit into which speech can be sequentially decomposed, has been most popular (Foss & Gernsbacher, 1983; Marslen-Wilson & Welsh, 1978; Pisoni & Luce, 1987). However, other units have been proposed, including units above the phoneme level such as syllables (Mehler, Dommergues, Frauenfelder, & Segui, 1981), demisyllables (i.e., a vowel plus a preceding syllabic onset or following coda; Fujimura & Lovins, 1978; Samuel, 1989), diphones (i.e., speech segments affected by two consecutive phonemes; Klatt, 1979; Marcus, 1981) or stress units (Grosjean & Gee, 1987), and feature units below the phoneme level (McClelland & Elman, 1986b; Stevens, 1986; Stevens, Manuel, Shattuck-Hufnagel, & Liu, 1992) (see Nygaard and Pisoni, Chapter 3, this volume, for further discussion).

The issue of prelexical representations connects with the issue of lexical segmentation of continuous speech. Understanding speech requires recognition of individual words (more exactly: lexically represented units), since the number of possible complete utterances is infinite. Yet speech signals do not necessarily contain robust and reliable cues to word boundaries. Several classes of solution have been proposed for the problem of segmenting continuous speech into words. One is that words are recognized in sequential order, and that the point of onset of a word is identified by virtue of successful recognition of the preceding word (Cole & Jakimik, 1978; Marslen-Wilson & Welsh, 1978). Another is that alternative, possibly overlapping, word candidates compete for recognition (this is the mechanism embodied in TRACE: McClelland & Elman, 1986b). The third class of solution proposes an explicit segmentation procedure (e.g., Cutler & Norris, 1988). Explicit segmentation may presuppose units of segmentation at the prelexical level.

Experimental evidence supports all three types of proposal to some extent. Sequential recognition, however, is poorly suited to vocabulary structure, as described in Section IIB2, and competition is fully compatible with explicit segmentation. Evidence exists for explicit segmentation (1) into syllables: listeners detect target strings such as *ba* or *bal* more rapidly when the strings correspond exactly to a syllable of a heard word than when they constitute more or less than a syllable (Mehler et al., 1981; Zwitserlood, Schriefers, Lahiri, & van Donselaar, 1993); and (2) at stress unit boundaries:

recognition of real words embedded in nonsense bisyllables is inhibited if the word spans a boundary between two strong syllables (i.e., two syllables containing full vowels), but is not if the word spans a boundary between a strong and a weak syllable, since only the former is a stress unit boundary (Cutler & Norris, 1988).

A striking outcome of the explicit segmentation research is that segmentation units appear to be language specific. The evidence for syllables reported above comes from French and Dutch. Evidence of syllabic segmentation has also been observed in Spanish (Bradley, Sánchez-Casas, & García-Albea, 1993) and Catalan (Sebastian-Gallés, Dupoux, Segui, & Mehler, 1992). Other tasks confirm the robustness of syllabic segmentation in French (Kolinsky, Morais & Cluytens, 1995; Segui, Frauenfelder, & Mehler, 1981). However, target detection does not show syllabic segmentation in English (Cutler, Mehler, Norris & Segui, 1986) or in Japanese (Otake, Hatano, Cutler, & Mehler, 1993; Cutler & Otake, 1994). Cutler and Norris's (1988) observation that segmentation in English is stress based, by contrast, is supported by patterns of word boundary misperceptions (Cutler & Butterfield, 1992) and by evidence of activation of monosyllabic words embedded as strong syllables in longer words (e.g., *bone,* in *trombone;* Shillcock, 1990).

Stress-based segmentation in English and syllabic segmentation in French are similar in that in both cases segmentation procedures appear to reflect the basic rhythmic structure of the language; this parallel led Otake et al. (1993) to investigate segmentation in Japanese, the rhythm of which is based on a subsyllabic unit, the mora. Otake et al.'s results (see also Cutler & Otake, 1994) supported moraic segmentation in Japanese.

2. Constraints of Temporal Structure

Spoken words are temporal signals. The temporal nature of spoken word recognition is the basis of the Cohort Model of Marslen-Wilson and Welsh (1978), which models word recognition via bottom-up analysis of the input combined with top-down influence from knowledge-driven constraints. Each stored lexical representation is an active element, which responds to both bottom-up and top-down information. The initial portion of a spoken word activates all words beginning in that way. Thus /s/ activates, for example, *sad, several, spelling, psychology.* As more information arrives, processing elements that do not match the input drop out of this initial cohort of potential words. If the next phoneme is /p/, for example, the cohort is reduced to words beginning /sp/; an incoming /ɪ/ reduces it still further, to *spinach, spirit, spill,* and so on until only one candidate word remains. This may occur before the end of the word. Because no words other than *spigot* begin /spɪg/, those four phonemes suffice to reduce the cohort to one word.

The model capitalizes on the temporal nature of speech in that initial portions of words affect the recognition process first. Recognition is efficient in that a word can be recognized by that point at which it becomes unique from all other words in the language (the "uniqueness point"), which may (as in *spigot*) precede the word's end.

In support of the uniqueness point concept, Marslen-Wilson (1984) reported correlations between phoneme detection RT and the distance of target phonemes from uniqueness points, and between the point at which listeners confidently recognized gated words and the words' uniqueness points. Similarly, nonwords that are the first part of real words (e.g. [krɛd] as in *credit*) are rejected more slowly than are nonwords that cannot become words (e.g. [krɛn]; Taft, 1986); mispronunciations later in words are detected faster and more accurately than changes in initial sounds (Cole, 1973; Marslen-Wilson & Welsh, 1978). In support of the concept of an activated cohort, Marslen-Wilson (1987) found that presentation of either *captain* or *captive* initially activated words related to both (e.g., *ship, guard*), suggesting that both potential words were themselves activated; at the end of either word, however, only associates of the word actually presented were facilitated. Marslen-Wilson and Zwitserlood (1989) reported that words were not primed by other words with similar ending portions; thus recognition of *battle* was primed by *batter,* but not by *cattle.* However, Connine, Blasko, and Titone (1993) found that nonwords that differed from real words by only one or two phonological features of the initial phoneme primed associates of their base words (i.e., *deacher* primed *school*).

Other evidence also suggests that words are not necessarily recognized as early as possible, and that word-final information may be fully processed. Gated words are usually recognized after their uniqueness point, sometimes only after their acoustic offset (Bard, Shillcock, & Altmann, 1988; Grosjean, 1985). Lexical decision RTs to words with the same uniqueness point and same number of phonemes after the uniqueness point (e.g., *difficult, diffident*) differ as a function of frequency; and listeners' latency to reject nonwords with equal uniqueness points is affected by what follows this point (e.g., *rhythlic,* which has the same ending as *rhythmic,* is rejected more slowly than *rhythlen,* although both become nonwords at the /l/; Taft & Hambly, 1986; see also Goodman & Huttenlocher, 1988). Words in sentences can be identified either from word-initial or word-final information, and both types of information interact with higher-level contextual information (Salasoo & Pisoni, 1985); truncated words can be recognized from either initial or final fragments (Nooteboom, 1981); and beginnings and ends of synthesized words are equally effective recognition prompts when the rest of the word is noise masked (Nooteboom & van der Vlugt, 1988). Identification of spoken words is facilitated by prior presentation of rhyming items (Milberg, Blumstein & Dworetzky, 1988) and, under noise masking, by prior presentation of words overlapping either from onset or offset; recognition of *flock* is facilitated as much by *stock* or *block* as by *flap* or *flop* (Slowiaczek et al., 1987).

Indeed, the uniqueness point concept may have limited application, since most short words (in English) become unique only at their end (*starve, start*), or even after it (*star* could continue as *starve, start, starling*, etc.; Luce, 1986), and most words (even content words) in conversational speech are mono-syllabic (Cutler & Carter, 1987). Counterproposals consider instead the overall similarity of a word to other words (Luce, Pisoni, & Goldinger, 1990; Marcus & Frauenfelder, 1985). All-or-none rejection of candidate words due to early mismatch is also inconsistent with detection of word-initial mispronunciations (Cole, 1973), with word-initial phoneme restora-tion (Warren, 1970), and with recognition of improbable utterances such as puns (Norris, 1982). Marslen-Wilson (1987) revised the cohort model to cope with these problems. The later version of the model assumes that minor mismatches only downgrade a candidate word's activation rather than remove it entirely from the cohort. However, the model still gives highest priority to word-initial information.

3. The Limits of Interaction

a. Interactive Models of Spoken Word Recognition

The Logogen Model (Morton, 1969) is a model of how sources of informa-tion combine in word recognition, originally designed for visual recogni-tion, and for data just on visual recognition thresholds at that. But it has been treated as a general model of word recognition by many researchers. "Logogens," in this model, are active feature counters associated with indi-vidual lexical items, which tot up incoming positive evidence in their indi-vidual favor. Each logogen has a threshold, at which it outputs a recognition response. Not all logogens are equal: those for high-frequency words, for instance, start with higher resting levels than those for low-frequency words. As the input may come not only from auditory features but also from higher-level sources such as syntactic and semantic analysis of the preceding speech context, the logogen model is interactive. Probably be-cause it is less fully specified than more recent models, the logogen model has not played a major role in recent years.

In the first version of the Cohort Model, higher-level context could reduce the cohort: words inconsistent with the developing context drop out. Thus, strong contextual constraints would produce even earlier recog-nition. Consistent with this, recognition of gated words showed facilitatory effects of both syntactic and semantic constraints (Tyler, 1984; Tyler & Wessels, 1983); and in a shadowing task, predictable mispronounced words were fluently restored to correct pronunciation, as if listeners had not noticed the errors (Marslen-Wilson, 1975). Further, Marslen-Wilson and Welsh (1978) found that the tendency of mispronunciations late in a word to be more often fluently restored than word-initial mispronunciations was significantly stronger for predictable than for unpredictable words. In the revised cohort model, however, higher-level context does not act directly on cohort membership. A set of potential candidates generated by bottom-up input is evaluated and integrated with context; information from prior context flows down only to this integrative stage, not as far as lexical selection. By this latter change the cohort model is no longer strictly interactive, but essentially an application to auditory word recognition of Norris's (1986) noninteractive model of context effects in visual word recognition, and similar to proposals about spoken word recognition made by Luce et al. (1990).

The case for interactivity in spoken word recognition is put most strongly by the connectionist model TRACE. A miniversion of the model (McClelland & Elman, 1986a) takes real speech input, but is of limited scope (one speaker and a vocabulary of nine CV syllables). The better-known version (McClelland & Elman, 1986b) finesses front-end analysis problems in the interest of explicating the higher-level capabilities; the input is an explicit representation of acoustic features. Both versions of the model embody interactive activation. On a series of levels are processing elements (nodes), each with (1) a current activation value, (2) a resting level, toward which its activation decays over time, and (3) a threshold, over which its activation spreads to connected nodes. Bidirectional connections exist between nodes within each level and at adjacent levels. TRACE mimics the temporal nature of speech by representing each node separately in each one of successive time slices.

Connections between nodes at the same level can be excitatory (e.g., connection at the phoneme level between /t/ and phonemes in adjacent time slices that can precede or follow /t/, such as vowels), or inhibitory (e.g., connection between /t/ and other phonemes in the same time slice). Between-level connections (e.g., from /t/ to all features at the feature level, below, which occur in /t/, or to all words containing /t/ at the word level, above) are always facilitatory. Connections are assigned weights (positive for excitatory connections, negative for inhibitory). Interactive activation is the process of constantly adjusting connection weights, and hence the activation of nodes, according to signals received from other nodes, on the same, lower, or higher levels. The input is a pattern of activation of feature nodes, presented sequentially across time slices. Activation spreads upward from the feature level, while within the feature level inhibition is exerted toward features incompatible with those activated by the input. As higher-level nodes are excited from the bottom up, their increasing activation leads them to exert influence from the top down, which in turn increases activation from the bottom up, and so on. Recognition occurs (at any output level) when a node's activation reaches some arbitrary level. A decision can in principle be made at any time, the current most highly activated node being deemed the output (McClelland & Elman, 1986b, p. 20). Alternatively, output could occur at a preset time rather than at a preset activation level.

An advantage of TRACE is its exploitation of variability in cues to phonemes. For instance, the fact that acoustic cues for stop consonants vary with the identity of the following vowel is represented in the miniversion of TRACE by connections that allow feature nodes for vowels to adjust the weights of feature nodes for prevocalic consonants. TRACE's major limitation, however, is that it deals ineffectively with the temporal nature of speech; multiplication of the entire network across time slices is a highly implausible proposal. Subsequent connectionist models of speech recognition exploited techniques better adapted to deal with temporal variation, such as simple recurrent networks (Elman, 1990; Norris, 1990). According to Klatt (1989), current connectionist models also provide only limited and implausible solutions to the problems of variability in speech.

Note that simultaneous consideration of input and higher-level information does not presuppose interactivity. In Massaro's (1987) Fuzzy Logical Model of Speech Perception (FLMP), multiple sources of information about speech input are simultaneously but independently evaluated in a continuous manner, and are integrated and compared as to the relative support they offer for stored prototypes. It is called a fuzzy logical model because continuous truth values are assigned to each source of information as a result of the evaluation process. The FLMP offers a way of integrating information from input and context without positing interaction: the information from each source is evaluated independently, and one does not modify the processing of the other. Massaro (1989) has argued that in signal detection theory terms, his model predicts top-down effects only on bias (β), not sensitivity (d'), whereas TRACE, which allows activation from higher levels of processing to feed back to and alter lower levels of processing, predicts that top-down effects will alter sensitivity; Massaro reported results consistent with the FLMP's predictions.

b. Lexical and Phonetic Processing

Evidence of word/nonword differences in the earliest stages of speech perception would argue strongly for interaction. Three main lines of research have addressed this issue. The first, using the phonetic categorization task, began with Ganong (1980), who asked listeners to identify CVC-initial consonants varying along a voicing continuum, one choice consistent with a word and the other with a nonword (e.g., *teak–deak* vs. *teep–deep*). The crossover point of listeners' identification functions shifted, such that more choices were lexically consistent. The lexical shift was largest in the ambiguous region of the continuum, which Ganong interpreted as a top-down effect, arguing that response bias would have affected the entire continuum equally.

Fox (1984), however, found that fast categorization responses were unaffected by lexicality (also see Miller & Dexter, 1988). Fox proposed that phonetic and lexical representations are computed in parallel; activation of lexical representations takes longer than phonetic computation, but once lexical information is available, it dominates, with the result that only later responses are lexically biased. Connine and Clifton (1987) replicated Fox's RT result, but argued that if the lexical effect was indeed a postperceptual response bias, its effects should mimic those of another bias such as monetary payoff; they did not, renewing support for top-down interpretation of lexical effects on categorization. Also, TRACE successfully simulated (McClelland & Elman, 1986b) both Ganong's (1980) and Fox's (1984) findings, as well as effects of phonological legality in categorization (Massaro & Cohen, 1983).

An influential study by Elman and McClelland (1988) capitalized on one type of compensation for coarticulation, namely identification of alveolar and velar stops after dental versus palatal fricatives. Lip rounding for the palatal [ʃ] elongates the vocal tract, while lip retraction for the dental [s] shortens it, resulting in changes in the articulation of any following stop; but listeners compensate for these: an ambiguous sound halfway between [t] and [k] tends to be reported as [t] if it occurs after [ʃ], but as [k] if it occurs after [s] (Mann & Repp, 1981). Elman and McClelland appended an ambiguous fricative between [ʃ] and [s] to words normally ending in [ʃ] (*foolish*) and [s] (*Christmas*), and had listeners judge an ambiguous stop consonant between [t] and [k], presented in word-initial position immediately following the ambiguous fricative. A compensation shift appeared in listeners' judgments after the ambiguous as well as after the unambiguous fricative. The ambiguous fricative provided no acoustic reason for compensation; Elman and McClelland therefore interpreted the shift in terms of top-down lexical influence inducing biased judgments about acoustic structure at the phonetic decision level.

In phonetic categorization experiments, of course, many stimuli are by definition unnatural, that is, not what speakers ever produce; this makes the segmental perception task both difficult and unrepresentative of natural recognition. Also, the same words are responded to repeatedly, which may preactivate lexical representations and hence make influence of lexical information more likely. Recent results with the task suggest that lexical effects are fragile and rather dependent on unnaturalness of the stimuli. Burton, Baum, and Blumstein (1989) found that lexical effects on [d]–[t] categorizations disappeared when the stimuli covaried burst amplitude with VOT (and were thus more like natural speech). Likewise, McQueen (1991) found no lexical effects in word-final [s]–[ʃ] categorizations with high-quality stimuli, though lexical effects appeared when the same stimuli were degraded by filtering. (Note that McQueen's finding of small and unreliable lexical effects on word-final phoneme categorization also contradicts TRACE, which predicts stronger lexical effects word-finally than word-initially; as word information accumulates, top-down feedback should strengthen.) Compare these inconsistent lexical status effects with effects of speaking rate, actual or inferred (e.g., Miller, 1981a, 1981b; Miller & Liberman, 1979). A continuum varying formant transition duration from [b] (short) to [w] (long) produces more [b] judgments before a long [a], more [w] judgments before a short [a], indicating that listeners compensate for (inferred) rate of articulation by computing transition duration in relation to stimulus duration (Miller & Liberman, 1979). This effect appears with severely filtered phonetic context (Gordon, 1988), suggesting that it operates at an early, coarse-grained, level of phonetic processing; moreover, the effect cannot be removed by, for instance, requiring fast responses (Miller & Dexter, 1988; Miller, Green, & Schermer, 1984). Thus, the rate effect seems to be automatic, and robust in a way that the effects of lexical status are not. The presence of lexical status effects, as Pitt and Samuel (1993) concluded from a comprehensive meta-analysis of the phonetic categorization studies, depends heavily both on position of the phoneme in the stimulus item, and on the phonetic contrast involved. In all, the pattern of variability suggests that the phonetic categorization task may not be the best way to study lexical–phonetic relationships.

In phoneme restoration studies (Warren, 1970), a phoneme is excised and replaced by noise; listeners report hearing noise simultaneous with an intact speech signal (something that they have often experienced). Their judgments of the location of the noise are imperfect, but the limits of illusory continuity correspond roughly to average word duration (Bashford, Meyers, Brubaker, & Warren, 1988; Bashford & Warren, 1987), suggesting that once lexical information is available, it supplants lower-level information. Samuel (1981a) compared listeners' judgments when noise actually replaced a phoneme (as it did in Warren's stimuli) or was overlaid on a phoneme (as listeners reported). Discriminability (d') of replaced versus overlaid stimuli was significantly worse in real words than in nonwords, and in high-frequency words than in low-frequency words (although Samuel, 1981b, failed to replicate the frequency effect). Discriminability was also worse when the distorted word was preceded by the same word, undistorted. Bias (β) showed no effects either of lexical status or of frequency. Samuel (1987) similarly found that words with early uniqueness points were less discriminable (at least for distortions late in the word) than words with late uniqueness points; and words with more than one completion (e.g., *-egion*) were less discriminable than words with a unique completion (*-esion*). Samuel interpreted his results in terms of top-down lexical influence upon phonetic decisions: previously activated or otherwise easily identifiable words are more speedily accessed and feedback from their lexical representations overrides the low-level discrimination, while nonwords remain discriminable because no lexical representations exercise influence. Real words are, however, no more detectable under noise than nonwords (Repp & Frost, 1988).

The third line of research uses phoneme-monitoring and asks whether responses are pre- or postlexical. Postlexical responding is suggested by findings that targets are detected faster on predictable than on unpredictable words (Eimas & Nygaard, 1992; Mehler & Segui, 1987; Morton & Long, 1976), targets may be detected faster on words than on nonwords (P. Rubin, Turvey, & van Gelder, 1976), and word targets are detected faster than phoneme targets on the same words (Foss & Swinney, 1973). Likewise, if subjects monitor for targets occurring anywhere in a word, not just word-initially, targets are detected faster on high- versus low-frequency words (Segui & Frauenfelder, 1986) and on contextually primed versus unprimed words (Frauenfelder & Segui, 1989). On the other hand, Foss and Blank (1980; also see Foss, Harwood, & Blank, 1980) found no RT effects of word–nonword status or frequency of occurrence of the target-bearing word; and when subjects monitored for word-initial phonemes only no effects of word frequency (Segui & Frauenfelder, 1986) or contextual priming appeared (Frauenfelder & Segui, 1989). Repeated findings that the level of match between target specification and response item affects RT in this task (Cutler, Butterfield, & Williams, 1987; Dijkstra, Schreuder, & Frauenfelder, 1989; Healy & Cutting, 1976; McNeill & Lindig, 1973; Mills, 1980a, 1980b; Swinney & Prather, 1980; Whalen, 1984, 1991) are consistent with prelexical responses, as is the interference effect of phonemes phonologically similar to the target (Newman & Dell, 1978). Newman and Dell argued that a phonological representation constructed postlexically should allow a simple yes–no decision on match of input to target; but RT in their study showed a gradient of interference as a function of number of shared phonological features. Further, this interference effect is as strong in predictable as in unpredictable words (Dell & Newman, 1980; Stemberger, Elman, & Haden, 1985).

The apparently conflicting phoneme-monitoring findings can be accounted for by assuming that responses can be made either pre- or postlexically, as in the Race Model of phoneme detection proposed by Cutler and Norris (1979; also see Foss & Blank, 1980; Newman & Dell, 1978). In this model, parallel processes compute an explicit phonemic representation and access the lexicon, with a phoneme detection response possible on the basis of whichever representation is available first; the model contrasts with TRACE, which allows phonemic responses only from the phonemic level. Whether or not lexical effects on phoneme detection RT are observed depends on characteristics of the materials and of the subjects' task (Cutler, Mehler, Norris, & Segui, 1987; Foss & Gernsbacher, 1983); these can affect the level of response at which subjects' attention is focused and, in turn, which process wins the phoneme response race. TRACE successfully simulated (McClelland & Elman, 1986b) both Foss and Gernsbacher's (1983) failure to find lexical effects on word-initial phoneme detection, and Marslen-Wilson's (1980) finding that phoneme detection *did* show lexical influence late in a word. Counter to TRACE's predictions, however, is a finding by Frauenfelder, Segui, and Dijkstra (1990) on phoneme detection in nonwords. In TRACE, incoming phonetic information consistent with a particular word facilitates all phonemes in that word, which in turn leads to inhibition of phonemes not in the word. Thus TRACE predicts that RT to [t] in *vocabutary* will be slow (compared with RT to [t] in, say, *socabutary*), because incoming information will be consistent with the word *vocabulary*, which contains no [t]. The prediction was not borne out: RTs for the two types of nonword did not differ. This finding is consistent with the Race Model, which assumes a prelexical focus of attention with nonword input.

Attentional accounts have similarly been offered for RT differences in word versus phoneme monitoring (Brunner & Pisoni, 1982), for the disappearance of top-down effects under speeded response conditions in phonetic categorization (Miller et al., 1984), and for changes in the relative weight of cues to phonemic identity (Gordon, Eberhardt, & Rueckl, 1993). In phonemic restoration, Samuel (1991; Samuel & Ressler, 1986) elicited significantly more accurate discriminations of replaced versus overlaid phonemes by telling subjects which phoneme to attend to, suggesting that subjects can switch attention from the lexical level (which normally mediates the restoration illusion) to the phonetic level. In phoneme monitoring, listeners can be induced to attend selectively to position in the word (Pitt & Samuel, 1990) or syllable (Pallier, Sebastian-Gallés, Felguera, Christophe, & Mehler, 1993). Eimas, Hornstein, and Payton (1990) found that listeners making a phoneme choice response (e.g., [b] or [p]) normally attended to the phonetic level, but addition of a secondary task requiring a lexical judgment resulted in attention switching to the lexical level, such that lexical effects upon RT appeared. In sentence contexts, however, the same items did not produce reliable lexical effects with or without a secondary task (Eimas & Nygaard, 1992; cf. Foss & Blank, 1980; Foss et al., 1980), suggesting that attention switching is less easy in coherent contexts than in word lists. This in turn suggests that in phoneme monitoring, as in phonetic categorization, lexical effects may be highly dependent on those characteristics of the experimental situation that least resemble natural recognition conditions.

c. Sentence and Word Processing

How far should top-down influences from syntactic and semantic context extend? No current models propose direct interaction between nonadjacent processing levels, and effects of sentence context on phonetic processing seem better explained as response bias than as perceptual effects. Phonetic categorizations can be shifted by contextual probability, so that a sound between [b] and [p] can be judged [b] in *hot water for the —ath* but [p] in *jog along the —ath* (Miller et al., 1984); however, the shift disappears in speeded responses, suggesting that it is not a mandatory perceptual effect. Similarly, Connine (1987) found that sentence context affected phonetic categorization RT for stimuli at the continuum end points but not at the category boundary, again indicative of response bias rather than an alteration of perceptual decisions; and Samuel (1981a) found that the bias measure in phonemic restoration (which showed no lexical status or frequency effects) *was* influenced by sentence context, but the discriminability measure was not. Both Samuel and Connine argued that sentential context does not constrain phonetic processing, though they held that it may affect it indirectly by constraining lexical processing.

Consistent with constraints of sentence context on lexical processing are faster word monitoring in syntactically and semantically acceptable contexts than in semantically anomalous or ungrammatical contexts (Marslen-Wilson, Brown, & Tyler, 1988; Marslen-Wilson & Tyler, 1980) and earlier recognition of gated words in constraining semantic and syntactic contexts (Grosjean, 1980; Tyler & Wessels, 1983). Prior presentation of associates of the target-bearing word facilitates phoneme-monitoring RT when the words are in the same sentence (though such effects are weak in lists: Blank & Foss, 1978; Foss, 1982; Foss & Ross, 1983). However, Foss explained this phoneme-monitoring facilitation in terms of ease of integration of the word meaning into a representation of the sentence meaning, and Marslen-Wilson et al. (1988) accounted similarly for the word-monitoring finding. Connine, Blasko, and Hall (1991) provide converging evidence of rapid and efficient integration mechanisms. Context effects in gating experiments may result from guessing (given that, after all, guessing on the basis of partial information is what the subject has to do). Thus, none of these findings entail that availability of lexical candidates is constrained by the sentence context. Pertinent evidence on this issue comes from the case of homophony.

When a listener hears an ambiguous string such as [wik], sentence context could constrain lexical processing such that only the contextually appropriate sense of the word is retrieved; alternatively, if lexical processing is independent of syntactic and semantic processing, all senses may be activated, and the appropriate one chosen by reference to the context. Using the cross-modal priming task, Swinney (1979) found that homophones such as *bug* primed words related to both their senses, even when prior context was consistent with only one of the senses; although after just a few syllables, only the contextually appropriate sense was active. Facilitation of words related to both senses occurs even when one reading of the ambiguous word is far more frequent than the other(s): *scale* primes both *weight* and *fish* (Onifer & Swinney, 1981), and even when there are word class differences and syntactic context permits only one reading: *week/weak* primes both *month* and *strong* (Lucas, 1987).

Similarly, a spoken homophone facilitates naming of a visually presented word related to either one of its senses, irrespective of form class; *flower* is named more rapidly after either *She held the rose* or *They all rose* than after control sentences, and again the multiple-sense activation is short lived (Tanenhaus, Leiman, & Seidenberg, 1979). The same methodology produces automatic activation of multiple senses for noun–verb as well as noun–noun ambiguities (Seidenberg, Tanenhaus, Leiman, & Bienkowski, 1982). Lackner and Garrett (1972) presented listeners with two competing messages, and required them to attend to one and to paraphrase it. Speech in the unattended channel (which subjects could not report) resolved ambiguities in the attended utterances; subjects' paraphrases reflected either sense, depending on the available disambiguation, again suggesting availability of all senses.

All these results suggest momentary simultaneous activation of all senses of a homophone, irrespective of relative frequency or contextual probability, with postaccess decision processes rapidly and efficiently selecting an appropriate sense and discarding inappropriate sense(s). This would imply that lexical access is *not* subject to top-down influence from syntactic and semantic processing. Note that Seidenberg et al. (1982) found that strong associates in the preceding context *could* constrain one sense of a homophone; but they interpreted this as an effect of lexical association rather than of syntactic or semantic context. Similarly, completely restrictive syntactic contexts fail to prevent activation of multiple senses of noun–verb homophones (e.g., *sink;* Oden & Spira, 1983; Tanenhaus & Donnenwerth-Nolan, 1984), although Oden and Spira found a greater degree of facilitation for contextually appropriate than for contextually inappropriate senses. Tabossi (1988a; also see Tabossi, Colombo, & Job, 1987) found that strongly constraining contexts could lead to only one sense being activated if that particular sense was highly dominant (e.g., the *harbor* sense of *port* in *ships in the port*). But again, these contexts effectively primed the relevant sense via occurrence of a related word, contexts that constrained one sense without priming it (e.g., *The man had to be at the port*) produced facilitation for all senses. Thus, a within-lexical explanation is again as viable as a top-down account. Exhaustive activation of the senses of an ambiguous word does *not* occur when the word is not focused in the sentence (Blutner & Sommer, 1988), suggesting that the kind of activation of related words that the cross-modal priming task taps may occur only when attention is directed to the part of the sentence containing the priming word.

Unambiguous words can also have senses of varying relevance to particular contexts. All attributes may be momentarily activated when a word is heard, irrespective of their relative dominance and of their contextual appropriateness (Whitney, McKay, Kellas, & Emerson, 1985); shortly after word offset, however, attributes that are dominant and/or contextually appropriate are still active, but contextually inappropriate nondominant attributes are not. Similarly, central properties of unambiguous words (e.g., that *ice* is *cold*) are activated irrespective of contextual appropriateness, but peripheral properties (e.g., that *ice* is *slippery*) are activated only when appropriate (Greenspan, 1986; this latter experiment had a delay between context and target, and thus resembles Whitney et al.'s postoffset condition).

Tabossi (1988b) found that sentence contexts *could* constrain activation of different aspects of an unambiguous word's meaning; HARD was primed after *The strong blow didn't crack the diamond,* but not after *The jeweler polished the diamond.* However, Williams (1988) found that even in neutral contexts there could be a failure of priming, so that TABLE is not primed after *The boy put the chair. . . .* (although *chair* reliably primes TABLE out of context). Williams argued that the relations between prime and target here involved schematic world knowledge rather than lexical associations; he proposed that activation of background knowledge during construction of the semantic representation of a sentence determined the kind of attribute to which the listener's attention would be directed. Only certain kinds of semantic relation, however, are subject to such attentional constraint; other kinds of relation produce truly context-independent priming effects. This argument suggests that the scope for sentence context effects on lexical processing may be limited to certain kinds of relationship between a word and its context. Even then, context effects are, as argued above, apparently located at a relatively late stage of processing. Zwitserlood (1989) showed that both contextually appropriate and inappropriate words are momentarily activated before sufficient input is available to select between them; thus context does not constrain the availability of lexical candidates per se.

4. Competition for Lexical Selection

First proposed in TRACE, the notion that candidate words actively compete for recognition is achieving wide popularity. Evidence of activation of words embedded within or across other words (Cluff & Luce, 1990; Shillcock, 1990; Tabossi, Burani & Scott, 1995), or of simultaneous activation of partially overlapping words (Goldinger, Luce, & Pisoni, 1989; Goldinger, Luce, Pisoni, & Marcario, 1992; Gow & Gordon, 1995; Marslen-Wilson, 1990; Zwitserlood, 1989) is consistent with the competition notion, but does not entail it. Inhibition of recognition as a function of the existence of competitors provides direct evidence. Taft (1986) observed that nonwords that form part of real words are hard to reject. Direct evidence of competition between word candidates comes from the finding that *mess* is harder to recognize when preceded by the syllable [də] (as in *domestic*) than when preceded by, say, [nə] (McQueen, Norris, & Cutler, 1994), and from the finding that recognition is affected by the number of other words potentially accounting for a portion of the input (Norris, McQueen & Cutler, 1995; Vroomen & de Gelder, 1995).

Analysis of patterns of competition depends crucially on precise knowledge of vocabulary structure. Studies of lexical structure have been revolutionized in recent years by the availability of computerized dictionaries; it is now easy to analyze the composition of the vocabulary in many languages, and arguments based on analyses of lexical databases have come to play an important role in theorizing about spoken word recognition (e.g., Cutler & Carter, 1987; Luce, 1986; Marcus & Frauenfelder, 1985). It should be noted, however, that substantial corpora of spoken language, and the estimates of spoken word frequency that could be derived from them, are still lacking; such spoken word frequency counts as do exist (e.g., G. D. A. Brown, 1984; Howes, 1966) are, for practical reasons, small in scale compared to written frequency counts.

Recent modeling initiatives have been designed to exploit vocabulary structure effects. In the Neighborhood Activation Model (Luce et al., 1990), word decision units are directly activated by acoustic/phonetic input, with no top-down information from context playing a role at this stage. Once activated, the decision units monitor both input information and the level of activity in the system as a whole; their activity levels are also heavily biased by frequency. Thus in this model, the probability of recognizing a spoken word is a function both of the word's own frequency and of the number and frequency of similar words in the language: high-frequency words with few, low-frequency neighbors are recognized rapidly and accurately, while low-frequency words with many high-frequency neighbors are much harder to recognize (Goldinger et al., 1989; Luce et al., 1990). So far, the model has been implemented only for monosyllabic words (indeed, CVC words only). The model is similar to the Cohort model in determining initial activation by bottom-up influence only, but differs from it both in the relative importance of word-initial information (in NAM, information pertaining to any part of a word is equally important) and in the central role of frequency. It is similar to TRACE in assuming that recognition is crucially dependent on the pattern of activity in the system as a whole.

Specifically incorporating the notion of competition is SHORTLIST (Norris, 1991, 1994), a hybrid connectionist model that has strong similarities with both the revised Cohort model and TRACE, but is burdened neither with the Cohort model's overdependence on initial information nor with TRACE's multiplication of the lexical network across time slices. Furthermore, unlike TRACE, it is a strictly autonomous model. SHORT-LIST's main feature is the separation of recognition into two distinct stages. In the first, bottom-up information alone determines the set of potential word candidates compatible with the input (the "short list"); the set may include candidates that overlap in the input. The initial stage can be implemented as a simple recurrent network (Norris, 1990), although it has been simulated as a dictionary search by Norris (1994). The short-listed candidates are then wired into a small interactive activation network, containing only as many connections as are needed for the particular set of words being processed; these words then compete for recognition. Because the competition stage is limited to a small candidate set, the model can be implemented with a realistic vocabulary of tens of thousands of words (Norris, 1994).

As noted earlier, the notion of competition provides a potential solution to the problem of word recognition in continuous speech; even without word boundary information, competing words may effectively divide up the input amongst themselves. However, competition can also co-exist with explicit segmentation. When interword competition and stress-based segmentation are compared in the same experiment, independent evidence appears for both (McQueen et al., 1994).

III. SPOKEN WORD PRODUCTION

A. Methodology

The laboratory study of word production raises formidable problems; ensuring that a particular word is produced may subvert the spontaneous production process, for example, by making the word available to the subject's *recognition* system prior to its production. Tasks in which subjects output on command a previously learned sequence (e.g., Sternberg, Knoll, Monsell, & Wright, 1988) or paired associate (Meyer, 1990) may preserve later stages of the production process but preempt earlier stages. Presumably because of this difficulty with designing laboratory studies, much research on production has exploited naturalistic data: slips of the tongue, tip-of-the-tongue (TOT) states, pausing, and hesitation patterns. Word production in particular has been investigated via slips and TOT, in other words, primarily via instances of processing failure. Even though well-controlled laboratory conditions have been devised to collect slips (Baars, Motley, & MacKay, 1975), and articulatory failure in tongue twisters (Shattuck-Hufnagel, 1992) and tip-of-the-tongue states (Kohn et al., 1987), the possibility that the processes inferred from production failures are not those of normal production still bedevils this field.

Word production has also been studied via the picture-naming task, which has a long history in psychology (see Glaser, 1992); in particular, picture naming under conditions of interference from simultaneously presented words (e.g., Lupker, 1979) has allowed inferences about connections within the lexicon (cf. the cross-modal priming task for recognition). In recent versions of this task subjects hear a word and see a picture, and the asynchrony of presentation of these two stimuli may be varied; the dependent variable may be a response to the picture (e.g., Meyer & Schriefers, 1991) or to the spoken word (e.g., Levelt et al., 1991). Again, drawing inferences about word production from these tasks requires assumptions about word recognition as well. Picture-naming experiments of any kind are further limited in that they are applicable only to the study of words that can be depicted: concrete nouns, plus a few readily encodable action verbs (e.g., Kempen & Huijbers, 1983). There are still large areas of vocabulary for which no experimental investigation technique has yet been devised.

B. Issues

1. Stages in Word Production

As Levelt (1989) points out, the conceptual formulation stages of production have attracted more attention from outside psychology (e.g., from AI approaches to language generation) than from within it. There is naturalistic and empirical work on propositional and syntactic formulation (see Bock, Chapter 6, this volume), but virtually none that specifically addresses the input to lexical processing.

Picture-naming studies that partially address the issue include Huttenlocher and Kubicek's (1983) observation that picture naming can be primed by prior presentation of pictures of related objects; they argued that, however, because the size of the priming effect is the same in picture naming as in object recognition without naming, what is primed is recognition of the picture only, and not retrieval of the appropriate name from the lexicon. Flores d'Arcais and Schreuder (1987) found that the naming of pictures (e.g., of a guitar) was facilitated both by prior presentations of other pictures having functional relations to the target picture (e.g., an accordion) and by pictures of objects physically similar to the target (e.g., a tennis racket); they argued for separate involvement of functional and physical aspects of a picture in specification of the relevant lexical input. As in Huttenlocher and Kubicek's study, however, their effects may be located in picture processing rather than in lexical retrieval.

Whatever the precise nature of the input, lexical access in production involves a mapping from semantic to phonological form; a lexical representation can act as a transcoding device that accomplishes this mapping (see Fromkin, 1971, for such a proposal, and see Bock, Chapter 6, this volume). However, separation of semantic/syntactic and phonological information even within the lexical system for production has been assumed by many models. In its simplest form (e.g., Butterworth, 1989) this proposal assumes that each word is associated with a conceptual node, which is accessed by input from message generation, and that this node is in turn connected to a separate phonological node that sends the output to the subsequent stage of the production process. The influential language production model of Garrett (1975) laid greatest emphasis on separation of two distinct levels of processing, corresponding closely to a distinction between two types of words, open-class (or lexical, or content) and closed-class (or grammatical, or function) words. At the "functional" level, only open-class items and their grammatical relations are specified. At the "positional" level all words in an utterance are specified, including inflectional endings that specify grammatical relations. The former level is held to contain no aspects of phonological structure (or at least none that are capable of exercising independent effect at that level); the latter, although still held to be a stage prior to full phonetic specification, "involves certain aspects of sound structure." Although this proposal is not formulated in terms of lexical processing, it is compatible with a two-stage model of lexical processing in which syntactic and phonological forms are separately accessed.

A two-stage proposal for lexical access in production was made by Kempen and Huijbers (1983), and the word production part of Levelt's (1989) model of utterance production is likewise two stage. The conceptual nodes accessed in the first stage of lexical processing these authors call *lemmas*, the phonological nodes, *word forms*. Although Levelt (1989) is neutral as to whether lemmas and word forms are accessed together or separately, he subsequently (Levelt, 1992) proposed that the two stages are temporally sequential.

Corresponding to the notion of two stages, there are modeling efforts devoted principally to one or to the other. For the mapping from concept to lexicon, Oldfield (1966; Oldfield & Wingfield, 1964) proposed successive choice between binary semantic feature alternatives of increasing specificity (+/−*living*, +/−*animate*, +/−*human*, etc.). As Levelt (1989) points out, however, in any such decompositional system the semantic mapping that enables production of, for example, *terrier* will also suffice for production of *dog* (and indeed for more general terms at every level of the semantic hierarchy; *animal, creature,* etc.). Levelt terms this "the hyperonym problem." Semantic decomposition within lexical representations is proposed by Bierwisch and Schreuder (1992). In their model, the mapping from concepts to lemmas is mediated by the construction of an utterance semantic form that may allow alternative instantiations of a conceptual intention as sequences of lemmas; a verbalization function chooses the instantiation that will be mapped to the lexicon. The hyperonym problem is assumed to be solved by restricting lemma access to the closest match to the input semantic form. Roelofs (1992) proposes a spreading activation model of lemma access, in which lemma nodes receive activation from associated concept nodes, and the node with the highest activation level is "selected"; the lemma nodes are linked in turn to word-form nodes, so that selection of a lemma node presumably acts as the criterial stimulus for activation of the associated word-form node. Spreading activation solutions could in principle solve the hyperonym problem by ensuring that a specific input (*terrier*) will produce greater activation in more specific lemmas than in more general ones (*dog*). However, the problem does not arise in Roelofs's model because of the one-to-one mapping from concepts to lemmas. A decompositional process of concept access would, of course, merely shift the problem to the concept-node level. Roelofs (1993) argues, however, that decompositional acquisition of concepts is compatible with later chunking of the conceptual components to a unitary representation, such that concept access in production short-circuits the process of concept construction from semantic primitives.

The mapping from semantic to phonological structure in language production is reflected in slips at each level. In semantic misselection, a semantically related word may substitute for the target word (*the two contemporary* [T: *adjacent*] *buildings*), or two semantically related words may be simultaneously chosen and the output form may be a blend of both (*science fiction bookstops* [T: *stores/shops*]). In the latter case the two components of the blend are equally good alternative selections (in the particular context: Bierwisch, 1981). In phonological misselection, substitution errors may produce words with similarity of sound but not of meaning: *participate* for *precipitate* (Fay & Cutler, 1977). However, such pairs apparently do not blend (errors such as *partipitate* are not reported). Misselections that are only semantic or only phonological, and differing constraints on semantic versus phonological errors, are consistent with separation of semantic from phonological information in lexical access.

For word-form retrieval, Shattuck-Hufnagel (1979, 1983, 1986) proposes a model in which a suprasegmental framework, consisting of prosodically labeled syllable frames, is separately specified (presumably by extralexical considerations), and segmental components of the phonological forms of words are copied into it by a 'scan-copy" device. The latter selects and copies the segments in serial order. As each segment is selected it is checked off; the copied representation is constantly monitored. Shattuck-Hufnagel's model is primarily intended to account for patterns of phoneme slips: phoneme anticipations and exchanges occur when the scanner selects the wrong segment; perseverations are failures of check-off. Like other error-based models, Shattuck-Hufnagel's assumes that word forms consist of phoneme representations ordered in syllabic structure. Slips in the pronunciation of words preserve syllable structure: syllable-initial phonemes exchange with one another, syllable-final with one another, and so on. Patterns of error in tongue twisters reveal the same pattern (Shattuck-Hufnagel, 1992). However, slips at differing levels of syllable structure are possible: thus an initial consonant cluster can move as a unit (e.g., exchange with another syllable onset: *cledge hippers*), or one element of the cluster can move alone (*Sprench feaker*). Phonemes can be misordered, as in the above examples, or misselected (omitted, added, substituted: *overwelling* for *overwhelming, osposed* for *opposed, neasely* for *neatly*). Such slips involve movement or selection of whole phonemes, not of the phonological features in terms of which phonemes can be described (Shattuck-Hufnagel & Klatt, 1979). Slips are more likely when a sound occurs twice (e.g., *a lilting willy*); the two occurrences should have the same role in syllable structure (Dell, 1984). Slips are more likely between, and more likely to create, two words with the same pattern of syllable structure(s) (Stemberger, 1990).

Phoneme similarity can precipitate error: the likelihood of error increases with increasing similarity between phonemes, both in natural (Shattuck-Hufnagel, 1986; Shattuck-Hufnagel & Klatt, 1979) and in experimentally elicited slips (Levitt & Healy, 1985). Levitt and Healy also found that frequent phonemes tend to displace infrequent ones, and argued that the former have stronger output representations than the latter. However, no such asymmetry was observed in Shattuck-Hufnagel and Klatt's (1979) natural slips corpus; nor did they find that markedness was a relevant variable in error frequency (but see Stemberger, 1991). Similarity effects may occur in mapping a phonological to an articulatory code.

Speakers producing a learned word on command initiate production more rapidly if they are sure of the initial syllable of the word to be spoken, even more rapidly if they are sure of the initial two syllables, but knowledge of noninitial syllables alone cannot speed production (Meyer, 1990). Speakers naming a picture produce their response faster if just as they see the picture they hear a word with the same onset as the name, or just after they see the picture they hear a word with the same offset as the name (Meyer & Schriefers, 1991). Both results suggest that word encoding produces onsets before offsets rather than whole words at once.

2. Interaction between Stages of Production

a. Interactive Models of Word Production

Word production has been less systematically modeled than recognition. Morton's logogen model (1969), as a general theory of lexical representation and retrieval, is applicable equally to recognition and production. In the case of production, the evidence that raises a logogen's activation level will normally be conceptual input from the cognitive system, and the output once a logogen has reached threshold is an (unspecified) phonological code. Just as logogens are sensitive to semantics as well as phonology in recognition, they are sensitive to phonological as well as semantic information in production.

The model proposed by Dell (1986, 1988), in which lexical processing within sentence production is carried out by spreading activation within a network, contrasts most obviously with the noninteractive two-stage models of Levelt (1989) and others. Semantic, morphological, and phonological aspects of any lexical item's structure are represented separately within this network, but there is no division of the network to reflect this separation, with the result that activation can flow in either direction within any combination of these aspects of representation. Similar proposals for a lexical network have been made by Stemberger (1985) and MacKay (1987).

b. Sentence and Word Processing

Interaction between lexical and contextual processing in production would require the demonstration of feedback from lexical information to subsequent prelexical decisions about utterance content. Bierwisch and Schreuder (1992) propose that the matching of lexical representations to conceptual input involves distributed processing, but their model does not include feedback from lexicon to the input. Levelt and Maassen (1981) argued on the basis of a finding that word accessibility (as defined by naming latency) did not affect order of mention that there is *no* such feedback. Harley (1984) discusses speech errors in which recently activated words intrude into an utterance, for example, *I've eaten* (T:*read*) *all my library books,* spoken by a hungry person preparing to eat. But such errors do not imply that activation of, for example, food-related words in the lexicon has resulted in a change to the speaker's *plan* for the utterance; rather, as Garrett (1988) argues, they can be explained as high-level blend errors, in which multiple utterance plans, generated in parallel, may merge.

It has been argued that syntactic formulation precedes lexical selection (Fromkin, 1971), follows it (Bierwisch & Schreuder, 1992), or operates in parallel to it (Bock, 1982). Bock (1986) argued that phonological information cannot feed back to influence word availability during syntactic formulation. In her experiment, speakers were asked to describe pictures, for example, of a church being struck by lightning; prior presentation of a prime word tended to determine choice of subject noun when the prime was semantically related to one of the concepts in the picture (e.g., after the prime *thunder* speakers were more likely to start with *lightning*), but phonologically related primes (e.g., *frightening*) had no such effect. This result is compatible with models of lexical processing in which semantic and phonological information become available separately, and only the former is available to the syntactic formulator.

However, Bock (1987) found, using the same technique, that prior presentation of a prime word having maximal overlap from onset with a target word (e.g., *plan* for *plant*) inhibited choice of the target as first noun in a picture description. Bock argued that prior presentation of a close phonological neighbor makes word forms temporarily less accessible, which in turn prompts the syntactic formulator to choose a structure in which access of that form is delayed. Levelt and Maassen (1981) found that although word accessibility did not affect order of mention, it did affect syntactic formulation in that where nouns were less accessible, picture descriptions were spoken more slowly and contained less syntactic reduction (e.g., coordinate reduction). These findings could suggest feedback from word-form selection to syntactic formulation, but Levelt (1989) accommodates them within an autonomous framework by proposing that relative word-form inaccessibility causes an ongoing utterance production to grind to a halt, and the resulting (unspecified) distress signal prompts an earlier process (here, syntactic formulation) to start again with an alternative plan.

c. Lexical and Phonetic Processing

Natural phoneme misordering errors (Dell & Reich, 1981) and experimentally elicited phoneme slips (Baars et al., 1975) tend to result in real words (rather than nonwords) more often than chance would predict. Also, many word substitution errors show simultaneous semantic and phonological relationships (e.g., *typhoid;* T: *thyroid;* Aitchison & Straf, 1981). Baars et al. proposed a prearticulatory output monitor to explain the asymmetry, but Dell and Reich argued for simultaneous accessibility of semantic and phonological aspects of words (as proposed by Dell, 1986). As described above, this proposal conflicts with the autonomous two-stage models. Schriefers, Meyer, and Levelt (1990) asked subjects to name simple pictures (e.g., of a finger); naming time was slowed if subjects heard a semantically related word (e.g., *toe*) just before the picture appeared, but it was speeded if they heard a phonologically related word (e.g., *finch*) just *after* the picture appeared. Levelt et al. (1991) further adapted this paradigm such that the dependent variable became response time to make a lexical decision to the spoken word, presented just after the picture. When the spoken word was the name of the picture itself or was either semantically or phonologically related to this name, responses were inhibited in comparison to responses to a word unrelated to the picture. However, responses to words that were phonologically related to the picture's semantic associates (e.g., in the above example, *tone,* similar to *toe*) were not inhibited. Dell's (1986) spreading activation model would predict that any activation would be simultaneously semantic and phonological, counter to Levelt et al.'s results. Dell and O'Seaghdha (1991, 1992) propose a refinement of Dell's model, which brings it closer to the two-stage model; the access of semantic and of phonological information is modeled as separate stages subject to only limited interaction (presumed necessary to explain the speech error effects).

IV. RECOGNITION AND PRODUCTION

Apart from the obvious difference that the mapping between sound and meaning proceeds in opposite directions, what comparisons are appropriate between the processes of recognition and production of spoken words? Are the processes interdependent? Do they, for instance, draw on a single lexicon, or two? This issue has arisen regularly, despite the fact that most models address only one or the other system. In the logogen model, an exception to this separation, simultaneous sensitivity to both phonological and semantic input suggests a unitary lexical representation for each word; but later developments of the theory (Morton & Patterson, 1980) divided the lexicon into input versus output logogens, with the latter sensitive only to semantic information. Support for this view came from a finding by Shallice, McLeod, and Lewis (1985) that auditory name detection and reading words aloud can be performed simultaneously without cross-task interference. On the other hand, word substitution errors resembling the intended word in sound but not in meaning led Fay and Cutler (1977) to argue for a single lexical system, in which such production errors arise by misselection of a neighbor in an organization determined by the needs of recognition. This concluding section considers the similarities and differences in the structure of the recognition and production systems (via consideration, first, of some research issues that have arisen in both fields) (and see Bock, Chapter 6, this volume).

A. Some Common Issues in Recognition and Production Research

1. Frequency of Occurrence

Relative frequency of occurrence affects word recognition (see also Seidenberg, Chapter 5, this volume); for instance, accuracy of report of words in noise rises with frequency (Howes, 1957; Luce et al., 1990; Savin, 1963). However, because listeners produce many high-frequency erroneous responses, Savin (1963) ascribed this result to response bias rather than within-lexical effects; the same argument was made by Luce et al. (1990) because frequency effects on word identification were distinct from effects of neighborhood density (how many phonetically similar words could be confused with the target word), and by Connine, Titone, and Wang (1993) because frequency effects in a phonetic categorization task could be induced by manipulating overall list frequency. Luce et al. proposed that frequency effects occur at a late stage of word recognition, in which decision units, that can be biased by frequency, select among an initial set of candidates consistent with bottom-up information. (The revised cohort model uses a similar frequency mechanism: Marslen-Wilson, 1987.)

High-frequency words are recognized faster in auditory lexical decision (Connine, Mullenix, Shernoff, & Yelen, 1990; Dupoux & Mehler, 1990; Taft & Hambly, 1986; Tyler, Marslen-Wilson, Rentoul, & Hannay, 1988) but frequency effects are stronger with mono- than with polysyllabic words (Bradley & Forster, 1987); in phoneme monitoring, too, frequency effects appear only with targets on monosyllabic words (Dupoux & Mehler, 1990; Foss & Blank, 1980). Monitoring tasks are assumed to tap prelexical or access stages of processing. Where tasks tap later stages of processing, frequency effects are stronger, for example, in rhyme monitoring (McQueen, 1993). Frequency effects in gating disappear in constraining context (Grosjean & Itzler, 1984). The pattern of findings is thus consistent with models that place frequency effects at final decision rather than initial activation stages of lexical processing.

In production, frequency effects are stronger in picture naming than in naming a written word (Huttenlocher & Kubicek, 1983; Oldfield & Wingfield, 1965), but are not accounted for by object recognition time (Wingfield, 1968). Frequent words are less subject to phonological error than infrequent words (Dell, 1990; Stemberger & MacWhinney, 1986b). Word substitutions involving semantic associates tend to replace low-frequency with higher-frequency words (Levelt, 1989). TOT states are more common on low- than on high-frequency words (possibly better estimated by subjective than objective frequency; R. Brown & McNeill, 1966). The facilitatory effects of frequency suggested by these findings are instantiated in the logogen model (Morton, 1969) by differing levels of resting activation, in spreading-activation models by different weights on connections (e.g., MacKay, 1987), or by the number of connections to representations of possible contexts (Dell, 1990). However, frequency effects in homophones (*great/grate*) are determined by combined frequency rather than individual sense frequency (Dell, 1990; Jescheniak & Levelt, 1994), suggesting that they are located at word-form rather than lemma level. This in turn suggests that frequency effects in recognition and production have an ordering similarity (they arise late in word processing) but do not share a common location in a unitary system.

2. Morphological Structure

When two words exchange places in a speech error they frequently strand their inflectional affixes (e.g., *looking for boozes in his insect*); the affixes accommodate to their new stems (the plural inflection that would have been pronounced [s] on *insect* becomes [əz] on *booze*). This suggests separate representation of stem and inflectional affix in word production (Garrett, 1988; Stemberger & Lewis, 1986). Production of past-tense forms given infinitive verbs takes longer for irregular (*taught*) than for regular forms (*talked;* MacKay, 1976). Stems that end in the same phoneme as their inflection (e.g., *yield/yielded, doze/dozes*) are more subject to inflectional omission errors than stems ending in different phonemes (*grab/grabbed, change/changes;* Stemberger & MacWhinney, 1986a). Recognition of regularly inflected, but not irregularly inflected, forms facilitates later recognition of the stem (Kempley & Morton, 1982). Listeners perform same/different judgments faster on stems than on inflections (Jarvella & Meijers, 1983). These observations are all compatible with storage of inflected words in their base form. However, Stemberger and MacWhinney (1986b) argue that common inflected forms are stored as wholes, because they undergo error less often than uncommon inflected forms.

Inflectional affixes may therefore be stripped off in recognition; Taft, Hambly, and Kinoshita (1986) proposed the same for derivational prefixes, because RT to reject a nonword is longer if the nonword begins with a real prefix (e.g.,*dejouse* vs. *tejouse*). Against this suggestion are findings that RTs to detect mispronunciations in second versus first syllables are unaffected by whether or not the first syllable is a prefix (Cole & Jakimik, 1980), and that lexical decision RTs do not suggest that processing of prefixed words (e.g., *intention*) proceeds via processing of unrelated unprefixed words embedded in them (*tension;* Schriefers, Zwitserlood, & Roelofs, 1991; Taft, 1988; Tyler et al., 1988). A morphologically complex word such as *permit* is recognized more rapidly if subjects have just heard another word with the same stem, such as *submit,* but prior presentation of an affix does not have the same effect (Emmorey, 1989). Emmorey argued for a model of the lexicon in which words with the same stem are linked to one another, but having the same affix does not involve such links. Morphological structure is reflected in subjects' TOT guesses (D. C. Rubin, 1975); and when lexical stress is misplaced in production (e.g., *econOmists*), it virtually always falls on a syllable that does bear stress in a word morphologically related to the target (e.g., *economic;* Cutler, 1980), suggesting that lexical representations of morphologically related words are linked in production, too.

Garrett (1988) has argued that the separation of syntactic affixes from stems in production implies autonomy of syntactic from conceptual processing; the same argument was made for spoken word recognition by Katz, Boyce, Goldstein, and Lukatela (1987), who found that recognition time for inflectionally related Serbo-Croatian nouns was affected by syntactic form but not by frequency (which, it will be recalled, seems to be a late effect in recognition).

3. Phonological Structure

Proposals of the form of phonological representation in the recognition lexicon vary from the highly concrete, with contextual variation explicitly represented (e.g., Elman & Zipser, 1988) to the highly abstract, with all predictable information unspecified (Lahiri & Marslen-Wilson, 1991). In production, some sequencing errors apparently involve movement of elements postulated for underlying but not surface phonological representations (e.g., *swin and swaig;* T: *swing and sway;* Fromkin, 1973; the underlying representation of [ŋ] is hypothesized to be [ng]); others involve replacement of elements that would be underspecified in an abstract representation by elements that would be specified (Stemberger, 1991). Both these findings suggest that phonological representations for production may be in abstract form.

The phonological information in lexical entries includes syllable structure, in particular a division between onset and rime: speakers find it easier to play novel language games that require onset–rime division of words than games that require other divisions (Treiman, 1983, 1986); word blends most often involve division of component words between onset and rime (MacKay, 1972). Likewise, syllabic onsets exhibit perceptual integrity (Cutler, Butterfield, & Williams, 1987). Although the syllable per se is not a perceptual unit in English, it is in French and Dutch (see Section IIB1), and converging evidence for a role for the syllable in word production also comes from Dutch (Meyer, 1990). Similarly, studies in Japanese suggest that morae but not syllables play a role in recognition (Otake et al., 1993; Cutler & Otake, 1994) and production (Kubozono, 1989).

Lexical representation of word prosody in production has been proposed on the basis of TOT guesses that maintain stress pattern (R. Brown & McNeill, 1966), slips that maintain everything *but* stress pattern (Cutler, 1980), and stress priming effects in picture naming (Levelt, 1993). In recognition, lexical effects in phonetic categorization can be mediated by stress (Connine, Clifton, & Cutler, 1987) and by lexical tone (Fox & Unkefer, 1985). However, the purely prosodic correlates of stress pattern in English do not play a role in prelexical processing (Cutler, 1986), although misstressed words are hard to recognize if vowel quality alters (Bond & Small, 1983; Cutler & Clifton, 1984; Slowiaczek, 1990).

B. The Architecture of the System

The evidence on overlap between the production and recognition systems is inconclusive. If there are to be shared resources, the constraints of the two processes entail that the sharing must be at a central level; however, while the evidence outlined above is compatible with a shared-resource account, it also does not rule out separation of the two systems. There is clearly room for innovative research on this issue.

Similarly, no conclusive answer can as yet be given to the central issue in both recognition and production research: is the basic architecture of the processing system autonomous/modular or interactive (see Seidenberg,

Chapter 5, this volume)? Models of both types exist that can account for most existing evidence. However, there are reasons to prefer, at this point, an autonomous solution. First, a unidirectional flow of information presupposes a simpler architecture than bidirectional connections; if the explanatory power of each type of model is equivalent, then a choice can at least be made on the basis of simplicity. Second, autonomous models make clearer predictions about the sources of information accessible at each stage of processing, and hence are (at least in principle) more amenable to experimental test. Third, we have seen that many of the findings that have been regarded as favoring interactionist positions are far from robust. In production, phonological formulation is impervious to influence from semantic factors, and lexical accessibility does not strongly influence utterance formulation [in fact, in the only study that produced results apparently indicative of such influence (Bock, 1987), the significant priming effect was just 3% different from the chance prediction; in Levelt and Maassen's (1981) comparable study, an effect of similar size was not significant]. In recognition, the tasks that have been used to investigate the relationship between phonetic and lexical processing have proved to be subject to task-specific effects. In particular, the phonetic categorization task, which requires repeated responses to the same stimuli, seems unsuited to investigation of normal recognition. Of the other tasks, phonetic restoration has produced evidence that on balance favors an interactive account, while the evidence from phoneme monitoring more strongly supports an autonomous position. Likewise, the literature offers little evidence for strong determination of lexical recognition by higher-level context. Some a priori less-likely interpretations may be effectively ruled out by context; but context effects may simply be indications that integrative processes in recognition are extremely efficient. With efficient integration, does the system actually need top-down processes, which, by excluding improbable interpretations, might actually mislead?

Acknowledgments

Thanks for helpful comments on earlier versions of this text to Peter Eimas, David Fay, Pim Levelt, James McQueen, Joanne Miller, and Dennis Norris, and further thanks to Sally Butterfield, Francois Grosjean, David Pisoni, and Arthur Samuel.

References

Aitchison, J., & Straf, M. (1981). Lexical storage and retrieval: A developing skill? *Linguistics, 19,* 751–795.
Baars, B., Motley, M., & MacKay, D. G. (1975). Output editing for lexical status from artificially elicited slips of the tongue. *Journal of Verbal Learning and Verbal Behavior, 14,* 382–391.

Bard, E. G., Shillcock, R. C., & Altmann, G. T. M. (1988). The recognition of words after their acoustic offsets in spontaneous speech: Effects of subsequent context. *Perception & Psychophysics, 44,* 395–408.

Bashford, J. A., Meyers, M. D., Brubaker, B. S., & Warren, R. M. (1988). Illusory continuity of interrupted speech: Speech rate determines durational limits. *Journal of the Acoustical Society of America, 84,* 1635–1638.

Bashford, J. A., & Warren, R. M. (1987). Multiple phonemic restorations follow the rules for auditory induction. *Perception & Psychophysics, 42,* 114–121.

Bierwisch, M. (1981). Linguistics and language error. *Linguistics, 19,* 583–626.

Bierwisch, M., & Schreuder, R. (1992). From concepts to lexical items. *Cognition, 42,* 23–60.

Blank, M. A. (1980). Measuring lexical access during sentence processing. *Perception & Psychophysics, 28,* 1–8.

Blank, M. A., & Foss, D. J. (1978). Semantic facilitation and lexical access during sentence processing. *Memory & Cognition, 6,* 644–652.

Blutner, R., & Sommer, R. (1988). Sentence processing and lexical access: The influence of the focus-identifying task. *Journal of Memory and Language, 27,* 359–367.

Bock, J. K. (1982). Toward a cognitive psychology of syntax: Information processing contributions to sentence formulation. *Psychological Review, 89,* 1–47.

Bock, J. K. (1986). Meaning, sound and syntax: Lexical priming in sentence production. *Journal of Experimental Psychology: Learning, Memory, and Cognition, 12,* 575–586.

Bock, J. K. (1987). An effect of the accessibility of word forms on sentence structures. *Journal of Memory and Language, 26,* 119–137.

Bond, Z. S., & Small, L. H. (1983). Voicing, vowel and stress mispronunciations in continuous speech. *Perception & Psychophysics, 34,* 470–474.

Bradley, D. C., & Forster, K. I. (1987). A reader's view of listening. *Cognition, 25,* 103–134.

Bradley, D. C., Sánchez-Casas, R. M., & García-Albea, J. E. (1993). The status of the syllable in the perception of Spanish and English. *Language and Cognitive Processes, 8,* 197–233.

Brown, G. D. A. (1984). A frequency count of 190,000 words in the London-Lund Corpus of English Conversation. *Behavior Research Methods, Instrumentation and Computers, 16,* 502–532.

Brown, R., & McNeill, D. (1966). The "tip of the tongue" phenomenon. *Journal of Verbal Learning and Verbal Behavior, 5,* 325–337.

Brunner, H., & Pisoni, D. B. (1982). Some effects of perceptual load on spoken text comprehension. *Journal of Verbal Learning and Verbal Behavior, 21,* 186–195.

Burton, M. W., Baum, S. R., & Blumstein, S. E. (1989). Lexical effects on the phonetic categorization of speech: The role of acoustic structure. *Journal of Experimental Psychology: Human Perception and Performance, 15,* 567–575.

Butterworth, B. (1989). Lexical access in speech production. In W. D. Marslen-Wilson (Ed.), *Lexical representation and process* (pp. 108–135). Cambridge, MA: MIT Press.

Cluff, M. S., & Luce, P. A. (1990). Similarity neighborhoods of spoken two-syllable words: Retroactive effects on multiple activation. *Journal of Experimental Psychology: Human Perception and Performance, 16,* 551–563.

Cole, R. A. (1973). Listening for mispronunciations: A measure of what we hear during speech. *Perception & Psychophysics, 11,* 153–156.

Cole, R. A., & Jakimik, J. (1978). Understanding speech: How words are heard. In G. Underwood (Ed.), *Strategies of information processing* (pp. 67–116). London: Academic Press.

Cole, R. A., & Jakimik, J. (1980). How are syllables used to recognize words? *Journal of the Acoustical Society of America, 67,* 965–970.

Connine, C. M. (1987). Constraints on interactive processes in auditory word recognition: The role of sentence context. *Journal of Memory and Language, 26,* 527–538.

Connine, C. M., Blasko, D. G., & Hall, M. (1991). Effects of subsequent sentence context in auditory word recognition: Temporal and linguistic constraints. *Journal of Memory and Language, 30,* 234–250.

Connine, C. M., Blasko, D. G., & Titone, D. (1993). Do the beginnings of spoken words have a special status in auditory word recognition? *Journal of Memory and Language, 32*, 193–210.

Connine, C. M., & Clifton, C. E. (1987). Interactive use of lexical information in speech perception. *Journal of Experimental Psychology: Human Perception and Performance, 13*, 291–299.

Connine, C. M., Clifton, C. E., & Cutler, A. (1987). Lexical stress effects on phonetic categorization. *Phonetica, 44*, 133–146.

Connine, C. M., Mullenix, J., Shernoff, E., & Yelen, J. (1990). Word familiarity and frequency in visual and auditory word recognition. *Journal of Experimental Psychology: Learning, Memory, and Cognition, 16*, 1084–1096.

Connine, C. M., Titone, D., & Wang, J. (1993). Auditory word recognition: Extrinsic and intrinsic effects of word frequency. *Journal of Experimental Psychology: Learning, Memory, and Cognition, 19*, 81–94.

Cutler, A. (1980). Errors of stress and intonation. In V. A. Fromkin (Ed.), *Errors in linguistic performance: Slips of the tongue, ear, pen and hand* (pp. 67–80). New York: Academic Press.

Cutler, A. (1986). *Forbear* is a homophone: Lexical prosody does not constraint lexical access. *Language and Speech, 29*, 201–220.

Cutler, A., & Butterfield, S. (1992). Rhythmic cues to speech segmentation: Evidence from juncture misperception. *Journal of Memory and Language, 31*, 218–236.

Cutler, A., Butterfield, S., & Williams, J. N. (1987). The perceptual integrity of syllabic onsets. *Journal of Memory and Language, 26*, 406–418.

Cutler, A., & Carter, D. M. (1987). The predominance of strong initial syllables in the English vocabulary. *Computer Speech and Language, 2*, 133–142.

Cutler, A., & Clifton, C. E. (1984). The use of prosodic information in word recognition. In H. Bouma & D. G. Bouwhuis (Eds.), *Attention and performance X: Control of language processes* (pp. 183–196). Hillsdale, NJ: Erlbaum.

Cutler, A., Mehler, J., Norris, D. G., & Segui, J. (1986). The syllable's differing role in the segmentation of French and English. *Journal of Memory and Language, 25*, 385–400.

Cutler, A., Mehler, J., Norris, D. G., & Segui, J. (1987). Phoneme identification and the lexicon. *Cognitive Psychology, 19*, 141–177.

Cutler, A., & Norris, D. G. (1979). Monitoring sentence comprehension. In W. E. Cooper & E. C. T. Walker (Eds.), *Sentence processing: Psycholinguistic studies presented to Merrill Garrett* (pp. 113–134). Hillsdale, NJ: Erlbaum.

Cutler, A., & Norris, D. G. (1988). The role of strong syllables in segmentation for lexical access. *Journal of Experimental Psychology: Human Perception and Performance, 14*, 113–121.

Cutler, A., & Otake, T. (1994). Mora or phoneme? Further evidence for language-specific listening. *Journal of Memory and Language, 33*, 824–844.

Dell, G. S. (1984). Representation of serial order in speech: Evidence from the repeated phoneme effect in speech errors. *Journal of Experimental Psychology: Learning, Memory, and Cognition, 10*, 222–233.

Dell, G. S. (1986). A spreading-activation theory of retrieval in sentence production. *Psychological Review, 93*, 283–321.

Dell, G. S. (1988). The retrieval of phonological forms in production: Tests of predictions from a connectionist model. *Journal of Memory and Language, 27*, 124–142.

Dell, G. S. (1990). Effects of frequency and vocabulary type on phonological speech errors. *Language and Cognitive Processes, 5*, 313–349.

Dell, G. S., & Newman, J. E. (1980). Detecting phonemes in fluent speech. *Journal of Verbal Learning and Verbal Behavior, 19*, 609–623.

Dell, G. S., & O'Seaghdha, P. G. (1991). Mediated and convergent lexical priming in language production: A comment on Levelt et al. (1991). *Psychological Review, 98*, 604–614.

Dell, G. S., & O'Seaghdha, P. G. (1992). Stages of lexical access in language production. *Cognition, 42*, 287–314.

Dell, G. S., & Reich, P. (1981). Stages in speech production: An analysis of speech error data. *Journal of Verbal Learning and Verbal Behavior, 20,* 611–629.

Dijkstra, T., Schreuder, R., & Frauenfelder, U. H. (1989). Grapheme context effects on phonemic processing. *Language and Speech, 32,* 89–108.

Dupoux, E., & Mehler, J. (1990). Monitoring the lexicon with normal and compressed speech: Frequency effects and the prelexical code. *Journal of Memory and Language, 29,* 316–335.

Eimas, P. D., Hornstein, S. B. M., & Payton, P. (1990). Attention and the role of dual codes in phoneme monitoring. *Journal of Memory and Language, 29,* 160–180.

Eimas, P. D., & Nygaard, L. C. (1992). Contextual coherence and attention in phoneme monitoring. *Journal of Memory and Language, 31,* 375–395.

Ellis, L., Derbyshire, A. J., & Joseph, M. E. (1971). Perception of electronically gated speech. *Language and Speech, 14,* 229–240.

Elman, J. L. (1990). Representation and structure in connectionist models. In G. T. M. Altmann (Ed.), *Cognitive models of speech processing* (pp. 345–382). Cambridge, MA: MIT Press.

Elman, J. L., & McClelland, J. L. (1988). Cognitive penetration of the mechanisms of perception: Compensation for coarticulation of lexically restored phonemes. *Journal of Memory and Language, 27,* 143–165.

Elman, J. L., & Zipser, D. (1988). Learning the hidden structure of speech. *Journal of the Acoustical Society of America, 83,* 1615–1626.

Emmorey, K. D. (1989). Auditory morphological priming in the lexicon. *Language and Cognitive Processes, 4,* 73–92.

Fay, D., & Cutler, A. (1977). Malapropisms and the structure of the mental lexicon. *Linguistic Inquiry, 8,* 505–520.

Flores d'Arcais, G., & Schreuder, R. (1987). Semantic activation during object naming. *Psychological Research, 49,* 153–159.

Foss, D. J. (1969). Decision processes during sentence comprehension: Effects of lexical item difficulty and position upon decision times. *Journal of Verbal Learning and Verbal Behavior, 8,* 457–462.

Foss, D. J. (1982). A discourse on semantic priming. *Cognitive Psychology, 14,* 590–607.

Foss, D. J., & Blank, M. A. (1980). Identifying the speech codes. *Cognitive Psychology, 12,* 1–31.

Foss, D. J., & Gernsbacher, M. A. (1983). Cracking the dual code: Toward a unitary model of phonetic identification. *Journal of Verbal Learning and Verbal Behavior, 22,* 609–632.

Foss, D. J., Harwood, D., & Blank, M. A. (1980). Deciphering decoding decisions: Data and devices. In R. A. Cole (Ed.), *Perception and production of fluent speech* (pp. 165–199). Hillsdale, NJ: Erlbaum.

Foss, D. J., & Ross, J. (1983). Great expectations: Context effects during sentence processing. In G. B. Flores d'Arcais & R. J. Jarvella (Eds.), *The process of language understanding* (pp. 169–191) Chichester: Wiley.

Foss, D. J., & Swinney, D. A. (1973). On the psychological reality of the phoneme: Perception, identification and consciousness. *Journal of Verbal Learning and Verbal Behavior, 12,* 246–257.

Fox, R. A. (1984). Effect of lexical status on phonetic categorization. *Journal of Experimental Psychology: Human Perception and Performance, 10,* 526–540.

Fox, R. A., & Unkefer, J. (1985). The effect of lexical status on the perception of tone. *Journal of Chinese Linguistics, 13,* 69–90.

Frauenfelder, U. H., & Segui, J. (1989). Phoneme monitoring and lexical processing: Evidence for associative context effects. *Memory & Cognition, 17,* 134–140.

Frauenfelder, U. H., Segui, J., & Dijkstra, T. (1990). Lexical effects in phonemic processing: Facilitatory or inhibitory? *Journal of Experimental Psychology: Human Perception and Performance, 16,* 77–91.

Fromkin, V. A. (1971). The non-anomalous nature of anomalous utterances. *Language, 47,* 27–52.

Fromkin, V. A. (1973). *Speech errors as linguistic evidence.* The Hague: Mouton.

Fujimura, O., & Lovins, J. B. (1978). Syllables as concatenative phonetic units. In A. Bell & J. B. Hooper (Eds.), *Syllables and segments* (pp. 107–120). Amsterdam: North-Holland.

Ganong, W. F. (1980). Phonetic categorization in auditory word perception. *Journal of Experimental Psychology: Human Perception and Performance, 6,* 110–125.

Garrett, M. F. (1975). The analysis of sentence production. In G. H. Bower (Ed.), *The psychology of learning and motivation* (Vol. 9, pp. 133–177). New York: Academic Press.

Garrett, M. F. (1988). Processes in language production. In F. J. Newmeyer (Ed.), *The Cambridge Linguistic Survey: Vol. 3. Psychological and biological aspects of language* (pp. 69–96) Cambridge, UK: Cambridge University Press.

Glaser, W. R. (1992). Picture naming. *Cognition, 42,* 61–105.

Goldinger, S. D., Luce, P. A., & Pisoni, D. B. (1989). Priming lexical neighbours of spoken words: Effects of competition and inhibition. *Journal of Memory and Language, 28,* 501–518.

Goldinger, S. D., Luce, P. A., Pisoni, D. B., & Marcario, J. K. (1992). Form-based priming in spoken word recognition: The roles of competition and bias. *Journal of Experimental Psychology: Learning, Memory, and Cognition, 18,* 1211–1238.

Goodman, J. C., & Huttenlocher, J. (1988). Do we know how people identify spoken words? *Journal of Memory and Language, 27,* 684–698.

Gordon, P. C. (1988). Induction of rate-dependent processing by coarse-grained aspects of speech. *Perception & Psychophysics, 43,* 137–146.

Gordon, P. C., Eberhardt, J. L., & Rueckl, J. G. (1993). Attentional modulation of the phonetic significance of acoustic cues. *Cognitive Psychology, 25,* 1–42.

Gow, D. W., & Gordon, P. C. (1995). Lexical and prelexical influences on word segmentation: Evidence from priming. *Journal of Experimental Psychology: Human Perception and Performance, 21.*

Greenspan, S. L. (1986). Semantic flexibility and referential specificity of concrete nouns. *Journal of Memory and Language, 25,* 539–557.

Grosjean, F. (1980). Spoken word recognition processes and the gating paradigm. *Perception & Psychophysics, 28,* 267–283.

Grosjean, F. (1985). The recognition of words after their acoustic offset: Evidence and implications. *Perception & Psychophysics, 38,* 299–310.

Grosjean, F., & Gee, J. (1987). Prosodic structure and spoken word recognition. *Cognition, 25,* 135–155.

Grosjean, F., & Itzler, J. (1984). Can semantic constraint reduce the role of word frequency during spoken-word recognition? *Bulletin of the Psychonomic Society, 22,* 180–182.

Harley, T. A. (1984). A critique of top-down independent levels of speech production: Evidence from non-plan-internal speech errors. *Cognitive Science, 8,* 191–219.

Healy, A., & Cutting, J. (1976). Units of speech perception: Phoneme and syllable. *Journal of Verbal Learning and Verbal Behavior, 15,* 73–83.

Howes, D. (1957). On the relation between the intelligibility and frequency of occurrence of English words. *Journal of the Acoustical Society of America, 29,* 296–305.

Howes, D. (1966). A word count of spoken English. *Journal of Verbal Learning and Verbal Behavior, 5,* 572–604.

Huttenlocher, J., & Kubicek, L. F. (1983). The source of relatedness effects on naming latency. *Journal of Experimental Psychology: Learning, Memory, and Cognition, 9,* 486–496.

Jarvella, R. J., & Meijers, G. (1983). Recognizing morphemes in spoken words: Some evidence for a stem-organized mental lexicon. In G. B. Flores d'Arcais & R. J. Jarvella (Eds.), *The process of language understanding* (pp. 81–112). Chichester: Wiley.

Jescheniak, J.-D., & Levelt, W. J. M. (1994). Word frequency effects in speech production:

Retrieval of syntactic information and of phonological form. *Journal of Experimental Psychology: Learning, Memory and Cognition, 20,* 824–843.

Katz, L., Boyce, S., Goldstein, L., & Lukatela, G. (1987). Grammatical information effects in auditory word recognition. *Cognition, 25,* 235–263.

Kempen, G., & Huijbers, P. (1983). The lexicalisation process in sentence production and naming: Indirect election of words. *Cognition, 14,* 185–209.

Kempley, S. T., & Morton, J. (1982). The effects of priming with regularly and irregularly related words in auditory word recognition. *British Journal of Psychology, 73,* 441–454.

Klatt, D. H. (1979). Speech perception: A model of acoustic-phonetic analysis and lexical access. *Journal of Phonetics, 7,* 279–312.

Klatt, D. H. (1989). Review of selected models of speech perception. In W. D. Marslen-Wilson (Ed.), *Lexical representation and process* (pp. 169–226). Cambridge, MA: MIT Press.

Kohn, S. E., Wingfield, A., Menn, L., Goodglass, H., Gleason, J. B., & Hyde, M. (1987). Lexical retrieval: The tip-of-the-tongue phenomenon. *Applied Psycholinguistics, 8,* 245–266.

Kolinsky, R., Morais, J., & Cluytens, M. (1995). Intermediate representations in spoken word recognition: Evidence from word illusions. *Journal of Memory and Language, 34,* 19–40.

Kubozono, H. (1989). The mora and syllable structure in Japanese: Evidence from speech errors. *Language & Speech, 32,* 249–278.

Lackner, J. R., & Garrett, M. F. (1972). Resolving ambiguity: Effects of biasing context in the unattended ear. *Cognition, 1,* 359–372.

Ladefoged, P., & Broadbent, D. E. (1960). Perception of sequence in auditory events. *Quarterly Journal of Experimental Psychology, 12,* 162–170.

Lahiri, A., & Marslen-Wilson, W. D. (1991). The mental representation of lexical form: A phonological approach to the recognition lexicon. *Cognition, 38,* 245–294.

Levelt, W. J. M. (1989). *Speaking.* Cambridge, MA: MIT Press.

Levelt, W. J. M. (1992). Accessing words in speech production: Stages, processes and representations. *Cognition, 42,* 1–22.

Levelt, W. J. M. (1993). Timing in speech production with special reference to word form encoding. *Annals of the New York Academy of Sciences, 682,* 283–295.

Levelt, W. J. M., & Maassen, B. (1981). Lexical search and order of mention in sentence production. In W. Klein & W. J. M. Levelt (Eds.), *Crossing the boundaries in linguistics: Studies presented to Manfred Bierwisch* (pp. 221–252). Dordrecht: Reidel.

Levelt, W. J. M., Schriefers, H., Vorberg, D., Meyer, A. S., Pechmann, T., & Havinga, J. (1991). The time course of lexical access in speech production: A study of picture naming. *Psychological Review, 98,* 122–142.

Levitt, A. G., & Healy, A. F. (1985). The role of phoneme frequency, similarity and availability in the experimental elicitation of speech errors. *Journal of Memory and Language, 24,* 717–733.

Lucas, M. M. (1987). Frequency effects on the processing of ambiguous words in sentence contexts. *Language & Speech, 30,* 25–46.

Luce, P. A. (1986). A computational analysis of uniqueness points in auditory word recognition. *Perception & Psychophysics, 39,* 155–158.

Luce, P. A., Pisoni, D. B., & Goldinger, S. D. (1990). Similarity neighborhoods of spoken words. In G. T. M. Altmann (Ed.), *Cognitive models of speech processing* (pp. 122–147). Cambridge MA: MIT Press.

Lupker, S. J. (1979). The semantic nature of competition in the picture-word interference task. *Canadian Journal of Psychology, 36,* 485–495.

MacKay, D. M. (1972). The structure of words and syllables: Evidence from errors in speech. *Cognitive Psychology, 3,* 210–227.

MacKay, D. M. (1976). On the retrieval and lexical structure of verbs. *Journal of Verbal Learning and Verbal Behavior, 15,* 169–182.

MacKay, D. M. (1987). *The organization of perception and action.* New York: Springer.

Mann, V. A., & Repp, B. H. (1981). Influence of preceding fricative on stop consonant perception. *Journal of the Acoustical Society of America, 69,* 548–558.

Marcus, S. M. (1981). ERIS—Context-sensitive coding in speech perception. *Journal of Phonetics, 9,* 197–220.

Marcus, S. M., & Frauenfelder, U. H. (1985). Word recognition—uniqueness or deviation? A theoretical note. *Language and Cognitive Processes, 1,* 163–169.

Marslen-Wilson, W. D. (1975). Sentence perception as an interactive parallel process. *Science, 189,* 226–228.

Marslen-Wilson, W. D. (1980). Speech understanding as a psychological process. In J. D. Simon (Ed.), *Spoken language generation and recognition* (pp. 39–67). Dordrecht: Reidel.

Marslen-Wilson, W. D. (1984). Function and process in spoken word recognition. In H. Bouma & D. G. Bouwhuis (Eds.), *Attention and performance X: Control of language processes* (pp. 125–150). Hillsdale, NJ: Erlbaum.

Marslen-Wilson, W. D. (1985). Speech shadowing and speech comprehension. *Speech Communication, 4,* 55–73.

Marslen-Wilson, W. D. (1987). Parallel processing in spoken word recognition. *Cognition, 25,* 71–102.

Marslen-Wilson, W. D. (1990). Activation, competition and frequency in lexical access. In G. T. M. Altmann (Ed.), *Cognitive models of speech processing* (pp. 148–172). Cambridge MA: MIT Press.

Marslen-Wilson, W. D., Brown, C. M., & Tyler, L. K. (1988). Lexical representations in spoken language comprehension. *Language and Cognitive Processes, 3,* 1–16.

Marslen-Wilson, W. D., & Tyler, L. K. (1980). The temporal structure of spoken language understanding. *Cognition, 8,* 1–71.

Marslen-Wilson, W. D., & Welsh, A. (1978). Processing interactions and lexical access during word recognition in continuous speech. *Cognitive Psychology, 10,* 29–63.

Marslen-Wilson, W. D., & Zwitserlood, P. (1989). Accessing spoken words: The importance of word onsets. *Journal of Experimental Psychology: Human Perception and Performance, 15,* 576–585.

Massaro, D. W. (1987). *Speech perception by ear and eye: A paradigm for psychological inquiry.* Hillsdale NJ: Erlbaum.

Massaro, D. W. (1989). Testing between the TRACE model and the Fuzzy Logical Model of Speech Perception. *Cognitive Psychology, 21,* 398–421.

Massaro, D. W., & Cohen, M. M. (1983). Phonological context in speech perception. *Perception & Psychophysics, 34,* 338–348.

McClelland, J. L., & Elman, J. L. (1986a). Exploiting lawful variability in the speech wave. In J. S. Perkell & D. H. Klatt (Eds.), *Invariance and variability in speech processes* (pp. 360–385). Hillsdale, NJ: Erlbaum.

McClelland, J. L., & Elman, J. L. (1986b). The TRACE model of speech perception. *Cognitive Psychology, 18,* 1–86.

McNeill, D., & Lindig, K. (1973). The perceptual reality of phonemes, syllables, words, and sentences. *Journal of Verbal Learning and Verbal Behavior, 12,* 431–461.

McQueen, J. M. (1991). The influence of the lexicon on phonetic categorisation: Stimulus quality in word-final ambiguity. *Journal of Experimental Psychology: Human Perception and Performance, 17,* 433–443.

McQueen, J. M. (1993). Rhyme decisions to spoken words and nonwords. *Memory & Cognition, 21,* 210–222.

McQueen, J. M., Norris, D. G., & Cutler, A. (1994). Competition in spoken word recognition: Spotting words in other words. *Journal of Experimental Psychology: Learning, Memory and Cognition, 20,* 621–638.

Mehler, J., Dommergues, J.-Y., Frauenfelder, U., & Segui, J. (1981). The syllable's role in speech segmentation. *Journal of Verbal Learning and Verbal Behavior, 20,* 298–305.

Mehler, J., & Segui, J. (1987). English and French speech processing. In M. E. H. Schouten (Ed.), *The psychophysics of speech perception* (pp. 405–418). Dordrecht: Martinus Nijhoff.

Meyer, A. S. (1990). The time course of phonological encoding in language production: The encoding of successive syllables of a word. *Journal of Memory and Language, 29,* 524–545.

Meyer, A. S., & Schriefers, H. (1991). Phonological facilitation in picture-word interference experiments: Effects of stimulus onset asynchrony and types of interfering stimuli. *Journal of Experimental Psychology: Learning, Memory and Cognition, 17,* 1146–1160.

Milberg, W., Blumstein, S., & Dworetzky, B. (1988). Phonological factors in lexical access: Evidence from an auditory lexical decision task. *Bulletin of the Psychonomic Society, 26,* 305–308.

Miller, J. L. (1981a). Phonetic perception: Evidence for context-dependent and context-independent processing. *Journal of the Acoustical Society of America, 69,* 822–831.

Miller, J. L. (1981b). Some effects of speaking rate on phonetic perception. *Phonetica, 38,* 159–180.

Miller, J. L., & Dexter, E. R. (1988). Effects of speaking rate and lexical status on phonetic perception. *Journal of Experimental Psychology: Human Perception and Performance, 14,* 369–378.

Miller, J. L., Green, K., & Schermer, T. M. (1984). A distinction between the effects of sentential speaking rate and semantic congruity on word identification. *Perception & Psychophysics, 36,* 329–337.

Miller, J. L., & Liberman, A. L. (1979). Some effects of later-occurring information on the perception of stop consonant and semivowel. *Perception & Psychophysics, 25,* 457–465.

Mills, C. B. (1980a). Effects of context on reaction time to phonemes. *Journal of Verbal Learning and Verbal Behavior, 19,* 75–83.

Mills, C. B. (1980b). Effects of the match between listener expectancies and coarticulatory cues on the perception of speech. *Journal of Experimental Psychology: Human Perception and Performance, 6,* 528–535.

Morton, J. (1969). Interaction of information in word perception. *Psychological Review, 76,* 165–178.

Morton, J., & Long, J. (1976). Effect of word transitional probability on phoneme identification. *Journal of Verbal Learning and Verbal Behavior, 15,* 43–51.

Morton, J., & Patterson, K. E. (1980). A new attempt at an interpretation, or an attempt at a new interpretation. In M. Coltheart, K. E. Patterson, & J. C. Marshall (Eds.), *Deep dyslexia* (pp. 91–118). London: Routledge & Kegan Paul.

Newman, J. E., & Dell, G. S. (1978). The phonological nature of phoneme monitoring: A critique of some ambiguity studies. *Journal of Verbal Learning and Verbal Behavior, 17,* 359–374.

Nooteboom, S. G. (1981). Lexical retrieval from fragments of spoken words: Beginnings versus endings. *Journal of Phonetics, 9,* 407–424.

Nooteboom, S. G., & van der Vlugt, M. J. (1988). A search for a word-beginning superiority effect. *Journal of the Acoustical Society of America, 84,* 2018–2032.

Norris, D. G. (1982). Autonomous processes in comprehension: A reply to Marslen-Wilson and Tyler. *Cognition, 11,* 97–101.

Norris, D. G. (1986). Word recognition: Context effects without priming. *Cognition, 22,* 93–136.

Norris, D. G. (1990). A dynamic-net model of human speech recognition. In G. T. M. Altmann (Ed.), *Cognitive models of speech processing* (pp. 87–104). Cambridge MA: MIT Press.

Norris, D. G. (1991). Rewiring lexical networks on the fly. *Proceedings of EUROSPEECH 91, Genoa, 1,* 117–120.

Norris, D. G. (1994). SHORTLIST: A connectionist model of continuous speech recognition. *Cognition, 52,* 189–234.

Norris, D. G., McQueen, J. M., & Cutler, A. (1995). Competition and segmentation in spoken word recognition. *Journal of Experimental Psychology: Learning, Memory and Cognition, 21.*

Oden, G. C., & Spira, J. L. (1983). Influence of context on the activation and selection of ambiguous word senses. *Quarterly Journal of Experimental Psychology, 35,* 51–64.

Oldfield, R. C. (1966). Things, words, and the brain. *Quarterly Journal of Experimental Psychology, 18,* 340–353.

Oldfield, R. C., & Wingfield, A. (1964). The time it takes to name an object. *Nature (London), 202,* 1031–1032.

Oldfield, R. C., & Wingfield, A. (1965). Response latencies in naming objects. *Quarterly Journal of Experimental Psychology, 17,* 273–281.

Onifer, W., & Swinney, D. A. (1981). Accessing lexical ambiguities during sentence comprehension: Effects of frequency-of-meaning and contextual bias. *Journal of Verbal Learning and Verbal Behavior, 17,* 225–236.

Otake, T., Hatano, G., Cutler, A., & Mehler, J. (1993). Mora or syllable? Speech segmentation in Japanese. *Journal of Memory and Language, 32,* 358–378.

Pallier, C., Sebastian-Gallés, N., Felguera, T., Christophe, A., & Mehler, J. (1993). Attentional allocation within the syllabic structure of spoken words. *Journal of Memory and Language, 32,* 373–389.

Pisoni, D. B., & Luce, P. A. (1987). Acoustic-phonetic representations in word recognition. *Cognition, 25,* 21–52.

Pitt, M. A., & Samuel, A. G. (1990). Attentional allocation during speech perception: How fine is the focus? *Journal of Memory and Language, 29,* 611–632.

Pitt, M. A., & Samuel, A. G. (1993). An empirical and meta-analytic evaluation of the phoneme identification task. *Journal of Experimental Psychology: Human Perception and Performance, 19,* 699–725.

Repp, B. H., & Frost, R. (1988). Detectability of words and nonwords in two kinds of noise. *Journal of the Acoustical Society of America, 84,* 1929–1932.

Roelofs, A. (1992). A spreading-activation theory of lemma retrieval in speaking. *Cognition, 42,* 107–142.

Roelofs, A. (1993). Testing a non-decompositional theory of lemma retrieval in speaking: Retrieval of verbs. *Cognition, 47,* 59–87.

Rubin, D. C. (1975). Within-word structure in the tip-of-the-tongue phenomenon. *Journal of Verbal Learning and Verbal Behavior, 14,* 392–397.

Rubin, P., Turvey, M. T., & van Gelder, P. (1976). Initial phonemes are detected faster in spoken words than in non-words. *Perception & Psychophysics, 19,* 394–398.

Salasoo, A., & Pisoni, D. B. (1985). Interaction of knowledge sources in spoken word identification. *Journal of Memory and Language, 24,* 210–231.

Samuel, A. G. (1981a). Phonemic restoration: Insights from a new methodology. *Journal of Experimental Psychology: General, 110,* 474–494.

Samuel, A. G. (1981b). The role of bottom-up confirmation in the phonemic restoration illusion. *Journal of Experimental Psychology: Human Perception and Performance 7,* 1124–1131.

Samuel, A. G. (1987). Lexical uniqueness effects on phonemic restoration. *Journal of Memory and Language, 26,* 36–56.

Samuel, A. G. (1989). Insights from a failure of selective adaptation: Syllable-initial and syllable-final consonants are different. *Perception & Psychophysics, 45,* 485–493.

Samuel, A. G. (1991). A further examination of attentional effects in the phonemic restoration illusion. *Quarterly Journal of Experimental Psychology, 43A,* 679–699.

Samuel, A. G., & Ressler, W. H. (1986). Attention within auditory word perception: Insights from the phoneme restoration illusion. *Journal of Experimental Psychology: Human Perception and Performance, 12,* 70–79.

Savin, H. B. (1963). Word-frequency effect and errors in the perception of speech. *Journal of the Acoustical Society of America, 35,* 200–206.

Schriefers, H., Meyer, A. S., & Levelt, W. J. M. (1990). Exploring the time course of lexical access in production: Picture-word interference studies. *Journal of Memory and Language, 29,* 86–102.

Schriefers, H., Zwitserlood, P., & Roelofs, A. (1991). The identification of morphologically complex spoken words: Continuous processing or decomposition. *Journal of Memory and Language, 30,* 26–47.

Sebastian-Gallés, N., Dupoux, E., Segui, J., & Mehler, J. (1992). Contrasting syllabic effects in Catalan and Spanish. *Journal of Memory and Language, 31,* 18–32.

Segui, J., & Frauenfelder, U. H. (1986). The effect of lexical constraints upon speech perception. In F. Klix & H. Hagendorf (Eds.), *Human memory and cognitive abilities* (pp. 795–808). Amsterdam: North-Holland.

Segui, J., Frauenfelder, U. H., & Mehler, J. (1981). Phoneme monitoring, syllable monitoring and lexical access. *British Journal of Psychology, 72,* 471–477.

Seidenberg, M. S., & Tanenhaus, M. K. (1979). Orthographic effects on rhyme monitoring. *Journal of Experimental Psychology: Human Learning and Memory, 5,* 546–554.

Seidenberg, M. S., Tanenhaus, M. K., Leiman, J. M., & Bienkowski, M. (1982). Automatic access of the meanings of ambiguous words in context: Some limitations of knowledge-based processing. *Cognitive Psychology, 14,* 489–537.

Shallice, T., McLeod, P., & Lewis, K. (1985). Isolating cognitive modules with the dual-task paradigm: Are speech perception and production separate processes? *Quarterly Journal of Experimental Psychology, 37A,* 507–532.

Shattuck-Hufnagel, S. (1979). Speech errors as evidence for a serial-ordering mechanism in sentence production. In W. E. Cooper & E. C. T. Walker (Eds.), *Sentence processing: Psycholinguistic studies presented to Merrill Garrett* (pp. 295–342). Hillsdale, NJ: Erlbaum.

Shattuck-Hufnagel, S. (1983). Sublexical units and suprasegmental structure in speech production planning. In P. F. MacNeilage (Ed.), *The production of speech* (pp. 109–136). New York: Springer-Verlag.

Shattuck-Hufnagel, S. (1986). The representation of phonological information during speech production planning: Evidence from vowel errors in spontaneous speech. *Phonology Yearbook, 3,* 117–149.

Shattuck-Hufnagel, S. (1992). The role of word structure in segmental serial ordering. *Cognition, 42,* 213–259.

Shattuck-Hufnagel, S., & Klatt, D. H. (1979). The limited use of distinctive features and markedness in speech production: Evidence from speech error data. *Journal of Verbal Learning and Verbal Behavior, 18,* 41–55.

Shillcock, R. C. (1990). Lexical hypotheses in continuous speech. In G. T. M. Altmann (Ed.), *Cognitive models of speech processing* (pp. 24–49). Cambridge MA: MIT Press.

Slowiaczek, L. M. (1990). Effects of lexical stress in auditory word recognition. *Language & Speech, 33,* 47–68.

Slowiaczek, L. M., Nusbaum, H. C., & Pisoni, D. B. (1987). Acoustic-phonetic priming in auditory word recognition. *Journal of Experimental Psychology: Learning, Memory and Cognition, 13,* 64–75.

Stemberger, J. P. (1985). An interactive activation model of language production. In A. W. Ellis (Ed.), *Progress in the psychology of language* (Vol. 1, pp. 143–186). London: Erlbaum.

Stemberger, J. P. (1990). Wordshape errors in language production. *Cognition, 35,* 123–157.

Stemberger, J. P. (1991). Apparent anti-frequency effects in language production: The addition bias and phonological underspecification. *Journal of Memory and Language, 30,* 161–185.

Stemberger, J. P., Elman, J. L., & Haden, P. (1985). Interference between phonemes during phoneme monitoring: Evidence for an interactive activation model of speech perception. *Journal of Experimental Psychology: Human Perception and Performance, 11,* 475–489.

Stemberger, J. P., & Lewis, M. (1986). Reduplication in Ewe: Morphological accommodation to phonological errors. *Phonology Yearbook, 3,* 151–160.

Stemberger, J. P., & MacWhinney, B. (1986a). Form-oriented inflectional errors in language processing. *Cognitive Psychology, 18,* 329–354.

Stemberger, J. P., & MacWhinney, B. (1986b). Frequency and the lexical storage of regularly inflected forms. *Memory & Cognition, 14,* 17–26.

Sternberg, S., Knoll, R. L., Monsell, S., & Wright, C. E. (1988). Motor programs and hierarchical organization in the control of rapid speech. *Phonetica, 45,* 175–197.

Stevens, K. N. (1986). Models of phonetic recognition II: A feature-based model of speech recognition. In P. Mermelstein (Ed.), *Proceedings of the Montreal Satellite Symposium on Speech Recognition, Twelfth International Congress on Acoustics* (pp. 67–68). Montréal.

Stevens, K. N., Manuel, S. Y., Shattuck-Hufnagel, S., & Liu, S. (1992). Implementation of a model for lexical access based on features. *Proceedings of the Second International Conference on Spoken Language Processing, Banff, 1,* 499–502.

Swinney, D. A. (1979). Lexical access during sentence comprehension: (Re)consideration of context effects. *Journal of Verbal Learning and Verbal Behavior, 18,* 645–659.

Swinney, D. A., Onifer, W., Prather, P., & Hirschkowitz, M. (1979). Semantic facilitation across sensory modalities in the processing of individual words and sentences. *Memory & Cognition, 7,* 159–165.

Swinney, D. A., & Prather, P. (1980). Phonemic identification in a phoneme monitoring experiment: The variable role of uncertainty about vowel contexts. *Perception & Psychophysics, 27,* 104–110.

Tabossi, P. (1988a). Accessing lexical ambiguity in different types of sentential contexts. *Journal of Memory and Language, 27,* 324–340.

Tabossi, P. (1988b). Effects of context on the immediate interpretation of unambiguous nouns. *Journal of Experimental Psychology: Learning, Memory, and Cognition, 14,* 153–162.

Tabossi, P., Burani, C., & Scott, D. R. (1995). Word identification in fluent speech. *Journal of Memory and Language, 34.*

Tabossi, P., Colombo, L., & Job, R. (1987). Accessing lexical ambiguity: Effects of context and dominance. *Psychological Research, 49,* 161–167.

Taft, M. (1986). Lexical access codes in visual and auditory word recognition. *Language and Cognitive Processes, 1,* 297–308.

Taft, M. (1988). A morphological-decomposition model of lexical representation. *Linguistics, 26,* 657–667.

Taft, M., & Hambly, G. (1986). Exploring the cohort model of spoken word recognition. *Cognition, 22,* 259–282.

Taft, M., Hambly, G., & Kinoshita, S. (1986). Visual and auditory recognition of prefixed words. *Quarterly Journal of Experimental Psychology, 38A,* 357–366.

Tanenhaus, M. K., & Donnenwerth-Nolan, S. (1984). Syntactic context and lexical access. *Quarterly Journal of Experimental Psychology, 36A,* 649–661.

Tanenhaus, M. K., Leiman, J. M., & Seidenberg, M. S. (1979). Evidence for multiple stages in the processing of ambiguous words in syntactic contexts. *Journal of Verbal Learning and Verbal Behavior, 18,* 427–440.

Treiman, R. (1983). The structure of spoken syllables: Evidence from novel word games. *Cognition, 15,* 49–74.

Treiman, R. (1986). The division between onsets and rimes in English syllables. *Journal of Memory and Language, 25,* 476–491.

Tyler, L. K. (1984). The structure of the initial cohort: Evidence from gating. *Perception & Psychophysics, 36,* 417–427.

Tyler, L. K., Marslen-Wilson, W. D., Rentoul, J., & Hanney, P. (1988). Continuous and discontinuous access in spoken word recognition: The role of derivational prefixes. *Journal of Memory and Language, 27*, 368–381.

Tyler, L. K., & Wessels, J. (1983). Quantifying contextual contributions to word recognition processes. *Perception & Psychophysics, 34*, 409–420.

Vroomen, J., & de Gelder, B. (1995). Metrical segmentation and lexical inhibition in spoken word recognition. *Journal of Experimental Psychology: Human Perception and Performance, 21*.

Warren, R. M. (1970). Perceptual restoration of missing speech sounds. *Science, 167*, 392–393.

Whalen, D. H. (1984). Subcategorical mismatches slow phonetic judgments. *Perception & Psychophysics, 35*, 49–64.

Whalen, D. H. (1991). Subcategorical phonetic mismatches and lexical access. *Perception & Psychophysics, 50*, 351–360.

Whitney, P., McKay, T., Kellas, G., & Emerson, W. A. (1985). Semantic activation of noun concepts in context. *Journal of Experimental Psychology: Learning, Memory, and Cognition, 11*, 126–135.

Williams, J. N. (1988). Constraints upon semantic activation during sentence comprehension. *Language and Cognitive Processes, 3*, 165–206.

Wingfield, A. (1968). Effects of frequency on identification and naming of objects. *American Journal of Psychology, 81*, 226–234.

Zwitserlood, P. (1989). The locus of the effects of sentential-semantic context in spoken-word processing. *Cognition, 32*, 25–64.

Zwitserlood, P., Schriefers, H., Lahiri, A., & van Donselaar, W. (1993). The role of syllables in the perception of spoken Dutch. *Journal of Experimental Psychology: Learning, Memory and Cognition, 19*, 260–271.

CHAPTER 5

Visual Word Recognition: An Overview

Mark S. Seidenberg

The principal goal of visual word recognition research is to understand a process that is one of the basic components of reading, itself one of the remarkable expressions of human intelligence. This chapter provides an overview of current research in this area, focusing on issues concerning the types of processing mechanisms and knowledge representations that are involved. Granting that reading is an interesting skill to study, why focus on the process of word recognition in particular? Reading principally differs from other forms of language comprehension with respect to the medium in which processing occurs. Word recognition is the aspect of reading for which the use of the visual perceptual channel has the largest impact on the comprehension process. Whereas recognizing and pronouncing letter patterns are specific to this medium, most of the other capacities that are utilized in understanding a text are also used in comprehending spoken language. Thus, it is within the domain of word recognition that we find most of what is specific to reading comprehension rather than a reflection of more general linguistic factors, including the bases of reading-specific deficits and individual differences.[1]

Aside from helping us to understand how people read, word recognition research has provided insight into broader issues concerning the nature of human perceptual and cognitive capacities. Visual word recognition exists only because of the invention of writing systems, a relatively recently development in the span of human history. Reading exploits perceptual and cognitive capacities that did not evolve specifically for this function and provides an interesting domain in which to explore them.

The structure of the chapter is as follows. In the first section I discuss the theories of word recognition that have shaped research in the area. This material provides a framework for the discussion of specific topics in the sections that follow. The discussions of these topics are organized around a central issue that I term "division of labor." The main questions that have been the focus of word recognition research—how people pronounce words and nonwords, the effects of brain injury on performance, the role of phonological and morphological information in word recognition, the effects of differences among orthographies, the use of different decoding strategies, and the role of contextual information—turn out to be different realizations of this issue.

I. MODELS AND THEORIES IN WORD RECOGNITION RESEARCH

Word recognition research has been driven by various theoretical models that have been proposed over the years. The conception of "model" that has prevailed in this area is roughly comparable to Chomsky's (1965) notion of a descriptive theory: a model is a theoretical statement that rationalizes a set of phenomena and generates testable predictions (see Seidenberg, 1993, for discussion). These models have varied greatly in scope and detail. For example, there are models of the organization of the lexicon and the processing of words in different modalities, models of specific aspects of word processing such as frequency effects, and models of word processing tasks such as lexical decision. The goal of most models is to characterize what Coltheart (1987) and Caramazza (1984) term the "functional architecture" of the lexical processing system. In practice this involves building flow-chart style models that specify components of the system and transitions between them. One such model, the classic version of the dual-route model that provided the focus for the Patterson, Marshall, and Coltheart (1985) volume, is presented in Figure 1. These models have tended to be broad in scope but lacking specificity with regard to knowledge representations and processing mechanisms. Flow charts were originally used to represent the structure of implemented computer programs; the functional architecture approach adopted some of these diagraming conventions but not the underlying computer programs. This is a bit like having the table of contents of an unwritten book.

More recently there have been attempts to implement components of the lexical system as computer simulation models (see, e.g., Hinton & Shallice,

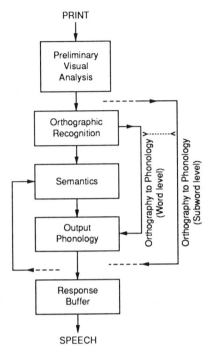

FIGURE 1   The version of the dual-route model from Patterson et al. (1985). Reprinted by permission of Lawrence Erlbaum Associates Ltd., Hove, UK.

1991; Kawamoto, 1986, 1993; Plaut & Shallice, 1993; Seidenberg & McClelland, 1989). These computational models tend to be narrower in scope than the kind of model illustrated in Figure 1 insofar as they deal with only parts of the word recognition process and apply to limited vocabularies, but they are acutely detailed. The differences in style and goals embodied by the functional and computational approaches lead to different problems in trying to assess them. The generality of claims pitched at the level of the functional architecture (e.g., "access the word's entry in the output phonological lexicon") makes them difficult to refute. Computational models, in contrast, are perhaps too easy to refute because simplifications are invariably introduced in the service of achieving the specificity that comes with implementation. Different criteria tend to be used in assessing the two types of models because they afford analyses and generate predictions at different levels of detail. For discussion of the merits and defects of these approaches, see Seidenberg (1988, 1993) and McCloskey (1991). In the remainder of this article I use the term "model" in the broader sense that encompasses both computational and functional architecture approaches, in keeping with the way it has been used in the field. However, trying to compare the two types of models is often like comparing the proverbial apples and oranges, although both are recognizably fruit.

A. Lexical Access Models versus Connectionist Models

The differences between computational and functional architecture-style models discussed above concern model-building methodology. There is also an important theoretical division between models that are based on the metaphor of a dictionarylike mental lexicon (e.g., Allport & Funnell, 1981; Coltheart, Curtis, Atkins, & Haller, 1993; Forster, 1976; Glushko, 1979) and those that are not (e.g., Seidenberg & McClelland, 1989; Plaut, McClelland, Seidenberg, & Patterson, in press). In the lexicon models, the theoretical constructs that are used in explaining specific phenomena are extensions of this central metaphor. Thus, the mental lexicon consists of "entries" corresponding to individual words, which are "searched." Recognizing a word involves successfully "accessing" its entry in this mental dictionary. The entry can be accessed by different "routes" or "access procedures." The kinds of research questions that follow from this approach have included: How is the dictionary organized (e.g., are there separate input and output representations)? What factors influence the latency of lexical access (e.g., frequency, phonological regularity, orthographic depth)? How many distinct word recognition routines are there? Is lexical access autonomous because the mental lexicon is an encapsulated module (Fodor, 1983), or is it influenced by contextual information? What kinds of information become available once lexical access is achieved and how is this information integrated with the preceding context?

The metaphor of a dictionarylike mental lexicon with entries that are accessed in recognition has dominated the field (see Cutler, Chapter 4, this volume). It has proved useful in understanding basic phenomena, it has provided a useful vocabulary for talking about these phenomena, and it is compatible with conscious intuitions about the nature of lexical knowledge. However, several phenomena that were discovered within the lexical access paradigm indicate the need for an alternative to it. For example, considerable research suggested that determining the meaning of a word in context is not like looking up a definition stored in a dictionary entry. Rather, the semantic features that are computed vary in contextually dependent ways (e.g., Anderson & Ortony, 1975; Barsalou, 1987; Merrill, Sperber, & MacCauley, 1981; Schwanenflugel & Shoben, 1985; Tabossi, 1988b). Thus, the fact that pianos are heavy might be activated in a furniture-moving scenario, but not in a context about a concert pianist (Barclay, Bransford, Franks, McCarrell, & Nitsch, 1974); the fact that cats have fur in a context about petting but the fact that cats have claws in a context about scratching (Merrill et al., 1981). Phenomena such as these seem to demand a different metaphor than that of "accessing" discrete lexical entries (Balota, 1990; Seidenberg, 1990).

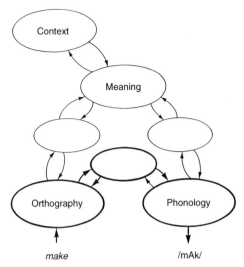

FIGURE 2   Seidenberg and McClelland's (1989) general framework. The part that was implemented is in bold outline. Copyright 1989 by the American Psychological Association. Reprinted by permission.

The distributed representations devised by Hinton (1981, 1986; McClelland, & Rumelhart, 1986) and others are compatible with these kinds of phenomena. They allow entities such as word meanings (or spellings, or pronunciations) to be encoded as patterns of activation over units encoding featural primitives. The exact pattern that is computed can vary depending on the availability of contextual information. In contrast to the lexical access models, there are no units dedicated to representing individual words; rather, the units represent sublexical features (graphemes, phonemes, sememes) each of which participates in many different words. Models such as the one illustrated in Figure 2 (from Seidenberg & McClelland, 1989) address issues in word recognition using distributed representations and other basic connectionist principles.[2]

According to the distributed view, patterns are computed over time rather than accessed at a discrete latency. Thus, there is no "magic moment" of lexical access (Balota, 1990); there can be partial activation of the information associated with a word (meaning, spelling, pronunciation), and the distributed patterns that are computed can vary in context-dependent ways, consistent with the phenomena noted previously. Characterizing the complex course of processing in a dynamical system becomes the central issue, not the series of steps leading to lexical access. Finally, a given pattern can develop on the basis of input from multiple sources. In reading, for example, the meaning pattern that is computed for a word might develop on the basis of input directly from orthography and from the context in which a word is perceived, and indirectly via phonology (see Figure 2). Van Orden and his colleagues describe basic properties of these parallel, interactive, "resonant" systems (Van Orden & Goldinger, 1994; Van Orden, Pennington, & Stone, 1990) that are incommensurate with the lexical access metaphor. There are useful ways to characterize the behavior of such highly interactive systems over time, but they bear little resemblance to the discrete stages and independent processing routines characteristic of earlier models. In short, the connectionist models differ from the lexical access models in terms of basic assumptions about how knowledge is represented and processed.

The two approaches also differ in terms of assumptions about where the explanations for word recognition phenomena are likely to be found. The lexical access approach attempts to explain word recognition in terms of knowledge representations and processing mechanisms that are largely specific to this domain rather than instantiating more general principles. For example, Coltheart et al. (1993) describe task-specific procedures for learning spelling–sound correspondences and applying them to generate pronunciations. In contrast, the distributed representations, learning through error correction, constraint satisfaction, and other concepts integral to the connectionist models were not created in order to explain facts about word recognition; rather they derive from a broader connectionist framework. The same concepts can therefore be used to explain phenomena in other domains. This approach is compatible with the earlier observation that reading makes use of capacities that did not evolve specifically for this task. Moreover, insofar as these concepts are independently motivated rather than domain or task specific, the connectionist approach holds out the possibility of developing an explanatory theory of the phenomena (Seidenberg, 1993). The lexical access approach is to a much greater degree an exercise in fitting models to behavioral data (see also Seidenberg, Plaut, Petersen, McClelland, & McRae, 1994).

Other aspects of the lexical access and connectionist approaches are discussed below as they bear on specific issues. This dichotomization of approaches serves to emphasize that while there are many specific models dealing with different aspects of word processing, they can be seen as instantiations of two general theoretical alternatives.

B. Division of Labor

The models illustrated in Figures 1 and 2 are alike in assuming that different types of information can be used in determining the meaning or pronunciation of a word from print. The division of labor issue concerns how the resources that are available in such systems are allocated. Division of labor may vary across words, individuals, or writing systems; it may be something that an individual can strategically alter; it may be the cause of different patterns of impairment following brain injury.

The principal lexical access-style model is the "dual-route" model introduced in a landmark paper by Marshall and Newcombe (1973), and subsequently elaborated by Coltheart (1978, 1987; Coltheart et al., 1993), Allport and Funnell (1981), and others. The dual-route model, like the Seidenberg and McClelland (1989) model, entails a general theory of word processing in reading but has been worked out in most detail with regard to the task of reading aloud. The two routes in the name originally referred to "lexical" and "nonlexical" mechanisms for pronouncing words and nonwords. The nonlexical mechanism involves the application of rules governing spelling-sound correspondences. (In Figure 1, this is the route labeled "Orthography to Phonology (Subword level)." The rules are nonlexical in the sense that they are general rather than word specific; they are "subword level" insofar as they apply to parts of words such as graphemes rather than entire words. The rules will generate correct pronunciations for rule-governed ("regular") words such as *gave* and nonwords such as *mave,* but not "exception" words such as *have.* The lexical mechanism involves pronunciations of individual words stored in memory ("Output Phonology" in Figure 1). Irregular words can be pronounced only by accessing these stored representations; nonwords can never be pronounced this way because their pronunciations are not stored; regular words can be pronounced this way, although the rules make this unnecessary. Thus, the division of labor in the dual-route model follows from the assumption that spelling-sound knowledge is encoded in terms of rules and the fact that English has minimal pairs such as *gave–have* and *leaf–deaf.* The rules cannot correctly specify both pronunciations; hence some words will have to be pronounced by looking up pronunciations stored in memory. That there are such rules is further suggested by the ability to pronounce nonwords.

Whereas for many years the dual-route model assumed a rule-based mechanism without identifying what the rules are, Coltheart et al. (1993) have recently described an algorithm for inducing grapheme–phoneme correspondence (GPC) rules. Applied to the 2897 word corpus described by Seidenberg and McClelland (1989), the algorithm induces 144 rules. The rules produce correct output for about 78% of the 2897 words in the corpus; the others are considered exceptions. The rules also generate plausible pronunciations for nonwords such as *nust, mave,* and *jinje* (see Seidenberg et al., 1994, for discussion).

Most versions of the dual-route model assume a third mechanism for pronouncing words. The lexical naming route involves accessing the pronunciations of individual words stored in memory. There are two suggestions for how this can be achieved. One involves accessing the meaning of a word from orthography and then accessing the phonological code from semantics, as in speech production. A lexical but nonsemantic pronunciation mechanism has also been proposed (e.g., Funnell, 1983; Schwartz, Saffran, & Marin, 1980), utilizing direct associations between orthographic and phonological codes for words. The evidence for this third mechanism (labelled "Orthography to Phonology-Word Level" in Figure 1) is provided by brain-injured patients who are able to read some words aloud despite severe semantic impairments but are unable to pronounce nonwords.

The division of labor issue is realized somewhat differently in the connectionist models. First, these models do not have parallel, independent processing "routes." Second, they do not utilize domain-specific types of knowledge representation such as grapheme–phoneme correspondence rules; the same types of knowledge representations (weighted connections between units) and processes (activation-based parallel constraint satisfaction) are used for all types of information. Third, a lexical code (e.g., the meaning of a word) is a pattern that builds up over time, based on input from different parts of the lexical system and from context.

Given that these models do not employ pronunciation rules, the principal factor that determined the division of labor in the dual-route model— whether a word's pronunciation is rule governed or not—does not apply. Seidenberg and McClelland's model, for example, uses a single mechanism to generate correct pronunciations for both "rule-governed" items and exceptions. Moreover, these models do not enforce a strict differentiation between "lexical" and nonlexical types of knowledge or processes. Division of labor is instead a function of the settings of the weights, which are determined by the nature of the tasks the net is being asked to solve (e.g., mapping from orthography to phonology vs. orthography to semantics), properties of the learning algorithm that is used, and the architecture of the system (e.g., the number of units allocated to different components). These issues are discussed below; see also Van Orden et al. (1990), Plaut and Shallice (1993), Seidenberg (1989, 1992), and Plaut, McClelland, Seidenberg, and Patterson (in press).

II. WORD AND NONWORD NAMING

Although largely irrelevant to the usual goals of silent reading, the task of pronouncing words and nonwords aloud has provided important evidence concerning the acquisition, representation, and use of lexical knowledge, and the bases of dyslexia. The models make different predictions as to which factors influence naming performance. According to the dual-route model the principal factor is whether a word is rule governed or not. In the connectionist models, what matters instead is the degree of consistency in the mapping between spelling and sound. The Seidenberg and McClelland (1989) model, for example, learned to generate correct pronunciations for almost all 2897 words in their training corpus, including both "rule-governed" words and "exceptions." The model's performance on a given spelling pattern depended on how consistently it was pronounced across items in the training set. The pattern *ike,* for example, is very consistent because it has many "friends," other *-ike* words that rhyme. The pattern *ave* has about as many friends, but there is one "enemy," *have.* The pattern *ove* is highly inconsistent because it is associated with three pronunciations (*love, prove, cove*), each of which occurs in multiple words. A large number of behavioral studies (e.g., Glushko, 1979; Seidenberg, Waters, Barnes, & Tanenhaus, 1984; Taraban & McClelland, 1987) suggest that subjects' naming latencies for monosyllabic words reflect this degree of consistency factor. For example, Jared, McRae, and Seidenberg (1990) describe experiments in which naming latencies for words depended on the ratio of friends and enemies; they also provide an analysis of a large number of studies in the literature showing that they conformed to this generalization as well. A connectionist model such as Seidenberg and McClelland's is able to simulate these effects (and related phenomena concerning word frequency) as a natural consequence of how learning works in a feed-forward network using distributed representations and an error-correcting learning algorithm.

These effects are problematical for the dual-route approach, which predicts a dissociation between rule-governed words and exceptions, but no intermediate degrees of consistency (for discussion, see Henderson, 1982; Patterson & Coltheart, 1987). The dual-route model can handle these effects only by assuming that in generating the pronunciation of a rule-governed word such as *gave,* the phonological code for the enemy *have* is activated (e.g., by word-level orthography to phonology), which then conflicts with *gave.* To the extent that orthographic patterns such as *gave* tend to activate pronunciations associated with neighbors such as *save* and *have,* the dual-route model begins to approximate the "analogy" process developed by Glushko (1979) and the effects of exposure to inconsistent neighbors in a connectionist model. Also problematic are the consistency effects for nonwords: *bint* takes longer to pronounce than *bink* because of the inconsistency of *mint* and *pint* (Glushko, 1979). The dual-route model holds that nonwords are pronounced by rule; hence there is no basis for the irregular word *pint* to interfere with pronouncing *bint.* It could be assumed that presentation of the nonword *bint* activates the phonological code associated with *pint,* causing interference with normal application of the rules. Allowing lexical knowledge to influence nonword production involves adopting a major assumption of the connectionist models, however.

On the other hand, nonword pronunciation has presented other problems for the connectionist approach. The Seidenberg and McClelland (1989) model learned to generate correct pronunciations for 2897 words, but performed more poorly than people on nonwords (Besner, Twilley, McCann, & Seergobin, 1990). It generated correct output for simple nonwords such as *bint* or *nust* but produced more errors than did people on difficult items such as *jinje* and *faije.* This led to conjectures that there is a limit on the capacity of connectionist networks to pronounce both regular and irregular words while maintaining good nonword generalization (Besner et al., 1990; Coltheart et al., 1993). Subsequent research (Plaut & McClelland, 1993; Plaut et al., in press; Seidenberg et al., 1994) has indicated that nonword performance increases to levels comparable to people by using a better phonological representation. The model described in these papers performs as well on nonwords as Coltheart et al.'s pronunciation rules; moreover, it also pronounces both regular and irregular words correctly.

Simulations concerning the division of labor relevant to word and non-word naming within the connectionist framework have not been conducted because no one has yet implemented both orthographic-phonological and orthographic-semantic-phonological computations together. The Seidenberg and McClelland (1989) model did yield some suggestive findings concerning division of labor, however. Given the architecture that was used, the model was able to encode the correct pronunciations of about 97% of the words in the training corpus. The only items it missed were a small number of lower-frequency irregularly pronounced words (e.g., *bush, once*). In effect, the model arrived at a division of labor in which all common words and the higher-frequency irregular words were pronounced by means of an orthographic-phonological computation. Generating correct pronunciations for the remaining low-frequency irregular words would have required input from the orthographic-semantic-phonological computation, which was not available, of course, because this component was not implemented. There is some behavioral evidence consistent with this particular division of labor. Strain, Patterson, and Seidenberg (in press) report experiments in which subjects named aloud words varying in frequency, spelling-sound regularity, and imageability. Their main finding is that the "imageability" of the stimuli, as indexed by the Gilhooly and Logie (1980) norms, affected naming latencies only for lower-frequency words with irregular pronunciations. The longer latencies for nonimageable words compared to imageable ones were taken as evidence for the involvement of semantic information in the generation of the naming response (imageability ratings reflect perceptual properties assumed to be stored in semantic memory). Lower-frequency irregularly pronounced words show a large effect of this factor because naming these words requires input from the orthographic-semantics-phonology computation. Other words are named by using the orthographic-phonological computation, as in the Seidenberg and McClelland (1989) model.

III. ACQUIRED DYSLEXIAS

Brain injury, caused by stroke, Alzheimer's disease, and other forms of neuropathology, often results in partial impairments of visual word recognition (for overviews, see Coltheart, 1987; Patterson, 1981; Shallice, 1988). The study of these impairments has provided important evidence concerning the operation of the normal system. Data concerning these acquired dyslexias has played a central role in the development of the dual-route approach. Perhaps the most impressive aspect of the dual-route model is its account of the major patterns of impairment that are observed in terms of its basic assumptions about division of labor.

Much of the patient data involves the task of reading words and non-words aloud, which is the focus of the discussion here. Assuming that brain injury can selectively impair naming mechanisms, the dual-route model predicts the patterns termed *surface* and *phonological* dyslexia. The lexical naming mechanism provides the only way to generate pronunciations for irregular words. Hence damage to this route would produce impaired reading of irregular words, with nonword pronunciation unaffected. This is the surface dyslexic pattern (Patterson et al., 1985). Damage to the nonlexical mechanism would impair the ability to pronounce nonwords, but leave word reading intact. This is the phonological dyslexic pattern (Beauvois & Dérouesné, 1979). There is a third well-studied form of acquired dyslexia, deep dyslexia (Coltheart, Patterson, & Marshall, 1980), characterized by other word-naming errors including semantic paraphasias such as *chair* read "*table,*" and visual-then-semantic errors such as *sympathy* read "*orchestra*" (via misanalysis as "*symphony*"). This pattern of impairment can be derived by assuming there is damage in several parts of the lexical system simultaneously (Morton & Patterson, 1980). Thus, the dual-route model provides an elegant account of three patterns of acquired dyslexia. The application of the dual-route model to these reading impairments is quite important. The derivation of reading deficits from a theory of normal processing represents a powerful approach to explaining behavior. Research on reading disorders has played an essential role in the emergence of modern cognitive neuropsychology, and the approach that it represents is now being applied to many other types of cognitive impairments (see Ellis & Young, 1988, for examples).

Connectionist models offer an alternative approach to understanding such impairments. The effects of brain injury can be simulated by introducing different types of "damage" to the models—for example, eliminating units or connections, degrading input or output representations, or causing anomalies in the spread of activation. If the model of normal processing is correct, it should be possible to identify different sources of behavioral deficits, as well as the effects of different types and degrees of brain injury. Thus the approach should be well suited to explaining the variability that is observed among patients who might otherwise seem to fit a common syndrome (Caramazza, 1984).

Consider again surface dyslexia. In the dual-route model, this pattern

TABLE 1   Characteristics of Surface Dyslexic Subtypes

"Dysfluent" type	"Fluent" type
Errors on exception words	Errors on exception words
Some regularization errors, also "visual" errors	Errors almost all regularizations
Also makes errors on regular words	Very accurate on regular words
Errors are not frequency sensitive	Errors are frequency sensitive
Nonword reading is impaired	Nonword reading is accurate
Latencies abnormally long	Latencies within normal limits
Semantics is largely intact	Semantics is grossly impaired
Case study: JC (Marshall & Newcombe, 1973)	Case study: MP (Bub et al., 1985)

derives from impairment to the lexical pronunciation mechanism. Patterson, Seidenberg, and McClelland (1989) "lesioned" the Seidenberg and McClelland (1989) model by eliminating hidden units or connections between units. Both types of damage produced impaired performance similar to that seen in some surface dyslexic patients, including JC, a patient described in Marshall and Newcombe's (1973) original paper (see Table 1). In the "normal" simulations, the model's error scores, which index how well its output approximates the target pronunciations for words, were systematically related to subjects' naming latencies. Damaging the model caused these scores to increase greatly. The damaged model also generated a greater number of incorrect responses, for both regular and irregular words, both high- and low-frequency words, and nonwords. The model produced some regularization errors such as *been* pronounced "*bean*" as well as nonregularizations such as *skirt* pronounced "*skart.*" All of these characteristics correspond to ones seen in surface dyslexics such as JC.

   Surface dyslexia also illustrates the issue of variability within a deficit syndrome, insofar as it fractionates into two subtypes, the "dysfluent" type described above and a second type that Patterson et al. (1989) termed "fluent" surface dyslexia. The classic patient of the latter type is MP (Bub, Cancelliere, & Kertesz, 1985). Like the dysfluent patients, she mispronounced irregular words more than regular words or nonwords (see Table 1). In every other respect, however, her behavior was different. Her naming latencies were within normal limits for an older subject. Only irregular words were mispronounced; regular word naming was nearly perfect. Her errors were frequency sensitive, with only lower-frequency items affected. Finally, almost all errors were simple regularizations, for example, *have* pronounced "*haive*" and *deaf* pronounced "*deef.*"

   The Seidenberg and McClelland (1989) model provides an account of these two subtypes of surface dyslexia (see Plaut et al., 1994, for discussion). Whereas the dysfluent pattern can be simulated by damaging the orthographic-phonological (OP) computation as implemented, the fluent pattern cannot. This suggests that the two patterns have different sources. One possibility is that MP's performance reflects the intact operation of the OP computation; her brain injury has eliminated contributions from the orthography-semantics-phonology (OSP) computations. The division of labor in the Seidenberg and McClelland (1989) model is that OP produced correct output for both high- and low-frequency regular words and high-frequency irregular words. These are also the items that MP names correctly. The model's errors were restricted to lower-frequency irregular words; by hypothesis, correct pronunciation of these words normally requires input from the OSP component. These are the items that MP misses. Recall as well that the latter items also yielded semantic effects on naming in the Strain et al. (in press) study of younger normals. Thus, MP's performance appears to result from an intact OP computation with impaired input from OSP. Importantly, there is one further bit of data consistent with this account. All of the MP-type "fluent" patients observed to date have had severe semantic impairments. MP, for example, has a global semantic impairment and does not know the meanings of the words she pronounces correctly. This is consistent with the diagnosis of impaired input from OSP and an intact, fluently operating OP. All of the JC-type "dysfluent" patients had relatively intact lexical semantics. This is consistent with impaired operation of OP, with correct pronunciations haltingly pieced together using input from OSP.[3]

This analysis of surface dyslexia provides another illustration of the differences between the dual-route and connectionist approaches. In the dual-route model, the fluent and dysfluent surface dyslexics are categorized together because they both produce errors on irregular words. These words are normally pronounced by means of the lexical route; hence, surface dyslexia involves damage to this route. The differences between the two subtypes are accommodated by assuming that they differ in terms of secondary impairments. For example, only the dysfluent surface dyslexics might have the visual impairment thought to be the cause of errors such as *spy* read as "*shy.*" The connectionist models show that a given type of error can arise from multiple underlying causes. Thus, errors on irregular words arose from both damage to the OP computation itself and from damage to OSP, which has a debilitating effect on the lower-frequency irregular words that normally require input from it. The properties of the computations within different components of the connectionist network, and the division of labor between them, provide a basis for understanding two very different "surface dyslexic" profiles.

Whereas the surface dyslexia patterns raise issues about accounting for patient variability, deep dyslexia raises issues about the explanatory value of a model. Deep dyslexia is a dramatic form of reading impairment charac-

TABLE 2   Behaviors Associated with Deep Dyslexia

Semantic paralexias	*Table → chair*
Visual errors	*Tandem → tantrum*
Visual then semantic errors	*Sympathy → orchestra*
Morphological errors	*Walked → walking*
More errors on abstract words than on concrete words	
More errors on function words than on content words	
Nonword pronunciation is very impaired	

terized by the set of behavioral characteristics summarized in Table 2. This pattern can be explained within the dual-route framework by assuming impairments at multiple loci in the Figure 1 model (Patterson & Morton, 1985). However, this account fails to explain a central fact about the deep dyslexic pattern, namely the co-occurrence of the characteristics in Table 2. Patients who produce semantic errors in reading aloud invariably exhibit the other deficits as well (see Coltheart et al., 1980, for discussion). It is not clear from the dual-route account why this should be.

Hinton and Shallice (1991) and Plaut and Shallice (1993) have shown that the co-occurring behavioral deficits can be produced by damage at a single locus in the networks they implemented. The main architectural feature of their networks is that they included recurrent connections among the semantic units, which allowed the creation of so-called attractor basins. The set of deep dyslexic deficits can be simulated by forms of damage that degrade and distort these attractors. This case illustrates how connectionist models can provide nontransparent explanations for co-occurring behavioral deficits that would otherwise seem unrelated.[4]

In summary, the dual-route model has provided an account of several forms of acquired dyslexia in terms of assumptions about the division of labor for word and nonword naming. This was a pioneering attempt to explain cognitive impairments in terms of models of normal performance. The connectionist models provide alternative explanations for some of these impairments and suggest explanations for other aspects of acquired dyslexia such as patient variability in terms of degree of damage. The accounts of the subtypes of surface dyslexia and deep dyslexia are not "implementations" of any earlier theory (Pinker & Prince, 1988). Whereas most of the research on acquired dyslexia using connectionist models has been directed at showing that they are compatible with the classical deficit patterns, the models are beginning to provide accounts of patterns of behavioral impairment that would be quite unexpected on the dual-route account. For example, Patterson and Hodges (1992) have studied several patients with progressive aphasia who exhibit progressive loss of semantic memory. These patients are also fluent surface dyslexics. Patterson and Hodges established that their semantic memory and word naming impairments were related: patients with a larger degree of semantic impairment produced more errors in naming irregular words. Patterson and Hodges suggest that this pattern reflects the interconnections between phonological and semantic representations in the Figure 2 model. Damage to semantic representations has secondary effects on the integrity of phonological representations, causing word naming errors. These dependencies are consistent with the properties of highly interactive systems (Plaut et al., 1994; Van Orden et al., 1990).[5]

IV. ROLE OF PHONOLOGY IN WORD RECOGNITION

Another domain in which the division of labor issue arises concerns one of the oldest issues in reading research: the role of phonological information in visual word recognition (for reviews, see Jorm & Share, 1983; McCusker, Hillinger, & Bias, 1981; Wagner & Torgeson, 1987). The nature of the reading task does not demand that phonology be used at all; in principle, words could be recognized and sentences comprehended on a strictly visual basis. As we have seen, words could also be recognized by using knowledge of how orthographic patterns relate to phonological codes, which are themselves related to meaning. The issue as to whether word recognition is "direct" or "phonologically mediated" has been a source of seemingly endless controversy, with the pendulum swinging back and forth between the extremes with some regularity. The issue is not merely a theoretical one because of its implications concerning methods for teaching reading, itself a highly charged educational policy issue (see Adams, 1990).

The dual-route model has always offered a reconcilist position on this issue, insofar as both direct and phonologically mediated routes were thought to prevail for different types of words. Exception words were read by the direct route; regular words could be recognized by either route but skilled readers were thought to recognize more of them directly (Castles & Coltheart, 1993). There has long been evidence that phonological information is rapidly activated in silent reading under a broad range of conditions. For example, there are facilitative priming effects for visually presented rhyming pairs such as *stone–flown* compared to unrelated controls (e.g., Meyer, Schvaneveldt, & Ruddy, 1974). Tanenhaus, Flanigan, and Seidenberg (1980) observed this effect using the Stroop task, in which subjects name the color of the ink the target is printed in. Phonological similarity of prime–target pairs produces significant interference with color naming compared to unrelated controls. Thus, subjects cannot inhibit activating phonological information even when it has a negative impact on performance. Similarly, Pollatsek, Lesch, Morris, and Rayner (1992) provide evidence that phonological information is used to integrate information across saccadic movements. A long-standing question, however, concerns the time course of phonological activation vis-à-vis meaning. The current phase of the debate focuses on whether meanings are ever computed directly from orthographic information. Van Orden and his colleagues (1990) have challenged the existence of the direct route on the following bases:

1. They question the data taken as evidence for the direct route. Much of this evidence involves tasks such as lexical decision that invite alternative interpretations of the results and criticism concerning their relevance to normal reading. Van Order et al. also discount evidence from phonological dyslexia, the disorder in which words can be read despite severe damage to the phonological route. These patients' reading might reflect adaptation to severe brain injury rather than a component of the normal system; moreover, their preserved capacity does not support very fluent reading, suggesting that it probably was not a major part of the premorbid system.

2. They note that connectionist models invalidate the dual-route model's central assumption that the direct route provides the only means for recognizing words containing irregular spelling-sound correspondences. As the Seidenberg and McClelland (1989) model shows, a single process can generate correct phonological codes for both regular and irregular words. Thus, all words might be read through phonological mediation, not merely those that are "rule governed."

3. They provide clear evidence of phonological mediation in a silent reading task, semantic categorization (see Van Orden, 1987; Van Orden, Johnston, & Hale, 1988). The subject is given a target category such as *flower* and then must decide if a target word is an exemplar of the category or not. On critical trials, the target is a homophone of a category exemplar (e.g., *rows*). On a significant proportion of these trials, subjects make false positive responses. Phonologically recoding the target leads to the activation of the meaning associated with the category exemplar, and on some trials subjects falsely respond "yes." Pseudohomophones (e.g., *article of clothing: sute*) produce similar effects.

4. Finally, they note that poor reading is often associated with impairments in the use of phonological information (e.g., Bradley & Bryant, 1985; Liberman & Shankweiler, 1979), consistent with the claim that efficient use of phonological recoding facilitates word recognition, contrary to the earlier view that the direct route is the more efficient method.

These are important considerations and they have created momentum that has pushed the pendulum toward phonological mediation once again. The conclusion that phonological information plays a central role in word recognition is supported by a body of compelling evidence that is growing rapidly (see, e.g., Lesch & Pollatsek, 1993; Lukatela & Turvey, 1994; Pollatsek et al., 1992). However, it may be an overstatement to say that word recognition in reading necessarily and exclusively proceeds from spelling to sound to meaning (Van Orden et al., 1988). The methods used in these studies provide a way to detect the activation of phonological information in word recognition; however, it is also necessary to address the range of conditions under which such effects occur. It has been widely assumed that phonological mediation occurs; the question is under what conditions, for which kinds of words, and at what level of reading skill. It is also necessary to consider what else might be going on in parallel with the activation of phonology.

Studies by Jared and Seidenberg (1991) showed that the false positive effects (e.g., saying that *rows* is a kind of flower) depend on several factors. First, there is the specificity of the categories that are used. Van Orden has employed relatively specific categories such as *flower* and *part of a horse's harness,* which allow subjects to rapidly generate a small number of common exemplars (*rose, tulip; rein, bit*). The size of the false positive effect is greatly reduced when broader categories such as *inanimate object* are used, eliminating the possibility of generating targets in advance. Second, the effect depends on word frequency. With narrow categories such as Van Orden used, both high- and low-frequency targets, as well as pseudohomophones, produced larger false positive rates than nonhomophonic controls. With broader categories, only lower-frequency targets and pseudohomophones showed the effect.

These studies appear to indicate that use of phonological information in word recognition depends on frequency, with higher-frequency words recognized with little or no input from phonology (Seidenberg, 1985). These conclusions have been contested by Lesch and Pollatsek (1993), who suggest that high-frequency words activate phonology but failed to produce false positive responses in the Jared and Seidenberg (1991) experiments because subjects can rapidly determine that they are not spelled correctly. If this argument is correct, however, the Van Orden paradigm is completely uninformative, because both false positive errors and the absence of such errors are now taken as evidence for phonological mediation. Lesch and Pollatsek (1993) employed a different paradigm in which a prime such as *bare* is followed by a target such as *lion* that is semantically related to a homophone of the prime (*bear*). The prime was presented briefly and followed by a pattern mask. With a 50-ms prime exposure, there were priming effects for the targets related to prime homophones. With a 200-ms exposure, this priming disappeared. The former effect was taken as evidence for phonological activation of meaning. The longer exposure allowed sufficient time for a spelling check to occur, eliminating priming. Lesch and Pollatsek (1993) did not systematically manipulate word frequency, however (see also Lukatela & Turvey, 1994). Using a similar priming methodology, Jared and

Seidenberg (1991) observed priming only with lower-frequency homophones.

The debate about the role of phonological information in visual word recognition is continuing, although on a different footing than before insofar as robust effects of phonology have been reliably obtained using several methodologies. Four additional points should be noted before closing this overview of the phonology issue. First, every experimental paradigm introduces a new set of methodological questions that need to be tracked down; in the case of the masked priming experiments such as Lesch and Pollatsek (1993) and Perfetti, Bell, and Delaney (1988), there is a need to understand the effects of the mask on processing and how these conditions relate to normal reading.

Second, closure on the phonology issue cannot be achieved without gaining a better understanding of the properties of the putative OS computation. What are the factors that limit the efficiency of the OS computation, thereby forcing a sharing of effort with OPS? Van Orden et al. suggest that OS is less efficient than OPS because "covariant learning procedures" have difficulty mastering the mapping between the orthographic and semantic codes, which are uncorrelated. However, attractor networks are quite able to learn such arbitrary mappings (see Plaut & Shallice, 1993), and the limits on their capacities are not known. Moreover, it is possible that the extent to which this mapping is arbitrary may have been overstated because research has tended to focus on monosyllabic words. The morphological structure of more complex words can be seen as reflecting nonarbitrary correspondences between meaning and the sensory codes for words (orthography and phonology). It would also be useful to have experimental methods that could detect the use of OS if it occurs, analogous to those that Van Orden et al. developed for detecting the use of phonology.

Third, the issue as to whether the use of phonological information varies as a function of word frequency is important to resolve, because the type-token facts about languages dictate that a small amount of OS would go a long way (Seidenberg, 1992). The distribution of words by frequency is highly skewed, with a small number of lexical types accounting for a large proportion of the tokens. Some relevant statistics are summarized in Table 3. The 150 most frequent words in the Francis and Kucera (1967) corpus account for over 50% of the approximately 1 million tokens in that database. The 150 most frequent words account for 51.9% of these tokens. The distribution of these 150 words by length is given in the table. There are 64 words from one to three letters in length; they account for 387,108 tokens, which is 38.8% of the entire corpus. There are 116 words from one to four letters in length, yielding 478,265 tokens, which is 47.9% of the corpus. Thus, almost half the words in the corpus consist of the 116 most frequent one- to four-letter words. It does not stretch the bounds of plausibility to consider these words to be likely candidates for OS. Even recog-

TABLE 3   Data Concerning the Most Common Words in English[a]

| Length in letters | 150 most frequent words: | | |
	Number of types	Σ Frequency of tokens	Cumulative % of entire corpus
1	2	28,421	2.8
2	24	168,282	19.7
3	38	190,405	38.8
4	52	91,157	47.9
5	25	31,892	51.1
6	4	3584	51.5
7	5	3891	51.9
Total	150	517,632	51.9

[a]Entire Kucera and Francis (1967) corpus: tokens, 998,052; types, 46,369. These calculations are based on an on-line version of the Kucera and Francis corpus that contains 998,052 tokens.

nizing a relatively small number of high-frequency words on this basis would account for a great deal of what is actually read.

Finally, it should be observed that the issue as to whether word recognition is direct or phonologically mediated is more central to the dual-route, lexical access style of model than the connectionist alternative. The focus of the dual-route model is on the independent processing mechanisms and the race between them. In systems with feedback connections between units that create the "resonances" that Van Orden and colleagues have discussed at length, the processing of a word will involve input from all parts of the system (Van Orden & Goldinger, 1994). Indeed, Van Orden has always postulated a "spelling check" mechanism for disambiguating homophones such as *pair* and *pear,* which involves a computation from meaning to orthography; if the system is resonant, activation will also flow from orthography to semantics, what was formerly called the direct route. As noted earlier, these systems are incongruent with the idea of independent subsystems that is central to the dual-route model and to the information processing approach it exemplifies. It is therefore something of a category error to refer to the processing routes in a dynamical system. Perhaps the biggest advance concerning the issue of direct access versus phonological mediation over the past twenty years may have been the development of new theoretical concepts that eliminate this dichotomy entirely.

V. THE ORTHOGRAPHIC DEPTH HYPOTHESIS

Another way in which the division of labor issue has arisen is in connection with the orthographic depth hypothesis, which concerns the effects of differences among writing systems on the word recognition process (Frost, Katz, & Bentin, 1987; Katz & Feldman, 1981; see also the papers in Frost & Katz, 1992). The world's orthographies represent different solutions to the problem of representing spoken language in written form. One of the fundamental ways in which they differ is in the extent to which the written and spoken forms correspond. In "shallow" alphabetic orthographies (Turvey, Feldman, & Lukatela, 1984), the correspondences between graphemes and phonemes are entirely consistent. Serbo-Croatian provides a well-studied example. English, in contrast, is relatively "deep," because the correspondences between graphemes and phonemes are inconsistent. The orthographic depth hypothesis is that the extent to which readers use phonological information in recognizing words depends on the extent to which it is represented by the orthography of their language. In dual-route terms, the nonlexical route predominates in shallow orthographies, because the correspondences between spelling and sound are rule governed. The lexical route must be used in reading deep orthographies such as Chinese or unpointed Hebrew. English, which has both rule-governed items and exceptions, requires using both pathways.

The orthographic depth hypothesis has inspired a massive amount of research, much of it on Serbo-Croatian. Findings of the following sort have been reported (e.g., Lukatela, Popadič, Ognjenovič, & Turvey, 1980; Lukatela & Turvey, 1980). When skilled readers of Serbo-Croatian make lexical decisions (i.e., decide if letter strings form words or not), factors related to the pronunciations of the stimuli affect performance. For example, many studies have exploited the ambiguity between (but not within) the Roman and Cyrillic alphabets used in writing the language. A stimulus such as *betap* contains letters that appear in both alphabets. How it is pronounced depends on whether it is interpreted as Roman or Cyrillic, owing to the ambiguity of the letters *b* and *p*. Lexical decision latencies for these ambiguous strings are reliably longer than latencies for unambiguous strings such as *vetar* (Lukatela et al., 1980). This phonological ambiguity effect is taken as strong evidence that phonological mediation is the rule in reading Serbo-Croatian (Turvey et al., 1984). Taken with the assumption that phonologically mediated lexical access is not possible for exception words in English, Kanji words in Japanese, or Chinese characters in general, these findings seem to support the orthographic depth hypothesis.

Several developments have served to complicate this elegant picture. First, there is the data, reviewed in the previous section, suggesting that phonological mediation is obligatory in English. If this is correct, then the orthographic depth hypothesis as originally formulated is simply wrong: it would have to be concluded that phonological mediation is obligatory despite differences in orthographic depth. Moreover, similar findings have been obtained in even deeper writing systems than English, such as Japanese

Kanji (Wydell, Patterson, & Humphreys, 1993) and unpointed Hebrew (Frost & Bentin, 1992). Finally, as we have seen, connectionist models provided a mechanism that explains how there could be efficient orthographic to phonological conversion even in the deeper orthographies.

Exactly the same methodological, empirical, and theoretical issues that arose concerning division of labor in English have arisen in connection with orthographic depth. For example, the many demonstrations of phonological effects on lexical decision in Serbo-Croatian do not necessarily delimit the range of conditions under which such effects obtain. Alternatively, the orthographic depth hypothesis might be reformulated as a claim about the units over which phonological recoding occurs. In Serbo-Croatian, for example, they might be graphemes and phonemes; in English, spelling and sound units of varying sizes including rimes; in Japanese Kana, morae or syllables. A final possibility is that the orthographic depth hypothesis is essentially correct; there may be phonological input to the recognition process across a broad range of orthographies, but to a greater degree in the shallower ones. However, orthographic depth is only one of the several dimensions along which writing systems vary. It is possible that trade-offs among the design features of writing systems are such that they are processed similarly despite differences in orthographic depth (Seidenberg, 1992). For example, Serbo-Croatian is more transparent than English at the level of grapheme-phoneme correspondences, but less transparent with regard to the assignment of syllabic stress. Although research on the orthographic depth hypothesis has focused on questions concerning phonology, it may have opened the door to a much broader range of interesting questions about the reading process in different writing systems.

VI. WORD RECOGNITION STRATEGIES

The next area in which the division of labor issue has arisen concerns decoding strategies. Do readers flexibly vary the division of labor as an implicit response to properties of the material being read or other situation-specific factors? Both the dual-route and connectionist models afford these possibilities. In the dual-route model, strategies involve varying reliance on the alternative routes (e.g., whether words are named lexically or nonlexically; whether meanings are accessed directly or through phonological mediation). In the connectionist models, subjects might vary the amount of attention that is allocated to different sets of connections. Cohen, Dunbar, and McClelland (1990), for example, developed a model of the Stroop task with separate word and color processing channels. Instructions to name the ink color or the word itself were simulated using attentional units that gated the amount of activation within a channel. In a similar way, individuals might allocate attention to different components of the lexical system.

That readers can consciously and voluntarily alter their decoding strategies is obvious from their ability to do such things as read words aloud with an accent or vary their reading speed. Experimenters can also create conditions that force people to modify their normal reading habits. For example, subjects in studies by Kolers (1975) were asked to read texts that were presented in modified formats (e.g., upside down, backward, upside down and backward). These manipulations raise a basic question about strategy research: do the studies provide information about processes involved in normal reading, including ways in which such processes can be flexibly employed, or are the studies merely effective in providing information about the manipulations themselves? In principle, such manipulations can provide useful information about normal reading. Kolers, for example, was not interested in backward reading per se; he used the task to generate data that allowed him to draw interferences about the normal system. Making such inferences requires having a good understanding of the effects of the experimental manipulations themselves—what they introduce to the reading task and how they interact wit normal mechanisms. Otherwise the studies merely provide data concerning the many and varied ways in which subjects cope with an endless array of experimental circumstances.

The history of research using the lexical decision task offers a cautionary tale. After more than twenty years of use, the reputation of this task is somewhat tarnished. It was originally introduced as a way to study the role of factors such as phonological, frequency, and contextual information in word recognition (e.g., Rubenstein, Lewis, & Rubenstein, 1971). With regard to phonology, it is now widely accepted that performance on the task does not provide a basis for resolving the question (for discussion see Coltheart, Besner, Jonasson, & Davelaar, 1979; Henderson, 1982). Regarding frequency, it has been argued that it yields exaggerated effects (Balota & Chumbley, 1984); the same has been said about context effects (Seidenberg, Waters, Sanders, & Langer, 1984; Stanovich & West, 1979). The problem in all of these cases is that lexical decision latencies involve both more and less than what is involved in recognizing a word in normal reading. They involve less in the sense that the task does not necessarily require subjects to determine the meanings of words. Subjects merely have to find a basis for reliably discriminating words from nonwords, and this can often be achieved on a nonsemantic basis (e.g., properties of the nonwords). They involve more than normal reading in that latencies also reflect the process of making the lexical decision itself, which can itself be affected by the experimental variables.

Many studies have shown that the effects of aspects of lexical structure such as the number of pronunciations or meanings of a word on lexical decisions depend on task- and experiment-specific factors such as the proportions of items of different types and properties of the nonwords used.

For example, James (1975) found that the extent to which a semantic factor (the abstractness/concreteness of words) influenced decision latencies depended on the characteristics of the nonwords used in the experiment. This might indicate that subjects are able to strategically vary which route of the dual-route model is used in recognizing words. Other studies suggest that the use of phonology varies in the same way (Shulman, Hornak, & Sanders, 1978; Waters & Seidenberg, 1985). However, these studies may merely indicate that subjects vary their strategies for making lexical decisions, not that they strategically control the recognition process. Just as the exaggerated frequency effects in the Balota and Chumbley (1984) study derived from subjects' criteria for making their decisions, so may the variable effects of phonological or semantic factors in studies such as James (1975) and Waters and Seidenberg (1985). When the nonwords in the experiment are nonpronounceable, subjects can base their decisions on whether the target looks like a word; hence semantic and phonological factors have no effect. When the stimuli look very wordlike, subjects are forced to base their decisions on the other information.

These studies suggest that subjects' criteria for making lexical decisions are rationally established in response to the conditions that confront them. Subjects identify the dimensions of the stimuli that provide a reliable basis for discriminating words from nonwords. They respond when they have obtained sufficient information to make the decision with a high probability of being correct. Little follows from such studies about the ability to strategically control the use of recognition pathways, less still about how reading strategies vary in response to properties of actual texts. As a consequence, many researchers have turned to other tasks.

Among the other tasks that are available, of course, is naming. Naming typically eliminates the decision stage that was the source of many problems in interpreting lexical decision data. Like lexical decision, however, the task does not require subjects to identify the meanings of words. The Seidenberg and McClelland (1989) model, for example, generates pronunciations for words without using semantics at all. Hence the task is not an ideal tool for studying factors that influence determining the meanings of words. It has been widely used to study how people pronounce words and nonwords, as we have seen. However, recent studies have shown that, as with lexical decision, subjects' strategies for performing the task can be manipulated in experiment-specific ways.

Monsell and Patterson (1992), for example, simply instructed subjects to change their naming strategy by telling them to regularize the pronunciations of exception words such as *pint* (so that it would rhyme with *mint*). Subjects can produce these regularized pronunciations quite easily. One possibility is that the experimental manipulation is useful because latencies to regularize exception words indicate how long it would take the OP route to generate a pronunciation in the absence of interference from the lexical route. However, the experimental manipulation may induce additional strategies for performing the task that have little to do with normal reading. One strategy for rapidly producing regularizations would be to focus on smaller orthographic units than normal. For example, divide the word at the onset–rime boundary (e.g., *p–int*), compute the pronunciation of the rime ("*int*") and then combine it with the onset ("*p*"). This behavior would be less informative about properties of OP than about the way in which subjects adapt to task demands.

Paap and Noel (1989) attempted to manipulate subjects' naming strategies by interfering with the use of the nonlexical route. Subjects read regular and exception words aloud while performing a secondary task, remembering a list of digits. With a short digit list (a light memory load), subjects produced the usual frequency by regularity interaction (Seidenberg, Waters, Barnes, & Tanenhaus, 1984). A longer digit list (heavier memory load) slowed latencies on all types of words except lower-frequency exception words, which were named more rapidly than in the light load condition. Paap and Noel's interpretation is that the heavy memory load interferes with the use of nonlexical phonology, requiring the use of the lexical route, which is not sensitive to spelling-sound regularity. Without a conflict between the two routes, exception words can be named very rapidly. This result seems to indicate that subjects can alter their reliance on different routes. However, the result has been difficult to replicate. Previous attempts to use secondary task methodologies to study phonological effects in word recognition were also problematical (see Waters, Komoda, & Arbuckle, 1985).

Finally, subjects also vary their naming strategies in response to more subtle manipulations of the stimuli. For example, Monsell, Patterson, Graham, Hughes, and Milroy (1992) showed that latencies to read exception words depended on whether they were blocked or intermixed with nonwords. Including nonwords yields faster latencies and more regularization errors. It appears that research using the naming task is beginning to recapitulate the earlier experience with lexical decision: studies are beginning to focus more on the ways in which performance can be manipulated than on using the task to address central questions about normal reading. The question as to whether readers are able to change their word recognition strategies in response to properties of texts or naturalistic task demands nonetheless remains an important, and unresolved, one.

VII. READING COMPLEX WORDS

The research I have reviewed to this point was almost exclusively concerned with the processing of monosyllabic, monomorphemic words, an accurate reflection of the state of the field. Much less attention has been paid to issues that arise in connection with complex words: what people know about word structure, and how this knowledge is represented in memory and used in reading words. It might be thought that these questions would attract as much attention as, say, strategic effects in the lexical decision task, but that has not happened as yet. In part this is because some early attempts to address these questions within the lexical access framework were not very successful. However, insights that have been gained from recent models of the processing of simple words may revive interest in complex words.

The processing of morphologically complex words was initially a central topic within the "lexical access" framework. Taft and Forster (1975) proposed that recognizing a complex word required decomposing it into component parts. One of these parts would serve as the word's "access unit." Thus, reading a prefixed word such as *unlock* involved removing the prefix, which uncovered the stem *lock,* which then provided access to a file in lexical memory containing all of the *lock* words (*relock, locked, locksmith,* etc.). The goal of Taft's research was to identify the aspect of lexical structure that functioned as the "access unit." However, numerous studies comparing different possible units have failed to converge on one candidate. Taft himself favors a unit called the BOSS (basic orthographic syllable structure), but there are studies that clearly fail to support this proposal (e.g., Lima & Pollatsek, 1983; Seidenberg, 1987; Taft, 1987).

A more promising hypothesis is that the access units are morphological structures of the sort proposed within linguistic theory. Whereas sentence processing is traditionally thought to involve using grammatical rules to parse a sequence of words, word recognition could be assumed to involve using morphological rules to parse individual lexical items. Caramazza and his colleagues (for review, see Badecker & Caramazza, in press) have provided considerable evidence consistent with this view. Their studies show that aspects of both normal and disordered word recognition reflect the use of morphological knowledge.

It is at this point that the same issues arise as with the topics reviewed in earlier sections. In languages such as English, morphological structure is apparently rule governed but admits many exceptions. For example, the past tense is formed by a rule adding the inflection /d/ to a present tense root (*hike–hiked, walk–walked*) but there are exceptions such as *run–ran* and *ride–rode.* The same holds for plural formation (*dog–dogs* and *hen–hens* but *mouse–mice* and *sheep–sheep*). In the derivational domain, many words afford transparent decomposition (*hand, unhand, unhanded, two-handed*), and morphological theories attempt to characterize these systematic aspects of word structure; however there are obvious exceptions: *unlock* is the opposite of *lock* but *untoward* is not the opposite of *toward; deliver* is not related to *liver; sweetbreads* are neither sweet nor bread. Henderson (1985) provides many other examples. Morphological parsing rules that correctly analyze the "regular" forms will misanalyze the "exceptions." As in the case of spelling-sound correspondences, dual-route models have been proposed as the solution to this problem. The traditional view of inflectional morphology is that it consists of a rule component and a list of exceptions that must be learned by rote (Berko, 1958; Pinker & Prince, 1988). Pinker (1991) has proposed a "modified traditional theory" in which the rule is retained but the list is replaced by an "associative network." That the past tense is rule governed is taken as illustrating deep and essential properties of linguistic knowledge (Pinker, 1991, 1994). Marslen-Wilson, Tyler, Waksler, and Older (1994) have developed a related model of derivational morphology. Transparent forms such as *untie* are represented in memory in terms of their component morphemes (*un* + *tie*); opaque forms such as *untoward* are listed directly in the lexicon. Thus, both Pinker and Marslen-Wilson et al. assume that morphological structure governs the organization of the mental lexicon. Pinker proposes separate processing mechanisms for rule-governed items and exceptions; in contrast, Marslen-Wilson et al. propose a single processing mechanism that acts on representations that encode morphological structure.

As in the case of spelling-sound correspondences, connectionist models of the same phenomena present a different picture. As before there is a contrast between a dual-route approach proposing separate mechanisms for the rule-governed cases and exceptions, and a connectionist approach in which a single network is employed for all. Thus, for example, Daugherty and Seidenberg (1992; Daugherty, Petersen, MacDonald & Seidenberg, 1993) describe simple feed-forward networks that take present tenses as input and generate past tenses as output. These networks used essentially the same architecture as the Seidenberg and McClelland (1989) model of spelling-sound correspondences. Given *like* as input, the Daugherty and Seidenberg (1992) model generates *liked* as output. Given *bake,* it produces *baked.* Given *take,* however, it produces *took* and given *make* it produces *made.* Finally, given a nonword such as *mave,* it generates *maved.* This behavior is strictly analogous to that of the Seidenberg and McClelland (1989) model, which also used a single feed-forward network to generate pronunciations for "rule-governed" items, exceptions, and nonwords. Seidenberg (1992) points out other similarities between the spelling-sound and past tense phenomena. For example, when asked to generate the past tenses for verbs, subjects exhibit frequency, regularity, and consistency effects analogous to those in the spelling-sound domain.

Connectionist models of the processing of morphologically complex words are still at an early stage in development, and they have already generated considerable controversy. They are controversial because they raise fundamental questions about the nature of linguistic knowledge. In linguistic theory, the capacity to generalize is taken as classic evidence that linguistic knowledge is represented in terms of generative rules. Cases where the rules fail to account are excluded as exceptions. Thus, traditional treatments of linguistic knowledge are intrinsically committed to a dual-route approach (the competence–performance distinction itself can be seen as embodying the approach). The goal is to formulate abstract generalizations about linguistic phenomena, excluding exceptions and unclear cases as necessary. The fact that language can be described as rule governed is taken as an important discovery (Pinker, 1991), but there is a real sense in which this could not fail to be true given that the rules do not have to correctly apply in all cases (Seidenberg, 1992). Any body of knowledge can be described as rule governed as long as there is a second mechanism to handle the cases where the rules fail (e.g., a list of exceptions; an "associative net"; "performance"). Prior to the development of connectionist models, there was no obvious alternative to this dual-mechanism approach. Now, however, there is a kind of knowledge representation that uses the same mechanism to encode both rule-governed knowledge and exceptions. This forces us to reassess the kinds of evidence previously taken as implicating rules. This reassessment is under way, along with explorations of novel aspects of the new approach (see Seidenberg, in press, for an overview).

VIII. WORD RECOGNITION IN CONTEXT

The final topic to be considered is the processing of words in context. The studies of isolated words are concerned with how structural properties such as frequency and phonology influence recognition. The essential context question is: how are the word recognition processes discussed above influenced by information from the broader linguistic and extralinguistic contexts in which words normally appear? Or, in division of labor terms: to what extent is word recognition driven by lexical versus contextual types of information?

A. Modular versus Interactive Models of Context Effects

A central issue in 1980s word recognition research was whether the lexical processing system is an autonomous "module" of the mind. The role of prior knowledge in perception is a classic issue in psychology, and it figured prominently in the emergence of cognitive psychology as a field (see Neisser, 1967). Neisser summarized many demonstrations of the context dependency of perception that led to an emphasis on the constructive character of cognition. Some theorists viewed reading as an example of this type of behavior. For example, Hochberg (1970) emphasized the role of what later became known as "top-down" processing (Norman & Bobrow, 1975) in reading. Goodman (1968) provided the extreme statement of this view, concluding that reading is a "psycholinguistic guessing game" (i.e., words are read by guessing their identities from context), a conception that continues to exert considerable influence on educational policy (Adams, 1990). There were many studies of the role of schemas and other types of knowledge representations in reading (see, e.g., papers in Spiro, Bruce, & Brewer, 1980), reflecting the influence of research in artificial intelligence (Schank & Abelson, 1977). In 1979, Forster took a fresh look at the issue and published an article arguing that word recognition in reading is an autonomous, bottom-up process. Shortly thereafter, Fodor (1983) developed his account of mental "modules," using the lexicon as a prominent example.

Empirical evidence consistent with the view that the lexicon is an autonomous (or as Fodor termed it, "informationally encapsulated") module was provided by studies of lexical ambiguity. Ambiguous words such as *tire* and *watch* have multiple semantically unrelated meanings. Two 1979 studies (Swinney, 1979; Tanenhaus, Leiman, & Seidenberg, 1979) showed that immediately following a word such as *tire,* both common meanings are briefly activated, with the contextually appropriate reading selected briefly thereafter. These studies used a cross-modal priming paradigm in which a sentence (such as *John began to tire*) was followed by a target word related to one of the alternative meanings (e.g., *wheel, sleep*). Latencies to name the target (Tanenhaus et al., 1979) or make a lexical decision to it (Swinney) were compared to those on trials where the sentence and target were unrelated. Latencies were faster for targets related to both meanings of the ambiguous word than to unrelated controls. This effect was striking because it even occurred in sentences that could not be parsed using the alternative interpretation. Thus, *John began to tire* primed *wheel* even though *wheel* is related to a noun sense of *tire.* These studies suggested that the initial access of word meaning is not highly dependent on contextual information, consistent with the view that the lexicon is an autonomous processing module. Additional support was provided by studies such as Fischler and Bloom (1979) and Stanovich and West (1979) using other methodologies.

At roughly the same time, McClelland and Rumelhart were moving in exactly the opposite theoretical direction. Their 1981 article described a computational model of interactive processes in visual word recognition. This view emphasized the idea that perception is the result of the continuous flow of information both top-down and bottom-up (Rumelhart, 1977). The interactive-activation model provided a novel interpretation of "context effects" and was an important step in the development of what was to become the connectionist or parallel distributed processing paradigm in cognitive science (Rumelhart & McClelland, 1986). Ironically then, word recognition has played a prominent role in the development of both modular and connectionist approaches.

These developments set the stage for empirical tests of the modular and interactive accounts of word processing. Numerous studies assessed whether context did or did not affect lexical access (see, e.g., Burgess, Tanenhaus, & Seidenberg, 1989; Duffy, Morris, & Rayner, 1988; Glucksberg, Kreuz, & Rho, 1986; Simpson, 1981). Within the lexical access framework, however, it is important to establish the locus of contextual effects. Seidenberg, Waters, Sanders, and Langer (1984) distinguished between "prelexical" and "postlexical" effects of context. Prelexical effects were thought to reflect the influence of contextual information on the identification of a target word; "modularity" suggested these effects should be minimal. Postlexical effects reflect the integration of the word with the context once it had been recognized; these are completely compatible with modularity. Tasks such as lexical decision yield robust effects of contextual congruence, thought to largely reflect postlexical influences on the decision process itself, rather than the identification of the target word (Balota & Chumbley, 1984; Stanovich & West, 1979). Consistent with this interpretation, tasks such as naming, which do not include the decision component, yield much smaller contextual effects (Seidenberg, Waters, Sanders, & Langer, 1984; Stanovich & West, 1979). However, the distinction between pre- and postlexical loci of contextual effects is not preserved in the connectionist models, which lack a discrete moment of lexical access.

Along the same lines, Forster (1979) differentiated between "intralexical" versus "extralexical" sources of contextual effects. The intralexical effects reflect processes within lexical memory itself. The classic intralexical effect is semantic priming (Meyer & Schvaneveldt, 1971): one word primes another by means of spreading activation within the lexicon. These effects were thought to be compatible with the modular view (see Seidenberg, Waters, Sanders, & Tanenhaus, for discussion). Only the extralexical effects (e.g., the facilitative effect of a sentence context that did not contain any words that could produce semantic priming) were seen as violating modularity (see, e.g., Keenan, Potts, Golding, & Jennings, 1990; Morris, 1994). Thus, when contextual effects were observed it was not necessarily obvious whether they were incompatible with modularity or not.

It also became apparent that the lack of an effect of context does not necessarily indicate that the lexicon is modular. The Kawamoto (1986, 1993) model showed how the "multiple access" pattern that had been taken as diagnostic of an autonomous module could occur in a fully interactive processing system. In this model, recognizing a word involves computing its phonological and semantic codes. The model allowed contextual constraints to influence this process. The model exhibited the property that Marslen-Wilson (1989) termed "bottom-up priority:" the processing of a word was largely driven by the input code itself rather than by contextual information. Thus, the model would rapidly settle on the phonological and semantic patterns associated with words without much input from context. The lexicon that Kawamoto used included a number of heterophonic homographs such as *wind* and *bass*. The model was able to settle on one of the pronunciations of a homograph using information provided by the context; thus its behavior was constrained by contextual information. However, Kawamoto was able to examine the activation of different pronunciations over time (i.e., processing cycles). Initially the information associated with both alternative senses of the homograph was activated, even in "biasing" contexts. Later, the biasing contextual information was used to boost the activation of one meaning and suppress the alternatives. Thus, the model produced the multiple access pattern even though the system was not modular. This demonstration was important. However, it also raised additional questions. The *sine qua non* of interactive systems is their ability to rapidly exploit "soft," probabilistic constraints (Rumelhart, Hinton, & McClelland, 1986). The context *John began to* . . . might be seen as providing strongly biasing contextual information insofar as only one meaning of the target *tire* forms a grammatical continuation of the sentence. In Kawamoto's model, this constraint was too weak to overcome the initial bottom–up activation of both primary senses of *tire*. Yet one could imagine changing parameters in the model so as to magnify the effects of context, producing the selective access outcome.

B. Priming Effects

With these developments, attention began to move away from the broad question as to whether the lexicon is modular or interactive, and toward issues concerning the kinds of information that are provided by natural language contexts, how these types of information are represented, the mechanisms by which different sources of information are combined, and the factors that determine whether a given type of information does or does not influence lexical processing.

Consider, for example, the semantic priming phenomenon. Semantic priming is an effect: it refers to the fact that responses to a target word such as *nurse* are facilitated when preceded by a semantically or associatively related priming word (e.g., *hospital, doctor,* respectively). The effect has been widely studied, and it has found a broad range of applications. However, twenty years after its discovery, the effect is remarkably poorly understood. There are two completely dissimilar theories of the bases of these effects: spreading activation (Collins & Loftus, 1975; MacNamara, 1992) and the compound cue theory of Ratcliff and McKoon (1988). There has been considerable focus on how the magnitude of the effect varies as a function of experimental factors such as task, stimulus onset asynchrony and the proportion of related items (e.g., de Groot, 1984; Neely, 1977;

Seidenberg, Waters, Sanders, & Langer, 1984), but the types of semantic relations that reliably elicit priming effects are not known. Valiant attempts to address this question yielded little information; see, for example, Hodgson (1991) who found similar, small priming effects for several types of prime-target relations (e.g., synonyms, category-exemplar pairs, coordinate members of a category). Notice what a problem this creates for addressing the modularity question. Following Forster (1979), semantic priming effects have been seen as intralexical and therefore compatible with modularity. Yet because the scope of these effects has not been independently established, it cannot be determined whether the context effect in any given study is or is not due to semantic priming. Moreover, studies by Foss (1982) and Williams (1988) called into question whether semantic priming plays any role in sentence processing. Williams (1988), for example, found that whereas primes such as *cup* prime associated targets such as *saucer,* these effects do not obtain when the prime appears in a meaningful sentence context:

The doctor planted the seeds in an old cup. SAUCER

One step toward a theory of lexical processing that might explain priming and other types of contextual effects is provided by connectionist models in which semantic information is represented in terms of microfeatures (Hinton, 1981). Thus, Hinton and Shallice (1991) and Plaut and Shallice (1993) showed that errors in deep dyslexia could be explained in terms of simple assumptions about such distributed representations of meaning. McRae, de Sa, and Seidenberg (1994) provide the beginnings of an account of semantic priming effects in terms of an explicit computational theory of lexical representation. McRae et al. obtained feature norms from undergraduate subjects, which provide estimates of the features associated with concepts (e.g., *tiger: stripes, fur*) and their relative salience (*stripes:* very salient; *fur:* less salient). The norms were then used to construct stimuli for semantic priming experiments. For example, prime–target pairs consisting of a concept such as *tiger* and a feature such as *stripes* produced significant priming effects, and the magnitude of the effect was related to the degree of salience indicated by the norms. More interesting, the priming effect for a feature was boosted if the feature was itself highly correlated with other features also true of the concept. Thus, the feature *fur* gets a boost because it is correlated with features such as *tail* and *claws*. In addition, McRae et al. had some success in predicting the magnitudes of priming effects for "semantically related" concepts such as *car–train* and *tiger–bear*. For artifacts such as vehicles, the magnitude of the priming effect was related to the number of features shared by the prime and target. For biological kinds such as animals, effect size was related to the extent to which the prime and target overlapped in terms of intercorrelated features. This reflects the fact that biological kinds have more intercorrelated features than do artifacts (Keil, 1981). Finally, McRae et al. simulated these effects using a connectionist network (a modified Hopfield net) that learned to compute semantic features for concepts from orthographic input.

McRae et al. account for semantic priming effects in terms of different types and degrees of featural overlap between primes and targets. The effects in their studies may be related to phenomena identified by Tabossi (1988a, 1988b) concerning the effects of sentence contexts on word processing. Tabossi has conducted studies examining the effects of contextual information on the processing of both ambiguous and unambiguous words. She has been able to construct sentence contexts that yield "selective access" for ambiguous words (i.e., activation of only the contextually appropriate meaning). Her account of these effects is that the contexts affect the target words by activating some of their semantic features. Thus, the context *The violent hurricane did not damage the ships that were in the port, one of the best equipped along the coast* is thought to focus on features associated with the "dock" meaning of *port*. In both the Tabossi and McRae et al. accounts, contexts exert effects via the semantic features of an affected word.

These findings provide a basis for re-establishing the link between semantic priming and sentence context effects that had been broken by the Foss and Williams studies, but further data are needed before they can be taken as more than suggestive. Nonetheless, these studies suggest that it may be possible to explain at least some context effects in terms of relatedness of semantic features. This is a promising development.

C. Context Effects in a Unified Theory of Lexical and Syntactic Ambiguity Resolution

At roughly the same time as word recognition research became focused on the autonomy question, sentence processing research (studies of "parsing" operations in language comprehension) began to focus on a similar issue. Frazier and her colleagues (e.g., Ferreira & Clifton, 1986; Frazier, 1979; Frazier & Rayner, 1982) developed the view that the parser (syntactic analyzer) is an autonomous processing subsystem, guided by a principle called Minimal Attachment. This principle comes into play in resolving syntactic ambiguities that arise in sentences such as *John put the book on the table away* and *John saw the cop with binoculars*. Numerous empirical studies addressed whether contextual information could or could not override Minimal Attachment (see, e.g., Ferreira & Clifton, 1986; Trueswell, Tanenhaus, & Garnsey, 1994).

The studies of lexical and syntactic ambiguity resolution suggested that they are resolved by very different mechanisms (see Table 4). With respect to lexical ambiguity, the alternative meanings of words were thought to be

TABLE 4   Characteristics of Lexical and Syntactic Ambiguity Resolution

Lexical ambiguity	Syntactic ambiguity
Multiple alternatives initially considered	Single alternative initially considered
Parallel processing	Serial processing
Capacity free	Capacity limited
Context used to select appropriate meaning	Context used to confirm analysis or guide reanalysis
Meanings are stored and accessed	Syntactic structures constructed by rule

stored in memory and "accessed" in processing. Multiple meanings are initially accessed in parallel, with contextual information used shortly afterward to select the relevant one and suppress all alternatives. It was assumed that multiple meanings could be accessed in parallel because this process is automatic and capacity free (in the sense of Posner & Snyder, 1975, and others).

Syntactic ambiguity resolution has been viewed quite differently. According to Frazier and her colleagues' theory (Frazier, 1987; see also Chapter 1, this volume), the first stage in the comprehension process is the computation of the basic syntax (phrase structure) of the input. This analysis is the responsibility of a parser thought to have the capacity to compute only a single analysis at a time. The system is modular and therefore has access only to information about the grammatical categories of words (e.g., Determiner, Adjective, Noun, Verb), not their meanings. When the sequence of categories that the parser is analyzing is compatible with multiple phrase structure analyses, the path it follows is determined by the Minimal Attachment processing strategy, according to which the preferred syntactic interpretation is the syntactically simpler one, where simplicity is indexed by the number of nodes in a phrase structure tree. Other processing subsystems subsequently either confirm the initial syntactic analysis or detect anomalies, initiating a reanalysis. Frazier introduced a second parsing principle, Late Closure, that prevails in cases where Minimal Attachment does not adjudicate between two alternative analyses. The Late Closure principle also dictates that only a single analysis will be pursued.

Many of the differences between the lexical and syntactic ambiguity resolution mechanisms summarized in Table 4 derive from assumptions about the types of knowledge involved in each domain (Frazier, 1987; see also Chapter 1, this volume). Lexical ambiguity was thought to involve meanings that are stored in the lexicon. Processing involved accessing this information automatically and in parallel. Syntactic structures, in contrast, were thought to be constructed on the basis of grammatical rules rather than stored directly in memory. This computation is assumed to place demands on working memory and attentional resources that are limited in capacity. Because of these limitations, the parser can pursue only a single analysis at a time.

These views of lexical and syntactic ambiguity resolution have been called into question by developments in three areas. First, there is the fact that there were unexpected effects of context in both domains. In the lexical domain, there were studies that yielded selective access of meaning in biasing contexts (e.g., Simpson & Krueger, 1991). In the syntactic domain, there were studies in which biasing contextual information led subjects to pursue parses that were not the ones predicted by Minimal Attachment (e.g., Trueswell et al., 1994). Second, there were studies in both domains suggesting that frequency of alternatives plays an important role in ambiguity resolution (e.g., Duffy et al., 1988; MacDonald, 1993; Taraban & McClelland, 1987). Trueswell & Tanenhaus, 1991). Finally, several developments served to undermine the distinction between "accessing" a meaning and "computing" a syntactic structure. Connectionist models, as we have seen, abandon the concept of lexical entries that are accessed in word recognition. In contrast, most syntactic theories have abandoned the phrase structure rules that were the basis of parsing principles such as Minimal Attachment in favor of lexically based representations.

These developments have led to a view that provides a unified account of both lexical and syntactic ambiguity resolutions (for overviews, see Mac-Donald, Pearlmutter, & Seidenberg, 1994a, 1994b; Trueswell & Tanenhaus, in press; Tanenhaus & Trueswell, Chapter 7, this volume). The basic claim is that both lexical and syntactic ambiguity are governed by the same types of knowledge representations and processing mechanisms. As just noted, similar empirical, theoretical, and methodological issues have arisen in both the lexical and syntactic domains. The unified view suggests that these parallels between the domains derive from the fact that the syntactic ambiguities in question are based on ambiguities at the lexical level. The same ambiguity resolution mechanisms apply in both domains because both involve ambiguities over various types of lexical representations. Thus, for example, the main verb/reduced relative ambiguity that was the focus of numerous studies of Minimal Attachment (e.g., *The evidence examined by the lawyer was unconvincing;* Ferreira & Clifton, 1986) derives from ambiguities associated with the lexical item *examined*. The lexical representation for *examined* is assumed to contain information about more than just its spelling, sound, and meaning. The word is ambiguous in at least three other ways. First, there is an ambiguity of tense morphology: the -ed ending on the ambiguous verb is interpreted as a past tense in the main verb interpretation and as a past participle in the reduced relative interpretation. Second, there is an argument structure ambiguity: the reduced relative interpretation requires the transitive argument structure, whereas the main verb interpretation may take a variety of structures, transitive, intransitive, and so on. Finally, there is a voice ambiguity: the verb is interpreted in active voice in the main verb structure, passive in reduced relative.

Thus, whereas the "lexical ambiguity" studies examined ambiguities over one level of lexical representation, semantics, the "syntactic ambiguity" studies examined ambiguities over other levels of lexical representation. The "syntactic" ambiguities should then be affected by factors, such as the relative frequencies of alternatives, that have been shown to be relevant to "lexical" ambiguity resolution. MacDonald et al. (in press-a, b) summarize a broad range of evidence derived from studies of several types of syntactic ambiguities consistent with this prediction.

This view also provides a framework for thinking about contextual effects. According to MacDonald et al., contexts can be defined in terms of the extent to which they provide information relevant to resolving ambiguities at different levels of lexical structure. In Tabossi's (1988a, 1988b) studies of meaning ambiguity, for example, the contexts were informative because (by hypothesis) they provided information relevant to resolving ambiguities at the semantic level. Other contexts might be informative insofar as they provide evidence concerning tense, voice, argument structure, or any other level of lexical representation over which ambiguities are defined. The cues that figure centrally in the Bates and MacWhinney (1989) Competition Model can be construed in the same way. A cue is effective to the extent that it provides information relevant to resolving ambiguities at different levels of lexical representation.

These theoretical developments serve to increase the importance of the questions concerning word recognition in and out of context. The central issues in language comprehension research become the ones that have been the focus of lexical processing research for many years: what is the nature of lexical knowledge, how is this information represented in memory and used in recognizing words, what is the role of contextual information in recognition? But whereas word recognition research has focused on questions concerning orthography, phonology, and meaning, the sentence processing research introduces a much enriched conception of the lexicon in which it encodes all types of knowledge associated with words, as well as grammatical and probabilistic relationships among these types of knowledge. With this enriched conception of the lexicon in hand, word recognition research will continue to further the understanding of language comprehension.

Acknowledgments

Visual word recognition is an enormous field and I have not been able to discuss all the relevant issues or studies that might have been included in a longer article. Balota (1994) reviews many empirical phenomena not discussed here; Raichle & Posner (1994) discuss the evidence concerning brain bases of lexical representations; and the papers in Gough, Ehri and

Treiman (1992) provide an overview of reading acquisition and dyslexia research. My own research, including the preparation of this article, was supported by grants from NIMH (MH47556) and NIA (AG10109), which is gratefully acknowledged. The division of labor issue has been kicking around in discussions with Jay McClelland, David Plaut, and Karalyn Patterson for several years; this article is not a faithful transcription of those discussions but was greatly influenced by them. Michael Tanenhaus and Maryellen MacDonald also contributed greatly to my understanding of issues discussed herein, and I thank them. I am especially grateful to Karalyn Patterson for enormously helpful feedback on an earlier version.

Endnotes

1. Fingerspelling in sign languages also involves recognizing letters, although under different conditions than those in reading.
2. The implemented model was greatly simplified compared to the system illustrated in Figure 2. For example, practical limitations on computational resources at the time precluded implementing any of the feedback mechanisms that were envisioned. They have begun to be examined in subsequent work, however (e.g., Plaut, McClelland, Seidenberg, & Patterson, in press).
3. In order to be fully comparable to MP, the model would also have to pronounce nonwords more accurately, but as Plaut et al. (in press) show, that can be achieved by using an improved phonological representation.
4. Note that there are additional questions of fact that must be addressed before accepting either of these accounts. It could turn out, for example, that deep dyslexics really do have impairments in multiple components of the lexical system. This might be revealed, perhaps, by deficits on other tasks involving each of the impaired components. The fact that the deficits co-occur might be due to neuroanatomical caprice. The Plaut, Hinton, and Shallice account of deep dyslexia could be elegant but nonetheless incorrect. What their account does do is call into question the dual-route account and provide an alternative to it. Of course, it might also happen to be correct.
5. There is one other form of acquired dyslexia that has been widely studied within the dual-route approach, phonological dyslexia (Beauvois & Dérouesné, 1979). These patients are able to read words aloud correctly; when asked to read nonwords such as *mave* they typically either fail to respond or produce a lexicalization error (e.g., *move*). The dual-route model explains this pattern in terms of damage to the nonlexical spelling-sound rules with a preserved lexical naming mechanism (Coltheart, 1987). The connectionist account of this pattern is largely the same: damage to the OP mechanism produces errors on nonwords, which cannot be named by means of the intact OSP. The models differ insofar as the dual-route account includes a third, lexical but nonsemantic pronunciation mechanism (Schwartz et al., 1980). This additional route predicts that there could be a patient who (1) names words correctly, (2) does not know their meanings, and (3) cannot name nonwords. The patient reported by Funnell (1983) is said to fit this pattern. However, the patient's semantics, while impaired, was still at least partially intact. Thus, the extent to which OSP might have supported word naming is difficult to assess.

References

Adams, M. (1990). *Beginning to read*. Cambridge, MA: MIT Press.
Allport, D. A., & Funnel, E. (1981). Components of the mental lexicon. *Philosophical Transactions of the Royal Society of London, Series B 295*, 397–410.
Anderson, R. C., & Ortony, A. (1975). On putting apples into bottles: A problem of polysemy. *Cognitive Psychology, 7*, 167–180.

Badecker, W., & Caramazza, A. (in press). Morphology and aphasia. In A. Zwicky & A. Spencer (Eds.), *Handbook of morphology*. Oxford: Blackwell.

Balota, D. A. (1990). The role of meaning in word recognition. In D. A. Balota, G. B. Flores d'Arcais, & K. Rayner (Eds.), *Comprehension processes in reading*. Hillsdale, NJ: Erlbaum.

Balota, D. (1994). Word recognition: The journey from features to meaning. In M. Gernsbacher (Ed.), *Handbook of psycholinguistics* (pp. 303–358). San Diego: Academic Press.

Balota, D. A., & Chumbley, J. I. (1984). Are lexical decisions a good measure of lexical access? The role of word frequency in the neglected decision stage. *Journal of Experimental Psychology: Human Perception and Performance, 10,* 340–357.

Barclay, J. R., Bransford, J. D., Franks, J. J., McCarrell, N. S., & Nitsch, K. (1974). Comprehensive and semantic flexibility. *Journal of Verbal Learning and Verbal Behavior, 13,* 471–481.

Barsalou, L. W. (1987). *The instability of graded structure: Implications for the nature of concepts.* Cambridge, UK: Cambridge University Press.

Bates, E., & MacWhinney, B. (1989). Functionalism and the competition model. In B. MacWhinney & E. Bates (Eds.), *The crosslinguistic study of sentence processing.* Cambridge, UK: Cambridge University Press.

Beauvois, M. F, & Dérouesné, J. (1979). Phonological alexia: Three dissociations. *Journal of Neurology, Neurosurgery, and Psychiatry, 42,* 1115–1124.

Berko, J. (1958). The child's learning of English morphology. *Word, 14,* 150–177.

Besner, D., Twilley, L., McCann, R., & Seergobin, K. (1990). On the connection between connectionism and data: Are a few words necessary? *Psychological Review, 97,* 432–446.

Bradley, L., & Bryant, P. E. (1985). *Rhyme and reason in reading and spelling.* Ann Arbor: University of Michigan Press.

Bub, D., Cancelliere, A., & Kertesz, A. (1985). Whole-word and analytic translation of spelling to sound in a non-semantic reading. In J. C. Marshall, M. Coltheart, & K. Patterson (Eds.), *Surface dyslexia.* London: Erlbaum.

Burgess, C. Tanenhaus, M. K., & Seidenberg, M. S. (1989). Context and lexical access: Implications of onword interference for lexical ambiguity resolution. *Journal of Experimental Psychology: Learning, Memory, and Cognition, 15,* 620–632.

Caramazza, A. (1984). The logic of neuropsychological research and the problem of patient classification in aphasia. *Brain and Language, 21,* 9–20.

Castles, A., & Coltheart, M. (1993). Varieties of developmental dyslexia. *Cognition, 47,* 149–180.

Chomsky, N. (1965). *Aspects of the theory of syntax.* Cambridge, MA: MIT Press.

Cohen, J. D., Dunbar, K., & McClelland, J. L. (1990). On the control of automatic processes: A parallel distributed processing account of the stroop effect. *Psychological Review, 97,* 332–361.

Collins, A., & Loftus, E. (1975). A spreading-activation theory of semantic processing. *Psychological Review, 82,* 407–428.

Coltheart, M. (1978). Lexical access in simple reading tasks. In G. Underwood (Ed.), *Strategies of information processing* (pp. 151–215). New York: Academic Press.

Coltheart, M. (1987). Introduction. in M. Coltheart, G. Sartori, & R. Job (Eds.), *Cognitive neuropsychology of language.* London: Erlbaum.

Coltheart, M., Besner, D., Jonasson, J., & Davelaar, E. (1979). Phonological recoding in the lexical decision task. *Quarterly Journal of Experimental Psychology, 31,* 489–508.

Coltheart, M., Curtis, B., Atkins, P., & Haller, M. (1993). Models of reading aloud: Dual-route and parallel distributed processing approaches. *Psychological Review, 100,* 589–608.

Coltheart, M., Patterson, K. E., & Marshall, J. C. (Eds.). (1980). *Deep dyslexia.* London: Routledge & Kegan Paul.

Daugherty, K., Petersen, A., MacDonald, M. M., & Seidenberg, M. (1993). Why no mere mortal has ever flown out to left field, but people often say they do. In *Proceedings of the Fifteenth annual meeting of the Cognitive Science Society.* Hillsdale, NJ: Erlbaum.

Daugherty, K., & Seidenberg, M. S. (1992). Rules or connection? The past tense revisited. In *Proceedings of the 14th annual meeting of the Cognitive Science Society*. Hillsdale, NJ: Erlbaum.

de Groot, A. M. B. (1984). Primed lexical decision: Combined effects of the proportion of related prime-target pairs and the stimulus-onset asynchrony of prime and target. *Quarterly Journal of Experimental Psychology, 36A,* 253–280.

Duffy, S. A., Morris, R. K., & Rayner, K. (1988). Lexical ambiguity and fixation times in reading. *Journal of Memory and Language, 27,* 429–226.

Ellis, A. W., & Young, A. W. (1988). *Human cognitive neuropsychology.* London: Erlbaum.

Ferreira, F., & Clifton, C. (1986). The independence of syntactic processing. *Journal of Memory and Language, 25,* 348–368.

Fischler, I., & Bloom, P. (1979). Automatic and attentional processes in the effects of sentence contexts on word recognition. *Journal of Verbal Learning and Verbal Behavior, 18,* 1–20.

Fodor, J. A. (1983). *Modularity of mind.* Cambridge, MA: MIT Press.

Forster, K. I. (1976). Accessing the mental lexicon. In E. W. Walker & R. J. Wales (Eds.), *New approaches to language mechanisms.* Amsterdam: North-Holland.

Forster, K. I. (1979). Levels of processing and the structure of the language processor. In W. Cooper & E. Walker (Eds.), *Sentence processing: Psycholinguistic studies* presented to Merrill Garrett. Hillsdale, NJ: Erlbaum.

Foss, D. (1982). A discourse on semantic priming. *Cognitive Psychology, 14,* 590–607.

Francis, W. N., & Kucera, H. (1982). *Frequency analysis of English usage: Lexicon and grammar.* Boston: Houghton Mifflin.

Frazier, L. (1979). *On comprehending sentences: Syntactic parsing strategies.* Bloomington: Indiana University Linguistics Club.

Frazier, L. (1987). Sentence processing; A tutorial review. In M. Coltheart (Ed.), *Attention and performance XII: The psychology of reading.* Hillsdale, NJ: Erlbaum.

Frazier, L., & Rayner, K. (1982). Making and correcting errors during sentence comprehension: Eye movements in the analysis of structurally ambiguous sentences. *Cognitive Psychology, 14,* 178–210.

Frost, R., & Bentin, S. (1992). Reading consonants and guessing vowels: Visual word recognition in Hebrew orthography. In R. Frost & L. Katz (Eds.), *Orthography, phonology, morphology, and meaning.* Amsterdam: North-Holland.

Frost, R., & Katz, L. (Eds.). (1992). *Orthography, phonology, morphology, and meaning.* Amsterdam: North-Holland.

Frost, R., Katz, L., & Bentin, S. (1987). Strategies for visual word recognition and orthographical depth: A multilingual comparison. *Journal of Experimental Psychology: Human Perception and Performance, 13,* 159–180.

Funnell, E. (1983). Phonological processes in reading: New evidence from acquired dyslexia. *British Journal of Psychology, 74,* 159–180.

Gilhooly, K. J., & Logie, R. H. (1980). Age-of-acquisition, imagery, concreteness, familiarity, and ambiguity measures for 1944 words. *Behavior Research Methods and Instrumentation, 12,* 395–427.

Glucksberg, S., Kreuz, R. J., & Rho, S. (1986). Context can constrain lexical access: Implications for models of language comprehension. *Journal of Experimental Psychology: Learning, Memory, and Cognition, 12,* 323–335.

Glushko, R. J. (1979). The organization and activation of orthographic knowledge in reading aloud. *Journal of Experimental Psychology: Human Perception and Performance, 5,* 674–691.

Goodman, K. (1968). Reading: A psycholinguistic guessing game. *Journal of the Reading Specialist, 6,* 126–135.

Gough, P. Ehri, L., & Treiman, R. (1992). *Reading acquisition.* Hillsdale, NJ: Erlbaum.

Henderson, L. (1982). *Orthography and word recognition in reading.* London: Academic Press.

Henderson, L. (1985). Issues in the modelling of pronunciation assembly in normal reading. In J. C. Marshall, M. Coltheart, & K. Patterson (Eds.), *Surface dyslexia.* London: Erlbaum.

Hinton, G. E. (1981). Implementing semantic networks in parallel hardware. In G. Hinton & J. A. Anderson (Eds.), *Parallel models of associative memory*. Hillsdale, NJ: Erlbaum.

Hinton, G. E. (1986). Learning distributed representations of concepts. In *Proceedings of the Eighth annual conference of the Cognitive Science Society* (pp. 1–12). Hillsdale, NJ: Erlbaum.

Hinton, G. E., McClelland, J. L., & Rumelhart, D. E. (1986). Distributed representations. In D. E. Rumelhart & J. L. McClelland (Eds.), *Parallel distributed processing* (Vol. 1). Cambridge, MA: MIT Press.

Hinton, G. E., & Shallice, T. (1991). Lesioning an attractor network: Investigations of acquired dyslexia. *Psychological Review, 98*, 74–95.

Hochberg, J. (1970). Components of literacy. In H. Levin & J. P. Williams (Eds.), *Basic studies in reading*. New York: Basic Books.

Hodgson, J. M. (1991). Informational constraints on pre-lexical priming. *Language and Cognitive Processes, 6*, 169–264.

James, C. T. (1975). The role of semantic information in lexical decisions. *Journal of Experimental Psychology: Human Perception and Performance, 104*, 130–135.

Jared, D., McRae, K., & Seidenberg, M. S. (1990). The basis of consistency effects in word naming. *Journal of Memory and Language, 29*, 687–715.

Jared, D., & Seidenberg, M. S. (1991). Does word recognition proceed from spelling to sound to meaning? *Journal of Experimental Psychology: General, 120*, 358–394.

Jorm, A., & Share, D. (1983). Phonological recoding and reading acquisition. *Applied Psycholinguistics, 4*, 103–147.

Katz, L., & Feldman, L. B. (1981). Linguistic coding in word recognition: Comparisons between a deep and a shallow orthography. In A. M. Lesgold & C. A. Perfetti (Eds.), *Interactive processes in reading*. Hillsdale, NJ: Erlbaum.

Kawamoto, A. (1986). A connectionist model of lexical ambiguity resolution. In G. Cottrell, S. Small, & M. Tanenhaus (Eds.), *Lexical ambiguity resolution*. New York: Morgan Kauffman.

Kawamoto, A. (1993). A model of lexical ambiguity resolution. *Journal of Memory and Language, 32*, 474–516.

Keenan, J. M., Potts, G. R., Golding, J. M., & Jennings, T. M. (1990). Which elaborative inferences are drawn during reading? In D. A. Balota, G. B. Flores d'Arcais, & K. Rayner (Eds.), *Comprehension processes in reading*. Hillsdale, NJ: Erlbaum.

Keil, F. (1981). Constraints on knowledge and cognitive development. *Psychological Review, 88*, 197–227.

Kolers, P. A. (1975). Specificity of operations in sentence recognition. *Cognitive Psychology, 7*, 289–306.

Kucera, H., & Francis, W. N. (1967). *A computational analysis of present-day American English*. Providence, RI: Brown University Press.

Lesch, M. F., & Pollatsek, A. (1993). Automatic access of semantic information by phonological codes in visual word recognition. *Journal of Experimental Psychology: Learning, Memory, and Cognition, 19*, 285–294.

Liberman, I. Y., & Shankweiler, D. (1979). Speech, the alphabet, and teaching to read. In L. B. Resnick & P. A. Weaver (Eds.), *Theory and practice of early reading* (Vol. 2). Hillsdale, NJ: Erlbaum.

Lima, S., & Pollatsek, A. (1983). Lexical access via an orthographic code? *Journal of Verbal Learning and Verbal Behavior, 22*, 310–332.

Lukatela, G., Popadič, D., Ognjenović, P., & Turvey, M. T. (1980). Lexical decision in phonologically shallow orthography. *Memory & Cognition, 8*, 124–132.

Lukatela, G., & Turvey, M. (1980). Some experiments on the Roman and Cyrillic alphabets of Serbo-Croatian. In J. F. Kavanagh & R. L. Venezky (Eds.), *Orthography, reading and dyslexia*. Baltimore: University Park Press.

Lukatela, G., & Turvey, M. (1994). Visual lexical access is initially phonology. I. *Journal of Experimental Psychology: General, 123*, 107–128.

MacDonald, M. C. (1993). The interaction of lexical and syntactic ambiguity. *Journal of Memory and Language, 32,* 692–715.

MacDonald, M. C., Pearlmutter, N., & Seidenberg, M. S. (1994a). The lexical nature of syntactic ambiguity resolution. *Psychological Review, 101,* 676–703.

MacDonald, M. C., Pearlmutter, N., & Seidenberg, M. S. (1994b). Syntactic ambiguity resolution as lexical ambiguity resolution. In C. Clifton, L. Frazier, & K. Rayner (Eds.), *Perspectives on sentence processing.* Hillsdale, NJ: Erlbaum.

MacNamara T. (1992). Priming and constraints it places on theories of memory and retrieval. *Psychological Review, 99,* 650–662.

Marshall, J. C., & Newcombe, F. (1973). Patterns of paralexia: A psycholinguistic approach. *Journal of Psycholinguistic Research, 2,* 175–199.

Marslen-Wilson, W. D. (1989). Access and integration: Projecting sound onto meaning. In W. D. Marslen-Wilson (Ed.), *Lexical representation and process.* Cambridge, MA: MIT Press.

Marslen-Wilson, W. D., Tyler, L. K., Waksler, R., & Older, L. (1994). Morphology and meaning in the English mental lexicon. *Psychological Review, 101,* 3–33.

McClelland, J. L., & Rumelhart, D. E. (1981). An interactive activation model of context effects in letter perception: Part 1. An account of basic findings. *Psychological Review, 86,* 287–330.

McCloskey, M. (1991). Networks and theories: The place of connectionism in cognitive science. *Psychological Science, 2,* 387–395.

McCusker, L. X., Hillinger, M. L., & Bias, R. G. (1981). Phonological recoding and reading. *Psychological Bulletin, 89,* 217–245.

McRae, K., de Sa, V., & Seidenberg, M. S. (1994). *The role of correlated properties in accessing conceptual memory.* Manuscript submitted for publication.

Merrill, E. C., Sperber, R. D., & MacCauley, C. (1981). Differences in semantic encoding as a function of reading comprehension skill. *Memory & Cognition, 9,* 618–624.

Meyer, D. E., & Schvaneveldt, R. (1971). Facilitation in recognizing pairs of words: Evidence of a dependence between retrieval operations. *Journal of Experimental Psychology, 90,* 227–234.

Meyer, D. E., Schvaneveldt, R. W., & Ruddy, M. G. (1974). Functions of graphemic and phonemic codes in visual word recognition. *Memory & Cognition, 2,* 309–321.

Monsell, S., & Patterson, K. E. (1992). *Voluntary surface dyslexia.* Paper presented at the meeting of the Experimental Psychology Society.

Monsell, S., Patterson, K. E., Graham, A., Hughes, C. H., & Milroy, R. (1992). Lexical and sublexical translation of spelling to sound: Strategic anticipation of lexical status. *Journal of Experimental Psychology: Learning, Memory, and Cognition, 18,* 452–467.

Morris, R. K. (1994). Lexical and message-level sentence context effects on fixation times in reading. *Journal of Experimental Psychology: Learning, Memory, and Cognition, 20,* 92–103.

Morton, J., & Patterson, K. E. (1980). A new attempt at an interpretation, or, an attempt at a new interpretation. In M. Coltheart, K. E. Patterson, & J. C. Marshall (Eds.), *Deep dyslexia.* London: Routledge & Kegan Paul.

Neely, J. H. (1977). Semantic priming and retrieval from lexical memory: Roles of inhibition-less spreading activation and limited capacity attention. *Journal of Experimental Psychology: General, 106,* 226–254.

Neisser, U. (1967). *Cognitive psychology.* New York: Appleton-Century-Crofts.

Norman, D. A., & Bobrow, D. G. (1975). On data-limited and resource-limited processes. *Cognitive Psychology, 7,* 44–64.

Paap, K., & Noel, R. W. (1989). Dual-route models of print to sound: Still a good horse race. *Psychological Research, 53,* 13–24.

Patterson, K. E. (1981). Neuropsychological approaches to the study of reading. *British Journal of Psychology, 72,* 151–174.

Patterson, K. E., & Coltheart, M. (1987). Phonological processes in reading: A tutorial review. In M. Coltheart (Ed.), *Attention and performance XII: The psychology of reading.* Hillsdale, NJ: Erlbaum.

Patterson, K. E., & Hodges, J. (1992). Deterioration of word meaning: Implications for reading. *Neuropsychologia, 30,* 1025–1040.

Patterson, K. E., Marshall, J. C., & Coltheart, M. (1985). General introduction. In J. C. Marshall, M. Coltheart, & K. E. Patterson (Eds.), *Surface dyslexia.* Hillsdale, NJ: Erlbaum.

Patterson, K. E., & Morton, J. (1985). From orthography to phonology: An attempt at an old interpretation. In K. E. Patterson, J. C. Marshall, & M. Coltheart (Eds.), *Surface dyslexia.* Hillsdale, NJ: Erlbaum.

Patterson, K. E., Seidenberg, M., & McClelland, J. (1989). Dyslexia in a distributed, developmental model of word recognition. In R. Morris (Ed.), *Parallel distributed processing.* Oxford: Oxford University Press.

Perfetti, C. A., Bell, L., & Delaney, S. (1988). Automatic phonetic activation in silent word reading: Evidence from backward masking. *Journal of Memory and Language, 27,* 59–70.

Pinker, S. (1991). Rules of language. *Science, 253,* 530–534.

Pinker, S. (1994). *The language instinct.* New York: Morrow.

Pinker, S., & Prince, A. (1988). On language and connectionism: Analysis of a parallel distributed processing model of language acquisition. *Cognition, 28,* 73–194.

Plaut, D. C., & McClelland, J. L. (1993). Generalization with componential attractors: Word and nonword reading in an attractor network. In *proceedings of the 15th annual Conference of the Cognitive Science Society.* Hillsdale, NJ: Erlbaum.

Plaut, D. C., McClelland, J. L., Seidenberg, M. S., & Patterson, K. E. (in press). Understanding normal and impaired word reading: Computational principles in quasiregular domains. *Psychological Review.*

Plaut, D. C., & Shallice, T. (1993). Deep dyslexia: A case study of connectionist neuropsychology. *Cognitive Neuropsychology, 10,* 377–500.

Pollatsek, A., Lesch, M., Morris, R., & Rayner, K. (1992). Phonological codes are used in integrating information across saccades in word identification and reading. *Journal of Experimental Psychology: Human Perception and Performance, 18,* 148–162.

Posner, M., & Snyder, C. R. (1975). Attention and cognitive control. In R. L. Solso (Ed.), *Information processing and cognition: The Loyola Symposium.* Hillsdale, NJ: Erlbaum.

Raichle, M. E., & Posner, M. I. (1994). *Images of mind.* San Francisco: Freeman.

Ratcliff, R., & McKoon, G. (1988). A retrieval theory of priming in semantic memory. *Psychological Review, 95,* 385–408.

Rubenstein, H., Lewis, S. S., & Rubenstein, M. A. (1971). Evidence for phonemic recoding in visual word recognition. *Journal of Verbal Learning and Verbal Behavior, 10,* 645–657.

Rumelhart, D. E. (1977). Toward an interactive model of reading. In S. Dornic (Ed.), *Attention and performance VI.* Hillsdale, NJ: Erlbaum.

Rumelhart, D. E., Hinton, G. E., & McClelland, J. L. (1986). A general framework for parallel distribution processing. In D. E. Rumelhart & J. L. McClelland (Eds.), *Parallel distributed processing: Vol. 1. Explorations in the microstructure of cognition.* Cambridge, MA: MIT Press.

Rumelhart, D. E., & McClelland, J. L. (1986). On learning the past tenses of English verbs. In J. L. McClelland & D. Rumelhart (Eds.), *Parallel distributed processing: Vol. 2. Explorations in the microstructure of cognition.* Cambridge, MA: MIT Press.

Schank, R., & Abelson, R. (1977). *Scripts, plans, goals, and understanding.* Hillsdale, NJ: Erlbaum.

Schwanenflugel, P. J., & Shoben, E. J. (1985). The influence of sentence constraint on the scope of facilitation for upcoming words. *Journal of Memory and Language, 24,* 232–252.

Schwartz, M., Saffran, E., & Marin, O. (1980). Fractionating the reading process in dementia: Evidence for word-specific print-to-sound associations. In M. Coltheart, K. E. Patterson, & J. C. Marshall (Eds.), *Deep dyslexia.* London: Routledge & Kegan Paul.

Seidenberg, M. S. (1985). The time course of information activation and utilization in visual word recognition. In D. Besner, T. G. Waller, & E. M. MacKinnon (Eds.), *Reading research: Advances in theory and practice* (Vol. 5). New York: Academic Press.

Seidenberg, M. S. (1987). Sublexical structures in visual and word recognition: Access units or orthographic redundancy? In M. Coltheart (Ed.), *Attention and performance XII: The psychology of reading*. Hillsdale, NJ: Erlbaum.

Seidenberg, M. S. (1988). Cognitive neuropsychology and language: The state of the art. *Cognitive Neuropsychology, 5,* 403–426.

Seidenberg, M. S. (1989). Word recognition and naming: A computational model and its implications. In W. D. Marlsen-Wilson (Ed.), *Lexical representation and process*. Cambridge, MA: MIT Press.

Seidenberg, M. S. (1990). Lexical access: Another theoretical soupstone? In D. Balota, G. Florais d'Arcais, & K. Rayner (Eds.), *Comprehension processes in reading*. Hillsdale, NJ: Erlbaum.

Seidenberg, M. S. (1992). Dyslexia in a computational model of word recognition in reading. In P. Gough, L. Ehri, & R. Treiman (Eds.), *Reading acquisition* (pp. 243–274). Hillsdale, NJ: Erlbaum.

Seidenberg, M. S. (1993). Connectionist models and cognitive theory. *Psychological Science, 4,* 228–235.

Seidenberg, M. S. (in press). Lexical morphology. In M. A. Arbib (Ed.), *Handbook of brain theory and neural networks*. Cambridge, MA: MIT Press.

Seidenberg, M. S., & McClelland, J. L. (1989). A distributed, developmental model of word recognition and naming. *Psychological Review, 96,* 447–452.

Seidenberg, M. S., Plaut, D. C., Petersen, A., McClelland, J. L., & McRae, K. (1994). Nonword pronunciation and models of word recognition. *Journal of Experimental Psychology: Human Perception and Performance, 20,* 1177–1196.

Seidenberg, M. S., Waters, G. S., Barnes, M. A., & Tanenhaus, M. K. (1984). When does irregular spelling or pronunciation influence word recognition? *Journal of Verbal Learning and Verbal Behavior, 23,* 383–404.

Seidenberg, M. S., Waters, G. S., Sanders, M., & Langer, P. (1984). Pre- and post-lexical loci of contextual effects on word recognition. *Memory & Cognition, 12,* 315–328.

Shallice, T. (1988). *From neuropsychology to mental structure*. Cambridge, UK: Cambridge University Press.

Shulman, H. G., Hornak, R., & Sanders, E. (1978). The effects of graphemic, phonetic, and semantic relationships on access to lexical structures. *Memory & Cognition, 6,* 115–123.

Simpson, G. B. (1981). Lexical ambiguity and its role in models of word recognition. *Psychological Bulletin, 96,* 316–340.

Simpson, G. B., & Krueger, M. A. (1991). Selective access of homograph meanings in sentence context. *Journal of Memory and Language, 30,* 627–643.

Spiro, R., Bruce, B., & Brewer, W. (1980). *Theoretical issues in reading comprehension*. Hillsdale, NJ: Erlbaum.

Stanovich, K., & West, R. (1979). Mechanisms of sentence context effects in reading: Automatic activation and conscious attention. *Memory & Cognition, 7,* 77–85.

Strain, E., Patterson, K. E., & Seidenberg, M. S. (in press). Semantic effects in single-word naming. *Journal of Experimental Psychology: Learning, Memory, and Cognition.*

Swinney, D. A. (1979). Lexical access during sentence comprehension: (Re)consideration of context effects. *Journal of Verbal Learning and Verbal Behavior, 18,* 645–659.

Tabossi, P. (1988a). Accessing lexical ambiguity in different types of sentential contexts. *Journal of Memory and Language, 27,* 324–340.

Tabossi, P. (1988b). Effects of context on the immediate interpretation of unambiguous nouns. *Journal of Experimental Psychology: Learning, Memory, and Cognition, 14,* 153–162.

Taft, M. (1979). Lexical access via an orthographic code: The basic orthographic syllable structure (BOSS). *Journal of Verbal Learning and Verbal Behavior, 18,* 21–39.

Taft, M. (1987). Morphographic processing: The BOSS re-emerges. In M. Coltheart (Ed.), *Attention and performance XII: The psychology of reading*. London: Erlbaum.

Taft, M., & Forster, K. (1975). Lexical storage and retrieval of prefixed words. *Journal of Verbal Learning and Verbal Behavior, 14*, 638–647.

Tanenhaus, M. K., Flanigan, H., & Seidenberg, M. S. (1980). Orthographic and phonological code activation in auditory and visual word recognition. *Memory & Cognition, 8*, 513–520.

Tanenhaus, M. K., Leiman, J., & Seidenberg, M. S. (1979). Evidence for multiple stages in the processing of ambiguous words in syntactic contexts. *Journal of Verbal Learning and Verbal Behavior, 18*, 427–440.

Taraban, R., & McClelland, J. L. (1987). Conspiracy effects in word recognition. *Journal of Memory and Language, 26*, 608–631.

Treiman, R. (1992). The role of intrasyllabic units in learning to read and spell. In P. Gough, L. Ehri, & R. Treiman (Eds.), *Reading acquisition*. Hillsdale, NJ: Erlbaum.

Trueswell, J. C., & Tanenhaus, M. K. (1991). Tense, temporal context and syntactic ambiguity resolution. *Language and Cognitive Processes, 6*, 339–350.

Trueswell, J. C., & Tanenhaus, M. K. (1994). Toward a lexicalist framework of constraint-based syntactic ambiguity resolution. In C. Clifton, L. Frazier, & K. Rayner (Eds.), *Perspectives on sentence processing*. Hillsdale, NJ: Erlbaum.

Trueswell, J. C., Tanenhaus, M. K., & Garnsey, S. M. (1994). Semantic influences on parsing: Use of thematic role information in syntactic disambiguation. *Journal of Memory and Language, 33*, 285–318.

Turvey, M. T., Feldman, L. B., & Lukatela, G. (1984). The Serbo-Croatian orthography constrains the reader to a phonologically analytic strategy. In L. Henderson (Ed.), *Orthographies and reading*. London: Erlbaum.

Van Orden, G. C. (1987). A ROWS is a ROSE: Spelling, sound and reading. *Memory & Cognition, 15*, 181–198.

Van Orden, G. C., & Goldinger, S. D. (1994). Interdependence of form and function in cognitive systems explains perception of printed words. *Journal of Experimental Psychology: Human Perception and Performance, 20*, 1269–1291.

Van Orden, G. C., Johnston, J. C., & Hale, B. L. (1988). Word identification in reading proceeds from the spelling to sound to meaning. *Journal of Experimental Psychology: Learning, Memory, and Cognition, 14*, 371–386.

Van Orden, G. C., Pennington, B. F., & Stone, G. O. (1990). Word identification in reading and the promise of subsymbolic psycholinguistics. *Psychological Review, 97*, 488–522.

Wagner, R. K., & Torgesen, J. K. (1987). The nature of phonological processing and its causal role in the acquisition of reading skills. Psychological Bulletin, 101, 191–212.

Waters, G. S., Komoda, M., & Arbucke, T. Y. (1985). The effects of concurring tasks on reading: Implications for phonological recoding. *Journal of Memory and Language, 24*, 27–45.

Waters, G. S., & Seidenberg, M. S. (1985). Spelling-sound effects in reading: Time course and decision criteria. *Memory & Cognition, 13*, 557–572.

Williams, J. N. (1988). Constraints upon semantic activation during sentence comprehension. *Language and Cognitive Processes, 3*, 165–206.

Wydell, T. N., Patterson, K. E., & Humphreys, G. W. (1993). Phonologically mediated access to meaning for Kanji: Is a *Rows* still a *Rose* in Japanese Kanji? *Journal of Experimental Psychology: Learning, Memory, and Cognition, 18*, 491–514.

CHAPTER 6

Sentence Production: From Mind to Mouth

Kathryn Bock

I. TOWARD AN EXPLANATION OF LANGUAGE PRODUCTION

The study of sentence production is the study of how speakers turn messages into utterances. Messages are communicative intentions, the things a speaker means to convey. Utterances are verbal formulations. They may be complete sentences or fragments of sentences, well formed or errant, fluent or hesitant. To rephrase a famous formulation of Chomsky's (1965, p. 3), a theory of sentence production is concerned with real speakers who are vulnerable to memory limitations, distractions, shifts of attention and interest, and errors (random or characteristic) in applying their knowledge of the language.

The goal of a theory of sentence production is to explain how speakers use linguistic knowledge in the production of utterances. This requires a specification of the knowledge that speakers have and a specification of the information processing system in which the knowledge is put to use. Linguistic knowledge is a component of the speaker's long-term memory. As a practical matter, descriptions of language structure from linguistics are often taken as best guesses about the organization of speakers' knowledge of their language (see Frazier, Chapter 1, this volume). The chief issues in production therefore center on information processing, and include how and when the processing system retrieves different kinds of linguistic

Speech, Language, and Communication

knowledge, how the system uses the knowledge once it has been retrieved, how and when the system retrieves and uses nonlinguistic knowledge, and how the system is organized within and constrained by human cognitive capacities.

What is there to explain? Phenomenologically, talking is not hard. In a lecture delivered at the University of Illinois in 1909, Titchener claimed to be able to "read off what I have to say from a memory manuscript" (1909, p. 8), certainly caricaturing the usual experience, but perhaps not by much. Because of this apparent ease, the interesting problems of production are more readily appreciated, and most often studied, in terms of talk's typical failures.

The failures range widely. A psychologist reported a transient neurological episode in which he was able to form perfectly coherent messages, but could not express them:

> The thoughts can only be described in sentence-like form, because they were as complex, detailed, and lengthy as a typical sentence. They were not sentences, however. The experience was not one of merely being unable to articulate a word currently held in consciousness. Instead, it was one of being fully aware of the target *idea* yet totally unable to accomplish what normally feels like the single act of finding-and-saying-the-word. . . . The idea . . . was as complete and full as any idea one might have normally, but was not an unspoken mental sentence. . . . It was the unusual "gap" in this usually seamless process [of sentence production], a process taken completely for granted in normal circumstances, that amazes me. (Ashcraft, 1993, pp. 49, 54)

William James described the tip-of-the-tongue experience, in which a single circumscribed meaning comes to mind but the corresponding word does not:

> Suppose we try to recall a forgotten name. The state of our consciousness is peculiar. There is a gap therein: but no mere gap. It is a gap that is intensely active. A sort of wraith of the name is in it, beckoning us in a given direction, making us at moments tingle with the sense of our closeness, and then letting us sink back without the longed-for term. If wrong names are proposed to us, this singularly definite gap acts immediately so as to negate them. They do not fit into its mould. And the gap of one word does not feel like the gap of another, all empty of content as both might seem necessarily to be when described as gaps. (James, 1890, pp. 251–252)[1]

A professor on leave from his university, and looking forward to his return, expressed the opposite sentiment:

> "I miss being out of touch with academia."

A radio-talk-show host, querying a guest about a government official who was reportedly having an affair with a female subordinate, questioned the propriety of the official being "involved with someone who he works for."

A secretary, discussing the problems of home renovation and their depiction in a movie called "The Money Pit," said,

"Have you ever seen the money, 'The Movie Pit'?"

A lecturer, intending to make the point that verbs are inflected for number, said,

"The verb is afflicted for number."[2]

And finally, an umbrella-carrying colleague was asked,

"Is that your elevator?"

These cases and many others reveal that a lot can go wrong between the mind and the mouth. What a theory of sentence production has to explain, apart from such errors, is the course of events on those less notable but more frequent occasions when everything goes right.

When set against the backdrop of normal success in speech, failures of production hint at an information handling system of great complexity but considerable efficiency. Measurements of normal speech rates give average values of about 150 words/min (Maclay & Osgood, 1959) or 5.65 syllables/s (Deese, 1984). Yet syntactic errors are surprisingly rare. In a tape-recorded corpus of nearly 15,000 utterances, Deese (1984) counted only 77 syntactic anomalies, roughly one in every 195 utterances. Heeschen (in press) reported a similarly low incidence of syntactic errors in spoken German. Errors of lexical selection are even less common, with attested rates averaging under one per thousand words (Bock & Levelt, 1994).

Dysfluency is more pervasive, as is the jabberwocky most prominently associated with the 41st president of the United States:

> No, we've taken—we're taking steps to fund it. Because I think when you create more export market—OPIC—and that's exactly what it does—you create more jobs in this country. In this sick and anemic country, which has had—incidentally has grown for the last five [audio technical difficulties]—Hey, just a minute. I haven't finished yet. (remarks by George Bush in Collegeville, Pennsylvania, September 9, 1992)

Notoriety aside, dysfluency and jabberwocky must be distinguished from outright error. First, they can be consequences of changes to or uncertainty in the message, rather than disruptions in production mechanisms themselves (Goldman-Eisler, 1968; Schachter, Christenfeld, Ravina, & Bilous, 1991). Message uncertainty is more akin to a thinking problem than a talking problem. Second, dysfluency and jabberwocky both seem to display local well-formedness: dysfluencies typically interrupt or punctuate syntactically and phonologically well-formed stretches of speech (Levelt, 1983), and commonplace jabberwocky, like its literary namesake, is often syntactically well-formed at the same time that it is semantically or pragmatically incoherent.

This chapter surveys some contemporary views about the processes that produce the structural and lexical features of utterances, as well as errors and dysfluencies. The first section sketches a modal view of the processes of production as background for the second section, which highlights some current controversies. The third section looks at fluency and how it is linked to the information processing problems of production. The conclusion touches on some residual questions about the relationships between production and comprehension and between performance and competence.

The treatment of these things is too cursory to do them full justice. More comprehensive surveys and alternative analyses of some of the issues can be found in Levelt (1989) and Bock and Levelt (1994). Bock (1995) reviews the observational and experimental methods that are used in production research. For other topics, I offer directions to supplementary literature throughout the chapter.

II. AN ANALYSIS OF SENTENCE PRODUCTION

Behind most current work in language production there is a widely shared view about the broad outlines of the production system (for a divergent perspective, see McNeill, 1987). In this section I sketch those outlines, reserving until later a discussion of some of the disagreements that have developed within this framework.

Figure 1 gives an overview. It separates processing into three broad components, the message component, the grammatical component, and the phonological component. The vertical connections represent the staggered flow of information over time, with the message leading and phonological encoding trailing. The message captures features of the speaker's intended meaning and communicative perspective (see Clark and Bly, Chapter 11, this volume). The phonological component spells out the sound structure of the utterance, both in terms of the phonological segments of word forms and the prosody of larger units (see Cutler, Chapter 4, and Fowler, Chapter 2, this volume). In between lies the grammatical component. This is the heart of language production, serving to build the bridge from meaning to sound.

A. The Grammatical Component: An Overview

The processes within the grammatical component subdivide into *functional processing* and *positional processing*.[3] Functional processing associates message elements with grammatical functions on the one hand and with entries in the mental lexicon on the other. Positional processes associate grammatical

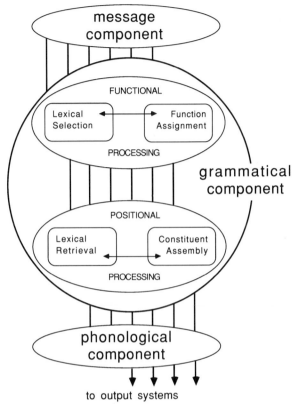

FIGURE 1   The components of the language production system (adapted from Bock & Levelt, 1994). The links among the components are staggered from left to right to represent the flow of information over time.

functions and lexical entries with sentence structures and word forms. Each of these subcomponents thus includes mechanisms that specify words or morphemes (lexical mechanisms) and mechanisms that create word order (structural mechanisms).

In functional processing, the lexical mechanism is lexical selection, which involves the identification of lexical entries that are suitable for conveying the speaker's meaning. These entries are often called *lemmas* in the production literature, and can be likened to the part of a dictionary entry that lists a word (i.e., indicates that an appropriate word exists) and gives its grammatical features. The structural mechanism is function assignment, which assigns and coordinates grammatical roles with features of lexical entries (ensuring, e.g., that the lexical entry destined to serve as the head of the subject phrase is a noun). Positional processing involves lexical retrieval (activating a schematic description of a word's phonological features) and the creation of a hierarchically structured, ordered set of word and morpheme slots (constituent assembly). In Dell's (1986) model, the lexical work is carried out in the lexical network and the structural work by *tactic frames*.

The grammatical component can be specified more concretely by going through the steps in generating a simple utterance and constructing problems or errors that might arise at each step. Suppose a speaker witnesses an event in which an unknown man gives a stick of licorice to a known boy. Later, in a conversation about the same boy, the speaker describes the event in this way: "A guy offered him some licorice." After the speaker had decided which features of the event to talk about (to encode in a message), what was required in order to convert the remembered event into this utterance?

1. Functional Processing

A major step in functional processing is lexical selection. The speaker must determine that words with the appropriate meanings exist (i.e., find lemmas corresponding to the intended meanings) and mark the lemmas for inclusion in the utterance. This marking, which constitutes selection, makes available the grammatical information that is associated with the word (e.g., whether it is a noun or verb). Several things can go wrong in this selection process. One is that a word is selected whose meaning does not quite match the intended meaning. This produces a kind of speech error called a semantic substitution (Hotopf, 1980), illustrated by our hypothetical speaker saying "A guy offered him some celery."[4] Another possibility is that two words with closely related meanings may be selected in tandem, creating a blend (Bolinger, 1961; MacKay, 1972) such as "A my offered him some celery" (*my* blending *man* and *guy*). A third problem is not strictly one of lexical selection, but offers some insight into its nature. Sometimes speakers select a word whose meaning they know but whose pronunciation eludes them. This yields a tip-of-the-tongue state (R. Brown & McNeill, 1966), which can be interpreted as successful lexical selection coupled with failed lexical retrieval or phonological encoding.

Another part of functional processing is function assignment, which determines what grammatical roles different phrases will play. It involves assigning syntactic roles such as nominative, accusative, dative, and so on to the rudiments of eventual phrases.[5] For example, during the formulation of "A guy offered him some licorice," provision must be made for associating individual referents (the known boy, the unknown man, the stick of licorice) with a nominative noun phrase (*a guy*), an accusative noun phrase (*some licorice*), a dative noun phrase (*him*), and a verb that unites them in the intended way (*offered*). Problems in function assignment manifest themselves in phrase exchange errors such as "I got into this guy with a discussion" when "I got into a discussion with this guy" was intended (Garrett, 1980). In such errors, phrases surface in the wrong syntactic role. So, in the error "He wants us to do something else" ("We want him to do something else" was intended), a plural first-person pronoun seems to have been assigned the accusative instead of the nominative function, and a singular masculine pronoun was assigned to the nominative instead of the accusative function. Notice that these are not simple exchanges of word forms, since the attested error is not "Him want we to do something else." A switch in the function assignments in the example utterance, erroneously assigning the dative to *a guy* and the nominative to the masculine pronoun, could yield "He offered a guy some licorice."

2. Positional Processing

The events of functional processing pave the way for positional processing, which retrieves certain specifications for the elements of the utterance and fixes their locations. Lexical retrieval consists of activating the lexical and grammatical morphemes that fill the slots in this structure. Lexical morphemes are customarily dubbed *lexemes* in the production literature, and they represent such word features as number of syllables, location of primary stress, and segmental (phonological) composition. For example, the lexeme for *licorice* might indicate that it has three syllables with stress on the first, along with a blueprint for its segmental phonology.

Common errors that can be traced to lexical retrieval are phonological word substitutions, in which a word that sounds the same as the intended word substitutes for it (Fay & Cutler, 1977). The intended utterance "make a funny face" turned into "make a fuzzy face" after a phonological substitution. These are sometimes called *malapropisms*. A hypothetical error of this sort in the example "A guy offered him some licorice" might yield "A guy offered him some limerick." A second type of error that is arguably due to a malfunction in lexical retrieval involves the exchange of individual words, as in "You remember . . . our Cambridge in kitchen?" (where the target utterance was "You remember . . . our kitchen in Cambridge?").

Grammatical morphemes consist of inflections and closed-class words. So, to construct "A guy offered him some licorice," the elements *a*, *-ed*, and *some* must be designated. Notably, these elements are rarely involved in errors like the substitutions and exchanges of lexemes (Garrett, 1982). Competing explanations for this apparent invulnerability to error fuel a controversy about whether these elements are retrieved in much the same way as lexemes (e.g., Stemberger, 1984) or are specified in a manner that, in effect, bypasses the need for lexical retrieval (Garrett, 1982).

The other subcomponent of positional processing is constituent assembly. This creates an implicit hierarchy for phrasal constituents and inflectional morphemes. The hierarchy controls the grouping and ordering of words during production, encoding various dependencies among syntactic functions.[6] For "A guy offered him some licorice," the hierarchy can be depicted in this way:

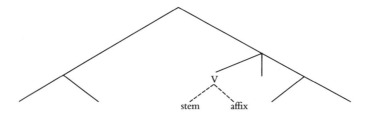

This structure is largely predictable from the types of syntactic functions that have to be represented and from the syntactic features of the selected lemmas. There are few errors that can be unambiguously attributed to the formation of these structures, although certain agreement errors (Bock & Eberhard, 1993; Bock & Miller, 1991) and word deletions are potential candidates. For example, a football broadcaster intoned the commercial message, "Formsby—No one woods as good" instead of "Formsby—No one knows wood as good." Since the utterance contains a verb slot (its presence can be inferred from the verb inflection -s) but lacks a direct object slot, one interpretation of this error (albeit not the only one) is that the direct object occupied the verb's place. A similar error might yield "A guy himmed some licorice." This sounds anomalous even as a mistake, in testimony to the fact that structural errors are very rare at all levels. In phonological encoding, as well, the structure of syllables is seldom deformed from acceptable English patterns.

One error feature that is more directly traceable to constituent assembly is known as *stranding* (Garrett, 1982). Stranding occurs because inflections are bound to other words in speech but, in processing, can be divorced from them. So, the past-tense feature on the verb *offered* requires the retrieval or generation of the inflectional morpheme *-ed*. Stranding is illustrated in the utterance of a speaker who intended to say "The dome doesn't have any windows" and instead said, "The window doesn't have any domes." In such errors, bound suffixes (here the plural *-s*) show up in their proper locations in the utterance but affixed to the wrong (often exchanged) word stems.

B. Monitoring

Not shown in Figure 1 is a component that has a major impact on ongoing speech. This is the monitor, which oversees the output of the production system and initiates self-repairs or redirects already-uttered speech. Levelt (1983, 1989) identified the monitor with the comprehension system, and construed its input as fully formed products of the production system. These products may be either inner speech (the voice in which we silently talk to ourselves) or overt speech. Monitoring should be distinguished from the potential for unconscious modification of the products of processing prior to production (see MacKay, 1987, chap. 9). The questions that have been asked about monitoring have to do with what speakers monitor, when they monitor, and how they repair their speech.

Levelt (1989, chap. 12) offers examples to suggest that speakers monitor every facet of speech for infelicity as well as outright error. Among clearly identifiable errors, there are differences in the likelihood of repair that may reveal something about where attention is directed during speech. Errors of word choice (saying "hot" instead of "cold") are surprisingly unlikely to be noticed: two studies have shown correction rates hovering around 50% (Levelt, 1983; Nooteboom, 1980). Sound errors may be caught more reliably. In one observational study, they were corrected at a rate of 75% (Nooteboom, 1980).

Blackmer and Mitton (1991) examined the timing of self-repairs in the spontaneous speech of callers to a radio talk-show. These speakers interrupted themselves an average of once every 4.8 s,[7] sometimes to repair speech errors. For speech-error repairs, the speakers halted 426 ms after the error, overall, and initiated corrections an average of 545 ms after the error. Revision (repairs for style or appropriateness) took significantly longer, averaging 1126 ms between the original utterance and the change. Although they did not break down the production errors, Blackmer and Mitton observed that most of the fastest (under 150 ms) error-to-cutoff times involved the production of aberrant phonemes. This reinforces the suggestion that speakers carefully monitor their articulation as well as the conceptual and pragmatic content of their messages.

How speakers repair their speech depends in part on the kinds of errors they detect. Levelt (1983) found that speakers often acknowledged their errors with the use of editing terms before correcting them (62% of speech errors were so marked vs. only 28% of revisions). The most common editing expression, according to Levelt (1989), is "er": it exists in many languages with only minor phonetic variations, and in Levelt's (1983) study of self-repairs, accompanied 30% of all repairs.

III. SOME POINTS OF CONTENTION

The foregoing sketch of the production system can be used to anchor a set of ongoing arguments about how the grammatical component is organized. I will proceed through the questions roughly as they arise within the organization shown in Figure 1, going from top to bottom, although in some cases the issues apply to the architecture of the entire system.

A. From Message to Language

1. Message to Word

The first controversy arises in the transition from the message component to the selection of lemmas. The presupposition behind the transition is that there is some point in processing that is nonverbal, the message, and another that is verbal (cf. Butterworth & Hadar, 1989, vs. McNeill, 1989). One difficulty with this conception arises because languages differ in the kinds of notions that are grammaticized, and therefore in the kinds of message information that will be relevant for grammatical encoding. For example, Chinese lacks the inflectional variation in noun number that is found in English, so there is no need for a Chinese speaker to represent number information in the message unless it is relevant to the communicative situation. English speakers have no such choice, since the vast majority of English nouns indicate number in some way. In the face of these language-conditioned variations in what must be represented in the message, is it defensible to suppose that the message is truly nonlinguistic or, more generally, that there is an abstract thought code ("mentalese") that is completely divorced from language (J. A. Fodor, Bever, & Garrett, 1974, chap. 7)? Put a different way, is there any sense in which an utterance is meaningful on its own (Murphy, 1991) and supposing so, are there limits to that meaning?

One view of these matters is represented in Whorfian claims that the forms of thought are in thrall to the grammatical forms of individual languages (for a wide-ranging review and new evidence, see Lucy, 1992a, 1992b). A compromise can be found in Slobin's (in press) proposal that speakers engage in something that he calls "thinking for speaking," a kind of mental activity whose goal is to package messages in a way that can be verbalized in the target language. So, an English speaker must "think number" in order to speak; Chinese speakers need not. Levelt (1989) endorses a similar view, suggesting that an important component of language learning is the discovery of what features of mentalese must be represented in messages. Levelt observed that once this learning is complete, there is no reason for the representation of the message to interact with the processes of grammatical encoding.

A related debate is over the format of mentalese, and specifically whether its elements, concepts, are wholes that are roughly isomorphic to the lexical vocabulary of language (J. A. Fodor, Garrett, Walker, & Parkes, 1980; Roelofs, 1992) or more primitive features that can be independently combined and separated (Bierwisch & Schreuder, 1992; McNamara & Miller, 1989). These *compositional* and *decompositional* views have a variety of implications for lexical access in production. Levelt (1989, 1992) has worked some of them out in what he terms the *hyperonym* problem, which arises most clearly in a decompositional framework. The problem is that the semantic conditions for a superordinate term (e.g., *dog*) should be satisfied whenever a subordinate (e.g., *poodle*) is conceptually represented. The solution demands something approximating a one-to-one relationship between concepts and lemmas, as in a compositional framework, or a requirement to use the most specific member of a set of satisfied lemmas (Levelt, 1992).

2. Message to Syntax

The mapping from messages to grammatical structures is equally poorly understood. It seems obvious that meanings and communicative functions somehow constrain the structures of utterances: languages have a tendency to group together syntactically things that belong together mentally (E. V. Clark & Clark, 1978), and speakers modify the structural organization of their utterances in response to subtle changes in the communicative context (Bock, 1977). However, it is unclear how message details serve to specify structural details in the course of normal processing and what the limits of these specifications are (for reviews of various perspectives, see Bates & MacWhinney, 1989; Bock, 1990; Newmeyer, 1992). Figure 2 depicts the leading possibilities in a Chinese-menu format.

The columns in the figure contain the basic choices that must be made in a theory of the mapping from messages to grammatical structures. The theory must include a specification of form–function correspondences (select one from Column A) and a specification of the architecture of the processing system (select one from Column B). Regarding form–function correspondence in Column A, the first position is that the grammatical

Column A FORM-FUNCTION CORRESPONDENCES	Column B ARCHITECTURE OF PROCESSING SYSTEM
ICONIC	INTERACTIVE
AUTONOMOUS	MODULAR

FIGURE 2   Theoretical options for specifying the mapping from messages to grammatical forms in production. To build a production theory, combine one option from Column A (form–function correspondences) with one option from Column B (architecture of processing system). Iconicity implies a tight relationship between messages and linguistic forms; autonomy implies a minimal or irrelevant relationship. Modularity implies a production system that imposes its own operating characteristics on its products independent of message specifications; interactivity implies a production system that updates message specifications in light of ongoing processes.

structure of an utterance is heavily constrained by communicative functions and intentions, both developmentally and in ongoing language use. New-meyer (1992) terms this *iconicity,* and Bates and MacWhinney (1989) call it level 4 functionalism. The alternative is *autonomy,* the position that the relationship between functions and structures is opaque or irrelevant to the explanation of form.

Moving to Column B, processing considerations are then factored into the theory. Because production processing itself creates constraints, over and above message constraints, certain structural details may be modified in the course of utterance formulation. For example, structures may be orga-nized to permit readily selectable words to be produced before inaccessible words (Bock, 1982; 1986a; 1987b) or to allow easily formulated structures to be produced in place of alternatives (Bock, 1986b; Bock & Kroch, 1989). To the degree that a processing system imposes its own unique constraints on its product, it can be said to be *modular.* If the imposition of these constraints involves modifying or updating the message, the system is in-stead *interactive.* The result in either case is an utterance structure that may be a compromise between the demands of the message, the demands of the grammar, and the demands of efficient encoding in real time.

In practice, theories of language processing tend to draw their options from the same rows in Figure 2. Theories combine iconic correspondences between form and function with interactive processing systems (e.g., Bates & MacWhinney, 1989), or combine autonomous grammatical components with modular processing systems (e.g., Frazier, 1987). In principle, how-ever, a theory could combine iconicity with modularity (e.g., a categorial grammar like the one discussed by Steedman, 1991, could be implemented in a modular processing system), or autonomy with interactivity (Mac-Donald, Pearlmutter, & Seidenberg, in press, lean in this direction). Al-though the full range of positions is currently approached only in theories of language comprehension, the same options are available to production theo-ries.

B. Debates about the Grammatical Component

1. Finding Words

Regarding the grammatical component itself, the central debates have to do with the discreteness of processing at each level. A strong force in these debates is the question of modularity (J. A. Fodor, 1983), particularly infor-mational encapsulation. Informational encapsulation implies that specific cognitive processes are heavily restricted in the kinds of representations that are accessible to them. On one side there is the bias that encapsulation is a property that serves to keep production efficient by restricting the passage of irrelevant noise from one process to the next (Levelt et al., 1991b). On the other side is the bias that the probabilistic sharing of different kinds of information can support efficient encoding through the use of redundancies (Dell & O'Seaghdha, 1991, 1992). Two specific questions will illustrate how these biases play out.

The first question is whether processing is completed at each level of the production system before activity ensues at the next. This point could be argued at every level of the system, but the focus of current attention is on lexical selection (locating a word's entry) and retrieval (getting sound information from the entry). Selection may be completed before retrieval commences (Butterworth, 1989; Levelt et al., 1991a, 1991b; Roelofs, 1992) or retrieval may be affected by partially activated but unselected lemmas (Dell & O'Seaghdha, 1991; Harley, 1993; Peterson, Shim, & Savoy, 1993). Figure 3 illustrates the difference in a simplified way. Discrete activity, shown in (A), activates only the sounds /kæt/ after selection of the lemma for *cat,* whereas cascaded activity (B) results in partial activation of sounds that belong to words related to *cat,* like the /r/ of *rat* and the /d/ of *dog.* The empirical focus of this debate is the *mixed error effect.* Mixed errors are word substitutions that resemble both the meanings and the sounds of an intended words (e.g., saying "rat" instead of "cat"). Mixed errors appear to be more probable than would be expected from a discrete system (Dell & Reich, 1981; Martin, Weisberg, & Saffran, 1989), lending support to the existence of cascaded activation.

The second question has to do with the existence of feedback between levels. A conservative view of production is that encoding proceeds in a strictly top-down fashion with no feedback from lower to higher levels (Garrett, 1976; Schriefers, Meyer, & Levelt, 1990). The alternative, worked out most thoroughly by Dell (1986), is that lower-level activity may influence higher-level processing. In Figure 3B, for example, the bidirectional arrows symbolize a two-way flow of information. At stake empirically is the explanation of a word superiority effect, or *lexical bias,* for sound errors: Sound errors are more likely to result in real words than chance would predict (Dell, 1986; Dell & Reich, 1981). Dell's explanation for this tendency involves the tuning created by interactive activation, which causes activity at lower levels to be modulated by rebounding activation from higher levels. In Figure 3, an erroneous /r/ is more likely to be retrieved than an erroneous /d/, although both sounds receive some activation from words related to *cat.* The /r/ reaps an additional benefit from the activation that rebounds from *rat.* This rebounding activation is a secondary consequence of the activation that feeds back from the /æ/ and /t/ shared by *cat* and *rat.* Because only real words produce this secondary effect, real words are a more likely product of sound errors than chance would predict.

The alternative to the interactive activation account for such errors is an

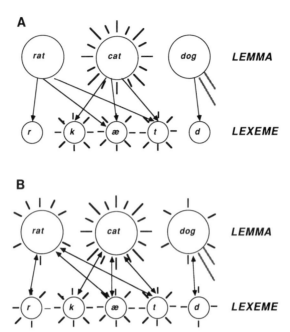

FIGURE 3 Simplified processing models for relating lemmas (word entries) to lexemes (word forms) in word production. Halos around nodes indicate activated information, and denser halos denote more activation. In (A), activation is discrete, so that selection at each level is all or none, and there is no feedback of activation from lower to higher levels. In (B), activation is cascaded, allowing partial activation of information related to unselected information at the level above, and activation feeds back from the lexeme to the lemma level. The probability of selection depends on relative amounts of activation. At the lemma level, *cat* is most likely to be selected, paving the way for selection at the lexeme level, where /k/, /æ/ and /t/ are most likely to be selected. An erroneous selection at the lemma level would tend to involve the *rat* lemma rather than the *dog* lemma, yielding a so-called mixed error. An erroneous selection at the lexeme level (given correct selection at the lemma level) would be more likely to involve the /r/ than the /d/ node, yielding a sound substitution that happens to create a word (*rat*).

editing mechanism that filters the products of processing. There is a wealth of different ways in which editing could work. The editor could be a gatekeeper that hands down only one decision from one level to the next. Alternatively, it could hand down all well-formed candidates, with well-formedness arbitrated by consistency with grammatical knowledge operating (in some unspecified way) outside of the performance system. There are also different loci at which editing could occur. There could be a form of editing at every level (MacKay, 1987; van Wijk & Kempen, 1987), at some subset of levels, or only prior or subsequent to final output (Levelt, 1989).[8] An editor that serves as a gatekeeper at every level of the production system, passing only one candidate unit or structure from each level to the next, creates a completely discrete, top-down processing system like the one in Figure 3A. Within this framework, the lexical bias in sound substitutions results from editorial biases. The editor may be more likely to accept real word than nonword errors (see Baars, Motley, & MacKay, 1975, for supporting evidence). Mixed errors in word substitutions constitute a bigger challenge, so far not satisfactorily addressed.

2. Finding Places for Words

The preceding questions about grammatical encoding concern the "vertical" relationships in Figure 1. There is another set of questions, less well developed in the literature, that have to do with "horizontal" relationships between the lexical and structural processes at each level. Broadly stated, the problem is that words must find places within structures, and not just any place will do. Bock (1987a) called this the *coordination problem*.[9] A common theoretical solution is a slot and filler mechanism (Dell, 1986; Garrett, 1988; Shattuck-Hufnagel, 1979) in which a structural frame provides slots into which words or sounds must be inserted, and the words and sounds carry information about the kinds of slots they require. Coordination is then a simple matter of fitting pieces into place. After the manner of Dell (1986), Figure 4 shows a simple slot and filler arrangement accompanying a lexical network.

Constraints on speech errors make this kind of mechanism plausible, because exchange errors of all kinds usually involve units of the same lin-

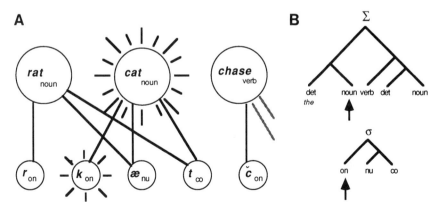

FIGURE 4   A slot and filler scheme for utterance (Σ) and syllable (σ) structures. The units within the lexical network (A) are labeled according to filler type (noun, verb, on = syllabic onset, nu = syllabic nucleus, co = syllabic coda). The structural frames (B) have matching labels to constrain the types of fillers that may be inserted into each terminal position or slot. The pointers beneath each structure indicate the slot currently being filled from the network. See Dell (1986) for detailed discussion of a model of this kind.

guistic type. However, the mechanism can be notoriously ungainly. The features of the frames are stipulated rather than generated, information is multiply represented, and representations are sometimes taken apart only to be put back together again. For example, in Shattuck-Hufnagel's (1979) model, a word is retrieved from the lexicon with its sounds properly ordered, but the sounds are then copied, one by one, into an independently generated frame. The emergence of more elegant theoretical alternatives to the slot and filler approach (e.g., Dell, Juliano, & Govindjee, 1993) should serve to fuel interest in alternative processing mechanisms for solving various coordination problems in production. So far, however, these mechanisms do not go far enough on their own to solve the coordination problem for syntax (see Dell & O'Seaghdha, 1993, for discussion).

a. Incrementality and Parallelism in Coordination

One issue that is latent in the coordination problem concerns incrementality (V. Ferreira, 1993) and, intimately related to it, the scope of planning units in encoding. Incrementality refers to the word-by-word character of speech. This creates a challenge for speakers, because there is a certain amount of parallelism in thinking and in messages: one can seemingly hold in mind all at once a complex idea or a rich visual image. To communicate the information, it may have to be dissected into propositionlike elements (Levelt, 1981) and known concepts (Levelt, 1992) and the pieces arrayed in time. The tension between parallelism and incrementality shows up in various speech errors. Certain kinds of blends, exchanges, and anticipation errors might be taken as reflections of simultaneity in the preparation of elements that are asynchronous in the spoken utterance.

Where is linearity imposed? The most common solution puts a hierarchical frame in control of the sequencing of terminal elements, and calls in some fashion on slot and filler mechanisms. The frames impose an order on elements (words, sounds, etc.) that may be available in parallel (Dell, 1986; Garrett, 1988). Because the scope of the frame becomes smaller as an utterance develops from a message to an articulatory plan, the sizes of the planning units change across the levels of Figure 1. Although there is no requirement in such models that the planning of high-level units be completed before work on lower-level units can begin (Garrett, 1976), there is typically no account of when or how the frames themselves are constructed.

A somewhat different solution ties incrementality to the order in which words (technically, lemmas) become accessible in the mental lexicon (Bock, 1982, 1987a; Bock & Warren, 1985; Kelly, Bock, & Keil, 1986; Levelt, 1989; McDonald, Bock, & Kelly, 1993) and builds sentence structures around the words as they are selected (V. Ferreira, 1993; Kempen & Hoenkamp, 1987). The structures that are created are drawn from the possibilities licensed by the language, but their assembly is opportunistic and carried out in ongoing time. For instance, a speaker might tend to say "The bird fed a worm to the nestling" if the word *worm* is selected earlier than *nestling,* but say "The bird fed the nestling a worm" if the lemma for *nestling* is selected first.

The attraction of this solution is that it accounts at once for the seriality of speech and for the intuition that words normally emerge as they are retrieved, often without logjams or temporal chasms. Still, there must be mechanisms that implement grammatical constraints at the same time that they juggle words, and these mechanisms must be explicit within a production theory.[10] The theory must also explain how word order in an utterance is negotiated with respect to the elements of a message, a problem with a long history: Levelt (1989, p. 26) attributes to Wundt the view that "word order follows the successive apperception of the parts of a total conception," and notes the difficulties that this hypothesis confronts when it is faced with word-order constraints in languages. Any general solution to the problem will require accounts of whether and how the dissection of messages is constrained so as to deliver chunks for grammatical encoding on a manageable schedule, whether and how choices among competing realizations are made in the (possibly frequent) event that several words are available at the same time, and whether and how information is buffered when it is delivered ahead of schedule. This leads directly to the issue of minimal units of preparation.

b. The Scope of Coordination

The contrast between incrementality and parallelism in coordination has obvious implications for utterance preparation. The larger the minimal units of coordination (e.g., word, phrase, clause), the wider the scope of planning must be, and the greater the simultaneity in processing. In slot and filler approaches, differences in the sizes of planning units at different processing levels are explicitly linked to differences in linguistic units. For example, Garrett (1988) suggested that the scope of functional planning is roughly two clauses, and that of positional planning roughly a phrase, as reflected, respectively, in the spans of word exchange errors and sound exchange errors. Other work has also pointed toward clauselike units of higher-level planning (Bock & Cutting, 1992; Ford, 1982; Ford & Holmes, 1978).

However, the scope of preparation need not be tied strictly to linguistically defined units. An alternative, one that is more consistent with lexically driven incrementalism, envisions a flexible deployment of information processing capacity across linguistic levels (Bock, 1982; Huitema, 1993; Levelt, 1989). The presumption is that variations in the construction and use of structural frames reflect changes in cognitive capacity and general constraints on the size or complexity of individual structural realizations (e.g., the length of an individual phrase or word), as well as hierarchically defined variations in structural units. So, the scope of preparation might sometimes encompass an entire simple utterance (e.g., "here it is") and sometimes no more than one complicated word (e.g., "eponymously").

3. Positional Processing

a. Lexical Retrieval

There are two hot spots in work on lexical retrieval in production, both of them related to the role of word frequency. One has to do with the precise locus of word-frequency effects in production, mirroring a related controversy in the study of reading (Balota & Chumbley, 1985, 1990; Monsell, 1990, in press; Monsell, Doyle, & Haggard, 1989; Savage, Bradley, & Forster, 1990), but with a different set of concerns. There is evidence that the production of words in the course of naming pictures is affected by word frequency (Huttenlocher & Kubicek, 1983; Oldfield & Wingfield, 1965), recently confirmed in detail by Jescheniak & Levelt (1994). Frequency also affects the likelihood of speech errors in words and sounds (Dell, 1990; del Viso, Igoa, & García-Albea, 1991; Kelly, 1986; Levitt & Healy, 1985; Stemberger & MacWhinney, 1986b), word order (Fenk-Oczlon, 1989), the spoken durations of words (Wright, 1979), and word length (Landauer & Streeter, 1973).

The question is where the effects of frequency arise. One theoretical view links the impact of frequent use most tightly to those components of processing that require the retrieval of stored information rather than inference, construction, or application of grammatical rules (Pinker, 1991). A different answer, implicit in connectionist views of language processing, is that frequency affects everything (Seidenberg & McClelland, 1989). Although the question is far from settled, some observations (del Viso et al., 1991; Kelly, 1986) and experimental results (Jescheniak & Levelt, in press) favor lexeme retrieval as the locus of frequency effects. This makes sense from the standpoint that lexeme retrieval is, in fact, retrieval, whereas lemma selection may demand inference in order to abstract a message from the communicative context, dissect a message into meanings that can be lexicalized, and map meanings to lemmas (as in a meaning-postulates framework; J. D. Fodor, Fodor, & Garrett, 1975).

Other evidence, however, points indirectly toward the lemma as a source of frequency effects. Using an error-eliciting procedure, Dell (1990) found that sound errors were more likely to occur on low-frequency than on high-frequency words, and that the occurrence of errors involving homophones like *by* and *buy* was related to the combined frequency of the words. The homophone result showed that low-frequency homophones inherit the benefits of having a high-frequency twin. This implies a lexeme locus for the frequency effect, since homophones share the same lexeme but have different lemmas. Paradoxically, however, frequency did not reliably affect the strength of lexical bias: high-frequency words were not significantly more likely to be the byproducts of sound error than low-frequency words. The absence of this frequency difference is inconsistent with the lexeme hypothesis, if lexical bias results from rebounding activation between lexemes and segments. Simulating all of these effects, Dell found that the best account was given by an interactive activation model in which frequency is represented at the lemma level. The same model readily explained homophone inheritance in terms of interactions between lemmas and lexemes.

Frequency is also at the center of a controversy over the closed-class vocabulary. As noted in Section IIA2, the closed-class elements of utterances are sometimes accorded a special status in generation, with the view being that they are inserted by grammatical mechanisms rather than lexical ones. One aspect of this view is a claim for syntactic immanence (see Bock, 1989): the constituent tree carries features that may uniquely specify a particular element (e.g., if a slot calls for a determiner that is indefinite and singular, English offers only one possibility[11]). A second aspect is a claim for special access: rather than being retrieved from the general lexicon, these elements come from a special store. A variant of this is Levelt's (1989) indirect access hypothesis: closed-class words are recruited by way of the syntactic information stored with the lemmas for open-class words. The evidence for a special encoding route comes from several sources, prominently including the vulnerability of the closed class to disruption in aphasia and its relative invulnerability to normal error (Garrett, 1982, 1992; Lapointe & Dell, 1989). Although the supposed invulnerability to error has been challenged by evidence that error probabilities are highly sensitive to frequency (Dell, 1990; Stemberger, 1984), the evidence from aphasia remains troublesome. As Garrett (1992) notes, many aphasics disproportionately lose the elements of the closed class, which are among the most frequent elements in the language. The paradox is that in the open-class vocabulary, the elements most likely to be lost are the infrequent ones.

b. Constituent Assembly

A different question about the effects of frequency arises with respect to constituent assembly. Bock (1986b, 1990; Bock, Loebell, & Morey, 1992) marshaled evidence that speakers tend to repeat constituent structures across successive utterances. For example, a speaker who employs a double-object dative in one utterance (perhaps, "The governess made the princess a pot of tea") is subsequently more likely to use a double-object dative than a prepositional dative, even in a completely unrelated utterance (so, "The woman is showing a man a dress" becomes relatively more likely than "The woman is showing a dress to a man"). There is suggestive but still inconclusive evidence that this effect strengthens with the repeated use of a structure (Bock

& Kroch, 1989), raising the possibility that the creation of sentence structures is a frequency-sensitive process. But since structural repetition does not appear to depend on the repetition of particular words (Bock, 1989) or thematic roles (Bock & Loebell, 1990) or features of word meaning (Bock et al., 1992), its explanation rests on the transient enhancement of general structural procedures rather than the enhanced retrieval or use of specific stored information. If this is so, it becomes difficult to use frequency effects as symptoms of simple retrieval processes. More broadly, it points to mechanisms of syntactic performance that undergo continuous modification with use, counter to the standard view of syntax as something whose use is fixed beyond childhood.

IV. FLUENCY

One issue that has yet to attain a sure foothold in the contemporary study of production is the question of what supports fluency. Although considerable attention is paid to the absence of fluency in errors and hesitations (Garrett, 1982, reviews these literatures together), the mere absence of trouble does not explain fluent speech. H. H. Clark and Clark (1977, pp. 261–262) characterized a hypothetical *ideal delivery* as one in which "people know what they want to say and say it fluently," with "most types of clauses . . . executed in a single fluent speech train under one smooth intonation contour" and pauses restricted to grammatical junctures. This characterization emphasizes a regular speech rate with fluid prosody. The grounds for this ideal might be placed either in the wants and needs of the listener (H. H. Clark & Clark, 1977) or in the speaker's own desire for proficient action. In either case, fluency is an ideal to which speakers aspire.

Two different explanatory traditions offer cognitive accounts of fluency. One emphasizes the salutary effects of an efficient mechanism, with efficiency achieved either by dint of an elegantly tailored architecture or by dint of practicing cognitive tasks. I will call these *mental skill* explanations. The other tradition stresses the role of attention or working memory resources in the creation of speech. I will call this a *mental energy* explanation. After reviewing some of the production work that falls into these two traditions, I briefly consider two other components of fluency that have so far gone mostly unmentioned, prosody and preparation.

A. Mental Skill and Mental Energy

Most current models of production offer a skill-based explanation of fluency that emphasizes efficiencies of architecture. Although the models differ over what creates an efficient architecture, whether it is something like informational encapsulation or the exploitation of informational redundancies, there has been little consideration from either standpoint of how the system comes to have the form that it does, or becomes as efficient as it is. Conceivably, the parser and production system are innate (Pinker, 1984), but just as conceivably, they organize themselves as the grammar is learned. There has likewise been little consideration of how the parameters of fluency (speech rate, prosody, preparation, etc.) change with experience, particularly across complete utterances (though see Wijnen, 1990). With the emergence of interest in developmental language performance problems (Gerken, 1991; Plunkett, 1993; Stemberger, 1989; Wijnen, 1990, 1992) and in production models that can change features of their organization with training, more emphasis may be laid on these issues.

A different, sometimes complementary tradition in cognitive explanation stresses mental capacity over the organization of mental skills. Some of the extensive research on hesitations in speech (filled and silent pauses) has been carried out in this framework. Garrett (1982; also see Goldman-Eisler, 1968) observed that hesitations may reflect normal advance planning and retrieval for an upcoming structural unit (Beattie, 1983; Boomer, 1965; Butterworth, 1980; Ford, 1982; Goldman-Eisler, 1972; Holmes, 1988; see Bock & Cutting, 1992, for review), or delay created by the momentary inaccessibility of a needed piece of information (Lounsbury, 1965; Smith & Clark, 1993), or transient increases in processing load. Garrett dubbed these three culprits "wait till the boat's loaded," "it's in the mail," and "don't bother me, I'm busy." The last of these implies that changes in fluency can be traced to transient variations in cognitive capacity that may affect production globally or locally. Experimental efforts to create variations of this kind have examined the effects on speech and writing of situational anxiety (Mahl, 1987; Reynolds & Paivio, 1968), secondary task demands (J. S. Brown, McDonald, Brown, & Carr, 1988; Power, 1985, 1986), and individual differences in working memory capacity (Daneman & Green, 1986). Errors can be analyzed from a similar perspective (Fayol, Largy, & Lemaire, 1994).

One intriguing relationship that has emerged within the capacity-limitations framework is a link between the duration of traditionally defined short-term memory traces and speech rate (Baddeley & Hitch, 1974; Schweickert & Boruff, 1986). Beginning with Baddeley, Thomson, and Buchanan (1975), evidence began to appear that the measured capacity of short-term memory is sensitive to the amount of time required to articulate words. Generally, people can immediately recall about as many items as they can pronounce in two seconds. This interacts with differences among languages in the normal sizes of the lexical units employed in short-term memory tasks (Cheung & Kemper, 1993; N. C. Ellis & Hennelly, 1980; Hoosain, 1982; Stigler, Lee, & Stevenson, 1986; Zhang & Simon, 1985) and with developmental differences in speech rate (Hulme, Thomson, Muir, &

Lawrence, 1984; Kynette, Kemper, Norman, & Cheung, 1990). The appearance is that various components of phonological encoding in normal language production may be closely identified with the components of verbal short-term memory, and are limited in similar ways (A. W. Ellis, 1980a, 1980b; see Cowan, 1992, and Schweickert, Guentert, & Hersberger, 1990, for qualifications).

B. Prosody

Integral to the ideal delivery is a smooth intonation contour. To achieve this, English speakers must control their speech rate, the relative timing of stressed and unstressed syllables, changes in amplitude, and changes in fundamental frequency. The determinants of these factors are of many kinds. According to Cutler and Isard (1980), they fall into four main categories: the stress patterns of individual words, the location of the main accent in an utterance (sentence accent), syntactic structure, and various pragmatic factors (including discourse structure, speech acts, speaker's attitude, and so on).

Interest in the production of prosody has centered on two of these factors. The first is the role of syntactic structure in determining prosodic boundaries. There is obviously a relationship between syntactic structure and prosodic structure, with pauses, slowing of speech, and drops in amplitude and fundamental frequency tending to occur at major syntactic breaks (Cooper & Paccia-Cooper, 1980; Cooper & Sorenson, 1981; Steedman, 1991). A question has been raised about whether these prosodic features are under the direct control of syntactic structures, or are instead created by an intermediate representation that makes its own contribution to prosody. F. Ferreira (1993) argued for the operation of an abstract prosodic structure, showing experimentally that changes in the durations of words and any pauses that follow them can reflect prosodic boundaries that are different from syntactic boundaries. Ferreira also reported striking evidence that the prosodic representation is not dependent on an utterance's specific speech sounds. She found that the combined duration of a word and any pauses that followed it was not predictable from the segmental contents of the words: longer words were followed by correspondingly shorter pauses and vice versa. This suggests that a prosodic structure can be created without reference to the sounds that comprise individual words (though data from Meyer, in press, dispute this possibility).

A second, related factor in the production of prosody is lexical stress and how it is distributed throughout an utterance. In English, words differ regarding whether they typically bear stress and, if they bear it, where. Function words commonly lack stress, but among content words in natural speech, nearly 90% are monosyllabic (i.e., stress bearing) or have stress on the first syllable (Cutler & Carter, 1987). There is a long-standing view (e.g., Pike, 1945) that English speakers try to space these stresses relatively evenly over time. Although this appears to be far from accurate (see Levelt, 1989, chap. 10), a grosser kind of rhythmicity is created by a tendency to alternate strong and weakly stressed syllables. To achieve this, speakers subtly shift the stress pattern of words (Kelly, 1988; Kelly & Bock, 1988) or arrange words to avoid long sequences of weak or strongly stressed syllables (Kelly & Rubin, 1988).

Errors involving stress and intonation sometimes occur, and these, too, have been examined for what they reveal about the production of prosody. In line with the evidence for rhythmic alternation, Cutler (1980b) showed that syllable deletion errors (e.g., "Next we have this biCENtial rug" instead of "bicenTENnial") tend to improve the rhythm of utterances, as do erroneous movements of lexical stress ("we do think in SPEcific terms," instead of "speCIFic"). Perhaps the best-known observation about prosody in speech errors is that sentence intonation tends to be preserved in the face of other errors: Garrett (1975) gives as an example the error, "stop beating your BRICK against a head wall" (produced in place of "stop beating your HEAD against a brick wall"). However, Cutler (1980a) contended that this holds only for open-class (content) words. When closed-class words move, they tend to carry sentence accent with them, if they bear it, as in, "you can turn it ON back now" (instead of "you can turn it back ON now"). Levelt (1989) interpreted these contrasting patterns as reflecting differences in when the accent-bearing elements actually move. On this view, open-class movement errors occur during grammatical encoding, and do not change the syntactic structure over which prosody is calculated, whereas closed-class elements move after their metrical patterns are specified, during phonological encoding.

C. Preparation

Speakers engage in a certain amount of preparation before they begin to talk. They take longer to initiate long utterances than short ones, and fundamental frequency is higher at the beginning of long utterances than short ones (Cooper, Soares, & Reagan, 1985). Oddly, despite the considerable attention given to hesitation and other forms of dysfluency in connection with questions about speech planning, comparatively little is known about changes in fluency as a consequence of variations in preparation. An utterance that is fully prepared (phonologically encoded into inner speech) can probably be uttered more fluently than an utterance whose preparation falls short of this (see Sternberg, Knoll, Monsell, & Wright, 1988). However, most utterances undergo less than full preparation because of the limit on the amount of fully formulated material that can be held in immediate memory, and because utterances can be launched before this limit is reached. Speakers often begin talking not too long after they formulate the first content word in the subject phrase (Huitema, 1993; Lindsley, 1975).

Between the extremes of maximal and minimal preparation, differences in the amount and type of preparation may have consequences for fluency. Huitema (1993) showed that about 95% of a set of simple descriptive utterances were produced fluently when speakers had a minimum of 1550 ms of pure planning time, versus 60% when the minimum planning time was 600 ms. Huitema also found that complex subject noun phrases consume planning resources to the point that speakers hesitate or slow their speech after producing them, presumably to prepare the rest of the utterance. With regard to lexical planning, Butterworth (1980, 1989) argued that content words are produced more fluently (with fewer pauses) when their lemmas have already been selected than when both the lemma and the lexeme must be prepared. Similarly, Deese (1980) suggested that speech whose content (but not form) is planned in advance displays less disruptive hesitation patterns than completely extemporaneous speech.

Less explicit kinds of preparation come in the form of contextual priming and interference, caused either by one's own prior speech or that of an interlocuter. Relationships of similarity or identity across the elements of sentences may affect the speed with which utterances are initiated (Dell & O'Seaghdha, 1992; Schriefers, 1992, 1993), the fluency with which they are produced (Bock & Loebell, 1990; Sevald & Dell, 1992; Sevald, Dell, & Cole, 1993), their word order (Bock, 1986a, 1987a; Bock & Irwin, 1980), their syntactic structure (Bock, 1986b, 1990), the ease of lexical selection and phonological encoding (Meyer & Schriefers, 1991; Roelofs, 1992, 1993; Schriefers et al., 1990; Wheeldon & Monsell, 1994), and the likelihood of error (Baars et al., 1975; Dell, 1984; Harley, 1990; Martin et al., 1989; Stemberger, 1985; Stemberger & MacWhinney, 1986a).

D. Summary

Because of the traditional emphasis on errors and dysfluency in production research, the positive components of fluency have received little direct attention. In some cases, explanations of error and dysfluency will help to shed light on their fluent speech counterparts. This seems particularly likely for hesitant speech, where fluency is the background against which hesitations are assessed. Likewise, the study of speech errors may help to disclose the joints in the architecture of normal language production. In other ways, however, fluency is more than the absence of dysfluency, and its explanation depends on characterizing how the disparate elements of language can be integrated into a smooth stream of speech.

V. CONCLUSION: THE PC PROBLEMS

From the broad standpoint of psycholinguistic theory, two overarching questions about language production have to do with how the processes of production (P_1) are related to the processes of comprehension (C_1), and how the processing theory for production (a performance theory, P_2) is related to a linguist's theory of language knowledge (a competence theory, C_2). These are the PC problems.

A. Production and Comprehension

Views of the relationship between production and comprehension run the gamut from close identification of the performance systems (MacKay, 1987; MacKay, Wulf, Yin, & Abrams, 1993) to substantial dissociations of them (Frazier, 1982; Shallice, McLeod, & Lewis, 1985). Although it may turn out that production is simply "comprehension turned upside down," in what follows I give some reasons for skepticism about this possibility. The main point is that differences in what a processing system has to do create differences in how the processing system works (Marr, 1982).

First, differences in the goals of the two systems make it reasonable to suppose that there may be differences in their normal functioning. The goal in comprehension is to create an interpretation of an utterance. In production, the speaker's immediate goal is simply to create an utterance. The utterance should be adequate to convey the speaker's meaning, but to do so, it must meet a range of constraints that are specified in the grammar of the language. This necessity gives the production problem a spin that Garrett put like this: "The production system must get the details of form 'right' in every instance, whether those details are germane to sentence meaning or not" (1980, p. 216). As a result, a general issue in a theory of production is to explain how speakers create linguistic structures at all levels. There can be no argument about whether syntax, for example, is "important" in production, because the speaker as a matter of course creates those features of utterances that we call their syntax. It is considerably less clear whether language comprehension requires that listeners reconstruct these features to the same level of detail.

Beyond this, differences in the starting points for production and comprehension also lead one to expect differences between them. Listeners must piece interpretations together from degraded and ambiguous input that arrives one syllable at a time. Speakers begin with an interpretation, in the form of a message. The message may be apprehended all at once, and without ambiguity. The hurdle is to assemble the linguistic pieces that convey the communicative intention.

Despite these differences, it is unlikely that the linguistic resources employed in comprehension are entirely independent of the resources for production. Communication is successful because words and their arrangements mean the same thing regardless of whether one's role is that of speaker or listener. One implication is that there is an important role in performance theories for general descriptions of the language knowledge that is called upon in comprehension and production. More controversial is the role that performance data can play in informing theories of linguistic knowledge.

B. Performance and Competence

One of the weightiest questions about the relationship between language knowledge and the systems that put that knowledge to use is whether the latter are in any important sense specialized for the implementation of the former (see Frazier, Chapter 1, this volume). The view that performance systems are linguistically neutral (and therefore linguistically uninteresting) is well entrenched in linguistics, inaugurated by Chomsky's (1965) famous formulation of the distinction between competence and performance. J. A. Fodor (1983) put forward a very different view, according to which the performance systems that subserve language are dedicated, largely segregated from other cognitive and perceptual systems, and innate. Dedicated performance systems, in turn, may be distantly related to the grammar of the language or may transparently encode it (J. D. Fodor, 1981, 1989).

Underlying the view that performance systems transparently encode the grammar is the *strong competence assumption,* which says that a linguistic theory captures knowledge as the speaker actually represents it. In some quarters (e.g., Bresnan & Kaplan, 1984; J. D. Fodor, 1989), this motivates an interest in language performance as one way of testing hypotheses about knowledge representation. On this view, when performance data diverge from the predictions of a linguistic theory, the data count against the theory.

In part because most psycholinguistic data reflect language comprehension, comprehension research has played a more substantial role than production research in informing competence theories. The undeniably linguistic nature of the input to comprehension also helps to drive interest: there is no need to grapple directly with the unknown commerce between language and thought. Moreover, the study of comprehension is closely tied to linguists' interest in language acquisition, insofar as the acquisition problem is in the first instance seen as a problem of making sense of linguistic input.

For several reasons, production data merit comparable weight in developing theories of linguistic knowledge. First, speakers are, in a sense, the proximate cause of the features of language. They create linguistic structure whenever they talk. Second, although variation in a speaker's use of structures is often ascribed to a concern for making comprehension easier, it is likely that some variations serve only to make production easier (P. M. Brown & Dell, 1987; Dell & Brown, 1991; Keysar, 1994; Schober, 1993). This means that linguistic explanations that incorporate performance constraints (e.g., Hawkins, 1990) cannot overlook the problems faced by speakers, which may be different from those faced by comprehenders and just as decisive in shaping the grammar. Third, questions about language acquisition motivate attention to production at least as much as attention to comprehension. Children's speech is the main source of current data about the course of language development, and because knowledge acquisition and skill acquisition are inextricably intertwined in this development, it is impossible to understand one without the other. Fourth, speaking is a cardinal facet of language ability: the commonsense test of skill in a language is not the ability to understand it, but the ability to speak it. And finally, production data can provide converging validation for competence explanations of comprehension evidence. This convergence is essential if linguistic theory is to be a theory of the knowledge that is used by all of the cognitive systems that perform language.

The problem of characterizing the conceptual input to production remains. However, with the advent of experimental methods that tap ongoing processes of production without changing a speaker's communicative intention (see Bock, 1995), it has become possible to temporarily bypass some of the thornier questions about relationships between language and thought. This makes the study of production more tractable and the prospects for satisfactory theoretical tests brighter.

One last cautionary point concerns the nature of the relationship between a production theory and linguistic theory (see Frazier, Chapter 1, this volume). There remains in some quarters a tendency to regard language production as the animation of a linguistic theory. This is a vestige of the early days of transformational generative grammar, when the mathematical term "generative" was sometimes confused with the processes of generation that production requires. The basic constructs of transformational theories (rewrite rules, transformations), linking abstract structures to concrete linguistic details, also appeared to trace a route for production. Efforts to use linguistic theory as a performance theory encouraged these misleading equations (see J. A. Fodor & Garrett, 1966, for review). It should be clear by now that production theory is a theory of using language, not an account of how language is represented, and that linguistic frameworks whose province is the static organization of language knowledge are unlikely to provide the theoretical machinery for explaining how that knowledge is deployed in time.

Acknowledgments

Several people aided in the preparation of this chapter, and I would like to acknowledge their help, with gratitude. In chronological order, they are Gary Dell, John Huitema, William F. Brewer, and Gregory Murphy. While writing the chapter, I received support from grants awarded by the National Science Foundation (BNS 90-09611) and the University of Illinois Research Board.

Endnotes

1. There are important differences between the "gap" that James describes and the "gap" that Ashcraft describes. Ashcraft's gaps seem to contain propositions, the elements of what I am here calling messages. James's gaps contain concepts, the meanings behind single words.
2. This error was reported in a scrawled note along with the annotation "poor verb."
3. The division into functional and positional processing generally corresponds to the *functional* and *positional* levels in Garrett's theory (1975, 1988), to *functional* and *constituent integration* in Bock (1978a), and to the top two levels of the lexical network with their associated tactic frames in Dell's (1986) model. Collectively, Levelt (1989) terms the processes *grammatical encoding*.
4. A genuine error of this sort occurred in a request for "one of those celery things" when the speaker meant to say "one of those licorice things."
5. These syntactic roles correspond roughly to the traditional roles of subject, direct object, and indirect object.
6. This conflates the constituent assembly and inflection processes discussed in Bock and Levelt (1994).
7. Because Blackmer and Mitton (1991) included filled pauses and repetitions in their repair classifications, not all of these interruptions represented actual corrections. Only a small minority were repairs of speech errors (3% of the sample), suggesting that many of the dysfluencies may have been something else (e.g., planning delays).
8. An editor that operates only on the final output is equivalent to the monitor discussed above.
9. The coordination problem is a species of the *binding* problem that afflicts connectionist approaches to language (J. A. Fodor & Pylyshyn, 1988).
10. DeSmedt (1990) and Kempen and Hoenkamp (1987) have developed computational models that satisfy these requirements, but as yet there have been few tests of their psycholinguistic implications.
11. The fact that this choice comes in two allomorphic variants (*a* and *an*) is not relevant here, since the variants are phonologically conditioned.

References

Ashcraft, M. H. (1993). A personal case history of transient anomia. *Brain and Language, 44,* 47–57.

Baars, B. J., Motley, M. T., & MacKay, D. G. (1975). Output editing for lexical status in artificially elicited slips of the tongue. *Journal of Verbal Learning and Verbal Behavior, 14,* 382–391.

Baddeley, A. D., & Hitch, G. J. (1974). Working memory. In G. H. Bower (Ed.), *The psychology of learning and motivation* (Vol. 8, pp. 47–90). New York: Academic Press.

Baddeley, A. D., Thomson, N., & Buchanan, M. (1975). Word length and the structure of short-term memory. *Journal of Verbal Learning and Verbal Behavior, 14,* 575–589.

Balota, D. A., & Chumbley, J. I. (1985). The locus of word-frequency effects in the pronunciation task: Lexical access and/or production? *Journal of Memory and Language, 24,* 89–106.

Balota, D. A., & Chumbley, J. I. (1990). Where are the effects of frequency in visual word recognition tasks? Right where we said they were! Comment on Monsell, Doyle, and Haggard (1989). *Journal of Experimental Psychology: General, 119,* 231–237.

Bates, E., & MacWhinney, B. (1989). Functionalism and the competition model. In B. MacWhinney & E. Bates (Eds.), *The crosslinguistic study of sentence processing* (pp. 3–73). Cambridge, UK: Cambridge University Press.

Beattie, G. (1983). *Talk: An analysis of speech and non-verbal behaviour in conversation.* Milton Keynes, England: Open University Press.

Bierwisch, M., & Schreuder, R. (1992). From concepts to lexical items. *Cognition, 42,* 23–60.

Blackmer, E. R., & Mitton, J. L. (1991). Theories of monitoring and the timing of repairs in spontaneous speech. *Cognition, 39,* 173–194.

Bock, J. K. (1977). The effect of a pragmatic presupposition on syntactic structure in question answering. *Journal of Verbal Learning and Verbal Behavior, 16,* 723–734.

Bock, J. K. (1982). Toward a cognitive psychology of syntax: Information processing contributions to sentence formulation. *Psychological Review, 89,* 1–47.

Bock, J. K. (1986a). Meaning, sound, and syntax: Lexical priming in sentence production. *Journal of Experimental Psychology: Learning, Memory, and Cognition, 12,* 575–586.

Bock, J. K. (1986b). Syntactic persistence in language production. *Cognitive Psychology, 18,* 355–387.

Bock, J. K. (1987a). Coordinating words and syntax in speech plans. In A. Ellis (Ed.), *Progress in the psychology of language* (Vol. 3, pp. 337–390). London: Erlbaum.

Bock, J. K. (1987b). An effect of the accessibility of word forms on sentence structures. *Journal of Memory and Language, 26,* 119–137.

Bock, J. K. (1989). Closed-class immanence in sentence production. *Cognition, 31,* 163–186.

Bock, J. K. (1990). Structure in language: Creating form in talk. *American Psychologist, 45,* 1221–1236.

Bock, J. K. (1995). *Language production: The methods and their theories.* Manuscript submitted for publication.

Bock, J. K., & Cutting, J. C. (1992). Regulating mental energy: Performance units in language production. *Journal of Memory and Language, 31,* 99–127.

Bock, J. K., & Eberhard, K. M. (1993). Meaning, sound, and syntax in English number agreement. *Language and Cognitive Processes, 8,* 57–99.

Bock, J. K., & Irwin, D. E. (1980). Syntactic effects of information availability in sentence production. *Journal of Verbal Learning and Verbal Behavior, 19,* 467–484.

Bock, J. K., & Kroch, A. S. (1989). The isolability of syntactic processing. In G. N. Carlson & M. K. Tanenhaus (Eds.), *Linguistic structure in language processing* (pp. 157–196). Dordrecht: Kluwer.

Bock, J. K., & Levelt, W. J. M. (1994). Language production: Grammatical encoding. In M. A. Gernsbacher (Ed.), *Handbook of psycholinguistics* (pp. 945–984). San Diego, CA: Academic Press.

Bock, J. K., & Loebell, H. (1990). Framing sentences. *Cognition, 35,* 1–39.

Bock, J. K., Loebell, H., & Morey, R. (1992). From conceptual roles to structural relations: Bridging the syntactic cleft. *Psychological Review, 99,* 150–171.

Bock, J. K., & Miller, C. A. (1991). Broken agreement. *Cognitive Psychology, 23,* 45–93.

Bock, J. K., & Warren, R. K. (1985). Conceptual accessibility and syntactic structure in sentence formulation. *Cognition, 21,* 47–67.

Bolinger, D. L. (1961). Verbal evocation. *Lingua, 10,* 113–127.

Boomer, D. S. (1965). Hesitation and grammatical encoding. *Language & Speech, 8,* 148–158.

Bresnan, J., & Kaplan, R. M. (1984). Grammars as mental representations of language. In W. Kintsch, J. R. Miller, & P. G. Polson (Eds.), *Method and tactics in cognitive science* (pp. 103–135). Hillsdale, NJ: Erlbaum.

Brown, J. S., McDonald, J. L., Brown, T. L., & Carr, T. H. (1988). Adapting to processing demands in discourse production: The case of handwriting. *Journal of Experimental Psychology: Human Perception and Performance, 14,* 45–59.

Brown, P. M., & Dell, G. S. (1987). Adapting production to comprehension: The explicit mention of instruments. *Cognitive Psychology, 19,* 441–472.

Brown, R., & McNeill, D. (1966). The "tip of the tongue" phenomenon. *Journal of Verbal Learning and Verbal Behavior, 5,* 325–337.

Butterworth, B. (1980). Evidence from pauses in speech. In B. Butterworth (Ed.), *Language production* (Vol. 1, pp. 155–176). London: Academic Press.

Butterworth, B. (1989). Lexical access in speech production. In W. D. Marslen-Wilson (Ed.), *Lexical representation and process* (pp. 108–135). Cambridge, MA: MIT Press.

Butterworth, B., & Hadar, U. (1989). Gesture, speech, and computational stages: A reply to McNeill. *Psychological Review, 96,* 168–174.

Cheung, H., & Kemper, S. (1993). Recall and articulation of English and Chinese words by Chinese-English bilinguals. *Memory & Cognition, 21,* 666–670.

Chomsky, N. (1965). *Aspects of the theory of syntax.* Cambridge, MA: MIT Press.

Clark, E. V., & Clark, H. H. (1978). Universals, relativity, and language processing. In J. H. Greenberg (Ed.), *Universals of human language: Vol. 1. Method and theory* (pp. 225–277). Stanford, CA: Stanford University Press.

Clark, H. H. & Clark, E. V. (1977). *Psychology and language: An introduction to psycholinguistics.* New York: Harcourt Brace Jovanovich.

Cooper, W. E., & Paccia-Cooper, J. (1980). *Syntax and speech.* Cambridge, MA: Harvard University Press.

Cooper, W. E., Soares, C., & Reagan, R. T. (1985). Planning speech: A picture's word's worth. *Acta Psychologica, 58,* 107–114.

Cooper, W. E., & Sorensen, J. M. (1981). *Fundamental frequency in sentence production.* New York: Springer-Verlag.

Cowan, N. (1992). Verbal memory span and the timing of spoken recall. *Journal of Memory and Language, 31,* 668–684.

Cutler, A. (1980a). Errors of stress and intonation. In V. A. Fromkin (Ed.), *Errors in linguistic performance: Slips of the tongue, ear, pen, and hand* (pp. 67–80). New York: Academic Press.

Cutler, A. (1980b). Syllable omission errors and isochrony. In H. W. Dechert & M. Raupach (Eds.), *Temporal variables in speech: Studies in honour of Frieda Goldman-Eisler* (pp. 183–190). The Hague: Mouton.

Cutler, A., & Carter, D. M. (1987). The predominance of strong initial syllables in the English vocabulary. *Computer Speech and Language, 2,* 133–142.

Cutler, A., & Isard, S. D. (1980). The production of prosody. In B. Butterworth (Ed.), *Language production* (Vol. 1, pp. 245–269). London: Academic Press.

Daneman, M., & Green, I. (1986). Individual differences in comprehending and producing words in context. *Journal of Memory and Language, 25,* 1–18.

Deese, J. (1980). Pauses, prosody, and the demands of production in language. In H. W. Dechert & M. Raupach (Eds.), *Temporal variables in speech* (pp. 69–84). The Hague: Mouton.

Deese, J. (1984). *Thought into speech: The psychology of a language.* Englewood Cliffs, NJ: Prentice-Hall.

Dell, G. S. (1984). Representation of serial order in speech: Evidence from the repeated phoneme effect in speech errors. *Journal of Experimental Psychology: Learning, Memory, and Cognition, 10,* 222–233.

Dell, G. S. (1986). A spreading-activation theory of retrieval in sentence production. *Psychological Review, 93,* 283–321.

Dell, G. S. (1990). Effects of frequency and vocabulary type on phonological speech errors. *Language and Cognitive Processes, 5,* 313–349.

Dell, G. S., & Brown, P. M. (1991). Mechanisms for listener-adaptation in language production: Limiting the role of the "model of the listener." In D. J. Napoli & J. A. Kegl (Eds.), *Bridges between psychology and linguistics: A Swarthmore festschrift for Lila Gleitman* (pp. 105–129). Hillsdale, NJ: Erlbaum.

Dell, G. S., Juliano, C., & Govindjee, A. (1993). Structure and content in language production: A theory of frame constraints in phonological speech errors. *Cognitive Science, 17,* 149–195.

Dell, G. S., & O'Seaghdha, P. G. (1991). Mediated and convergent lexical priming in language production: A comment on Levelt et al. (1991b). *Psychological Review, 98,* 604–614.

Dell, G. S., & O'Seaghdha, P. G. (1992). Stages of lexical access in language production. *Cognition, 42,* 287–314.

Dell, G. S., & O'Seaghdha, P. G. (1994). Inhibition in interactive activation models of linguistic selection and sequencing. In D. Dagenbach & T. H. Carr (Eds.), *Inhibitory processes in attention, memory, and language* (pp. 409–453). San Diego, CA: Academic Press.

Dell, G. S., & Reich, P. A. (1981). Stages in sentence production: An analysis of speech error data. *Journal of Verbal Learning and Verbal Behavior, 20,* 611–629.

del Viso, S., Igoa, J. M., & García-Albea, J. E. (1991). On the autonomy of phonological encoding: Evidence from slips of the tongue in Spanish. *Journal of Psycholinguistic Research, 20,* 161–185.

deSmedt, K. J. M. J. (1990). *Incremental sentence generation.* Unpublished doctoral dissertation, University of Nijmegen, The Netherlands.

Ellis, A. W. (1980a). Errors in speech and short-term memory: The effects of phonemic similarity and syllable position. *Journal of Verbal Learning and Verbal Behavior, 19,* 624–634.

Ellis, A. W. (1980b). Speech production and short-term memory. In J. Morton & J. C. Marshall (Eds.), *Psycholinguistics: 2. Structures and processes* (pp. 157–187). Cambridge, MA: MIT Press.

Ellis, N. C., & Hennelly, R. A. (1980). A bilingual word-length effect: Implications for intelligence testing and the relative ease of mental calculation in Welsh and English. *British Journal of Psychology, 71,* 43–51.

Fay, D., & Cutler, A. (1977). Malapropisms and the structure of the mental lexicon. *Linguistic Inquiry, 8,* 505–520.

Fayol, M., Largy, P., & Lemaire, P. (1994). When cognitive overload enhances subject-verb agreement errors: A study of French written language. *Quarterly Journal of Experimental Psychology, 47A,* 437–464.

Fenk-Oczlon, G. (1989). Word frequency and word order in freezes. *Linguistics, 27,* 517–556.

Ferreira, F. (1993). The creation of prosody during sentence production. *Psychological Review, 100,* 233–253.

Ferreira, V. (1994). *Is it better to give than donate? The consequences of syntactic flexibility in language production.* Manuscript submitted for publication.

Fodor, J. A. (1983). *The modularity of mind.* Cambridge, MA: MIT Press.

Fodor, J. A., Bever, T. G., & Garrett, M. F. (1974). *The psychology of language.* New York: McGraw-Hill.

Fodor, J. A., & Garrett, M. (1966). Some reflections on competence and performance. In J. Lyons & R. J. Wales (Eds.), *Psycholinguistics papers* (pp. 135–154). Edinburgh: Edinburgh University Press.

Fodor, J. A., Garrett, M. F., Walker, E. C. T., & Parkes, C. H. (1980). Against definitions. *Cognition, 8,* 263–367.

Fodor, J. A., & Pylyshyn, Z. W. (1988). Connectionism and cognitive architecture: A critical analysis. *Cognition, 28,* 3–71.

Fodor, J. D. (1981). Does performance shape competence? *Philosophical Transactions of the Royal Society of London, Series B, 295,* 285–295.

Fodor, J. D. (1989). Empty categories in sentence processing. *Language and Cognitive Processes, 4,* 155–209.

Fodor, J. D., Fodor, J. A., & Garrett, M. F. (1975). The psychological unreality of semantic representations. *Linguistic Inquiry, 6,* 515–531.

Ford, M. (1982). Sentence planning units: Implications for the speaker's representation of meaningful relations underlying sentences. In J. Bresnan (Ed.), *The mental representation of grammatical relations* (pp. 797–827). Cambridge, MA: MIT Press.

Ford, M., & Holmes, V. M. (1978). Planning units and syntax in sentence production. *Cognition, 6,* 35–53.

Frazier, L. (1982). Shared components of production and perception. In D. Caplan & J. C. Marshall (Eds.), *Neural models of language processes* (pp. 225–236). New York: Academic Press.

Frazier, L. (1987). Sentence processing: A tutorial review. In M. Coltheart (Ed.), *Attention and performance XII: The psychology of reading* (pp. 559–586). Hillsdale, NJ: Erlbaum.

Garrett, M. F. (1975). The analysis of sentence production. In G. H. Bower (Ed.), *The psychology of learning and motivation* (pp. 133–177). New York: Academic Press.

Garrett, M. F. (1976). Syntactic processes in sentence production. In R. J. Wales & E. C. T. Walker (Eds.), *New approaches to language mechanisms* (pp. 231–256). Amsterdam: North-Holland.

Garrett, M. F. (1980). Levels of processing in sentence production. In B. Butterworth (Ed.), *Language production* (pp. 177–220). London: Academic Press.

Garrett, M. F. (1982). Production of speech: Observations from normal and pathological language use. In A. Ellis (Ed.), *Normality and pathology in cognitive functions* (pp. 19–76). London: Academic Press.

Garrett, M. F. (1988). Processes in language production. In F. J. Newmeyer (Ed.), *Linguistics: The Cambridge survey: Vol. 3. Language: Psychological and biological aspects* (pp. 69–96). Cambridge, UK: Cambridge University Press.

Garrett, M. F. (1992). Disorders of lexical selection. *Cognition, 42,* 143–180.

Gerken, L. (1991). The metrical basis for children's subjectless sentences. *Journal of Memory and Language, 30,* 431–451.

Goldman-Eisler, F. (1968). *Psycholinguistics: Experiments in spontaneous speech.* London: Academic Press.

Goldman-Eisler, F. (1972). Pauses, clauses, sentences. *Language & Speech, 15,* 103–113.

Harley, T. A. (1990). Environmental contamination of normal speech. *Applied Psycholinguistics, 11,* 45–72.

Harley, T. A. (1993). Phonological activation of semantic competitors during lexical access in speech production. *Language and Cognitive Processes, 8,* 291–309.

Hawkins, J. A. (1990). A parsing theory of word order universals. *Linguistic Inquiry, 21,* 223–261.

Heeschen, C. (in press). Morphosyntactic characteristics of spoken language. In G. Blanken, J. Dittman, H. Grim, J. Marshall, & C. Wallesch (Eds.), *Linguistic disorders and pathologies.* Berlin: de Gruyter.

Holmes, V. M. (1988). Hesitations and sentence planning. *Language and Cognitive Processes, 3,* 323–361.

Hoosain, R. (1982). Correlation between pronunciation speed and digit span size. *Perceptual and Motor Skills, 55,* 1128.

Hotopf, W. H. N. (1980). Semantic similarity as a factor in whole-word slips of the tongue. In V. A. Fromkin (Ed.), *Errors in linguistic performance: Slips of the tongue, ear, pen, and hand* (pp. 97–109). New York: Academic Press.

Huitema, J. S. (1993). *Planning referential expressions in speech production.* Unpublished doctoral dissertation, University of Massachusetts, Amherst.

Hulme, C., Thomson, N., Muir, C., & Lawrence, A. (1984). Speech rate and the development of short-term memory span. *Journal of Experimental Child Psychology, 38,* 241–253.

Huttenlocher, J., & Kubicek, L. F. (1983). The source of relatedness effects on naming latency. *Journal of Experimental Psychology: Learning, Memory, and Cognition, 9,* 486–496.

James, W. (1890). *The principles of psychology* (Vol. 1). New York: Dover.

Jescheniak, J. D., & Levelt, W. J. M. (1994). Word frequency effects in speech production: Retrieval of syntactic information and of phonological form. *Journal of Experimental Psychology: Learning, Memory and Cognition, 20,* 824–843.

Kelly, M. H. (1986). *On the selection of linguistic options.* Unpublished doctoral dissertation, Cornell University, Ithaca, NY.

Kelly, M. H. (1988). Rhythmic alternation and lexical stress differences in English. *Cognition, 30,* 107–137.

Kelly, M. H., & Bock, J. K. (1988). Stress in time. *Journal of Experimental Psychology: Human Perception and Performance, 14,* 389–403.

Kelly, M. H., Bock, J. K., & Keil, F. C. (1986). Prototypicality in a linguistic context: Effects on sentence structure. *Journal of Memory and Language, 25,* 59–74.

Kelly, M. H., & Rubin, D. J. (1988). Natural rhythmic patterns in English verse: Evidence from child counting-out rhymes. *Journal of Memory and Language, 27,* 718–740.

Kempen, G., & Hoenkamp, E. (1987). An incremental procedural grammar for sentence formulation. *Cognitive Science, 11,* 201–258.

Keysar, B. (1994). The illusory transparency of intention: Linguistic perspective taking in text. *Cognitive Psychology, 26,* 165–208.

Kynette, D., Kemper, S., Norman, S., & Cheung, H. (1990). Adults' word recall and word repetition. *Experimental Aging Research, 16,* 117–121.

Landauer, T. K., & Streeter, L. A. (1973). Structural differences between common and rare words: Failure of equivalence assumptions for theories of word recognition. *Journal of Verbal Learning and Verbal Behavior, 12,* 119–131.

Lapointe, S. G., & Dell, G. S. (1989). A synthesis of some recent work in sentence production. In G. N. Carlson & M. K. Tanenhaus (Eds.), *Linguistic structure in language processing* (pp. 107–156). Dordrecht: Kluwer.

Levelt, W. J. M. (1981). The speaker's linearization problem. *Philosophical Transactions of the Royal Society of London, Series B, 295,* 305–315.

Levelt, W. J. M. (1983). Monitoring and self-repair in speech. *Cognition, 14,* 41–104.

Levelt, W. J. M. (1989). *Speaking: From intention to articulation.* Cambridge, MA: MIT Press.

Levelt, W. J. M. (1992). Accessing words in speech production: Stages, processes and representations. *Cognition, 42,* 1–22.

Levelt, W. J. M., Schriefers, H., Vorberg, D., Meyer, A. S., Pechmann, T., & Havinga, J. (1991a). The time course of lexical access in speech production: A study of picture naming. *Psychological Review, 98,* 122–142.

Levelt, W. J. M., Schriefers, H., Vorberg, D., Meyer, A. S., Pechmann, T., & Havinga, J. (1991b). Normal and deviant lexical processing: Reply to Dell and O'Seaghdha (1991). *Psychological Review, 98,* 615–618.

Levitt, A. G., & Healy, A. F. (1985). The roles of phoneme frequency, similarity, and availability in the experimental elicitation of speech errors. *Journal of Memory and Language, 24,* 717–733.

Lindsley, J. R. (1975). Producing simple utterances: How far ahead do we plan? *Cognitive Psychology, 7,* 1–19.

Lounsbury, F. G. (1965). Transitional probability, linguistic structure, and systems of habit-family hierarchies. In C. E. Osgood & T. A. Sebeok (Eds.), *Psycholinguistics: A survey of theory and research problems* (pp. 93–101). Bloomington: Indiana University Press.

Lucy, J. A. (1992a). *Grammatical categories and cognition: A case study of the linguistic relativity hypothesis.* Cambridge, UK; Cambridge University Press.

Lucy, J. A. (1992b). *Language diversity and thought: A reformulation of the linguistic relativity hypothesis.* Cambridge, UK: Cambridge University Press.

MacDonald, M. C., Pearlmutter, N. J., & Seidenberg, M. S. (in press). The lexical nature of syntactic ambiguity resolution. *Psychological Review.*

MacKay, D. G. (1972). The structure of words and syllables: Evidence from errors in speech. *Cognitive Psychology, 3,* 210–227.

MacKay, D. G. (1987). *The organization of perception and action: A theory for language and other cognitive skills.* New York: Springer-Verlag.

MacKay, D. G., Wulf, G., Yin, C., & Abrams, L. (1993). Relations between word perception and production: New theory and data on the verbal transformation effect. *Journal of Memory and Language, 32,* 624–646.

Maclay, H., & Osgood, C. E. (1959). Hesitation phenomena in spontaneous English speech. *Word, 15,* 19–44.

Mahl, G. F. (1987). *Explorations in nonverbal and vocal behavior.* Hillsdale, NJ: Erlbaum.

Marr, D. (1982). *Vision.* New York: Freeman.

Martin, N., Weisberg, R. W., & Saffran, E. M. (1989). Variables influencing the occurrence of naming errors: Implications for models of lexical retrieval. *Journal of Memory and Language, 28,* 462–485.

McDonald, J. L., Bock, K., & Kelly, M. H. (1993). Word and world order: Semantic, phonological, and metrical determinants of serial position. *Cognitive Psychology, 25,* 188–230.

McNamara, T. P., & Miller, D. L. (1989). Attributes of theories of meaning. *Psychological Bulletin, 106,* 355–376.

McNeill, D. (1987). *Psycholinguistics: A new approach.* New York: Harper & Row.

McNeill, D. (1989). A straight path—to where? Reply to Butterworth and Hadar (1989). *Psychological Review, 96,* 175–179.

Meyer, A. S., & Schriefers, H. (1991). Phonological facilitation in picture-word interference experiments: Effects of stimulus onset asynchrony and types of interfering stimuli. *Journal of Experimental Psychology: Learning, Memory, and Cognition, 17,* 1146–1160.

Monsell, S. (1990). Frequency effects in lexical tasks: Reply to Balota and Chumbley (1990). *Journal of Experimental Psychology: General, 119,* 335–339.

Monsell, S. (in press). The nature and locus of word frequency effects in reading. In D. Besner & G. W. Humphreys (Eds.), *Basic processes in reading: Visual word recognition.* Hillsdale, NJ: Erlbaum.

Monsell, S., Doyle, M. C., & Haggard, P. N. (1989). Effects of frequency on visual word recognition tasks: Where are they? *Journal of Experimental Psychology: General, 118,* 43–71.

Murphy, G. L. (1991). Meaning and concepts. In P. Schwanenflugel (Ed.), *The psychology of word meaning* (pp. 11–35). Hillsdale, NJ: Erlbaum.

Newmeyer, F. J. (1992). Iconicity and generative grammar. *Language, 68,* 756–796.

Nooteboom, S. G. (1980). Speaking and unspeaking: Detection and correction of phonological and lexical errors in spontaneous speech. In V. A. Fromkin (Ed.), *Errors in linguistic performance: Slips of the tongue, ear, pen, and hand* (pp. 887–95). New York: Academic Press.

Oldfield, R. C., & Wingfield, A. (1965). Response latencies in naming objects. *Quarterly Journal of Experimental Psychology, 17,* 273–281.

Peterson, R. R., Shim, M., & Savoy, P. (1993, November). *Time course of lexicalization in language production.* Paper presented at the meeting of the Psychonomic Society, Washington, DC.

Pike, K. (1945). *The intonation of American English.* Ann Arbor: University of Michigan Press.

Pinker, S. (1984). *Language learnability and language development.* Cambridge, MA: Harvard University Press.

Pinker, S. (1991). Rules of language. *Science, 253,* 530–535.

Plunkett, K. (1993). Lexical segmentation and vocabulary growth in early language acquisition. *Journal of Child Language, 20,* 43–60.

Power, M. J. (1985). Sentence production and working memory. *Quarterly Journal of Experimental Psychology, 37A,* 367–385.

Power, M. J. (1986). A technique for measuring processing load during speech production. *Journal of Psycholinguistic Research, 15,* 371–382.

Reynolds, A., & Paivio, A. (1968). Cognitive and emotional determinants of speech. *Canadian Journal of Psychology, 22,* 164–175.

Roelofs, A. (1992). A spreading activation theory of lemma retrieval in speaking. *Cognition, 42,* 107–142.

Roelofs, A. (1993). Testing a non-decompositional theory of lemma retrieval in speaking: Retrieval of verbs. *Cognition, 47,* 59–87.

Savage, G. R., Bradley, D. C., & Forster, K. I. (1990). Word frequency and the pronunciation task: The contribution of articulatory fluency. *Language and Cognitive Processes, 5,* 203–236.

Schachter, S., Christenfeld, N., Ravina, B., & Bilous, F. (1991). Speech disfluency and the structure of knowledge. *Journal of Personality and Social Psychology, 60,* 362–367.

Schober, M. F. (1993). Spatial perspective-taking in conversation. *Cognition, 47,* 1–24.

Schriefers, H. (1992). Lexical access in the production of noun phrases. *Cognition, 45,* 33–54.

Schriefers, H. (1993). Syntactic processes in the production of noun phrases. *Journal of Experimental Psychology: Learning, Memory, and Cognition, 19,* 841–850.

Schriefers, H., Meyer, A. S., & Levelt, W. J. M. (1990). Exploring the time course of lexical access in language production: Picture-word interference studies. *Journal of Memory and Language, 29,* 86–102.

Schweickert, R., & Boruff, B. (1986). Short-term memory capacity: Magic number or magic spell? *Journal of Experimental Psychology: Learning, Memory, and Cognition, 12,* 419–425.

Schweickert, R., Guentert, L., & Hersberger, L. (1990). Phonological similarity, pronunciation rate, and memory span. *Psychological Science, 1,* 74–77.

Seidenberg, M. S., & McClelland, J. L. (1989). A distributed, developmental model of word recognition and naming. *Psychological Review, 96,* 523–568.

Sevald, C. A., & Dell, G. S. (1994). The sequential cuing effect in speech production. *Cognition, 53,* 91–127.

Sevald, C. A., Dell, G. S., & Cole, J. (1993, November). *Syllable structure in speech production.* Paper presented at the meeting of the Psychonomic Society, Washington, DC.

Shallice, T., McLeod, P., & Lewis, K. (1985). Isolating cognitive modules with the dual-task paradigm: Are speech perception and production separate processes? *Quarterly Journal of Experimental Psychology, 37A,* 507–532.

Shattuck-Hufnagel, S. (1979). Speech errors as evidence for a serial-ordering mechanism in sentence production. In W. E. Cooper & E. C. T. Walker (Eds.), *Sentence processing: Psycholinguistic studies presented to Merrill Garrett* (pp. 295–342). Hillsdale, NJ: Erlbaum.

Slobin, D. I. (in press). From "thought and language" to "thinking for speaking." In J. Gumperz

& S. C. Levinson (Eds.), *Rethinking linguistic relativity*. Cambridge, UK: Cambridge University Press.

Smith, V. L., & Clark, H. H. (1993). On the course of answering questions. *Journal of Memory and Language, 32,* 25–38.

Steedman, M. (1991). Structure and intonation. *Language, 67,* 260–296.

Stemberger, J. P. (1984). Structural errors in normal and agrammatic speech. *Cognitive Neuropsychology, 1,* 218–313.

Stemberger, J. P. (1985). An interactive activation model of language production. In A. Ellis (Ed.), *Progress in the psychology of language* (pp. 143–186). London: Erlbaum.

Stemberger, J. P. (1989). Speech errors in early child language production. *Journal of Memory and Language, 28,* 164–188.

Stemberger, J. P., & MacWhinney, B. (1986a). Form-oriented inflectional errors in language processing. *Cognitive Psychology, 18,* 329–354.

Stemberger, J. P., & MacWhinney, B. (1986b). Frequency and the lexical storage of regularly inflected forms. *Memory & Cognition, 14,* 17–26.

Sternberg, S., Knoll, R. L., Monsell, S., & Wright, C. E. (1988). Motor programs and hierarchical organization in the control of rapid speech. *Phonetica, 45,* 175–197.

Stigler, J. W., Lee, S.-Y., & Stevenson, H. W. (1986). Digit memory in Chinese and English: Evidence for a temporally limited store. *Cognition, 23,* 1–20.

Titchener, E. B. (1909). *Lectures on the experimental psychology of the thought-processes.* New York: Macmillan.

van Wijk, C., & Kempen, G. (1987). A dual system for producing self-repairs in spontaneous speech: Evidence from experimentally elicited corrections. *Cognitive Psychology, 19,* 403–440.

Wheeldon, L. R., & Monsell, S. (1994). Inhibition of spoken word production by priming a semantic competitor. *Journal of Memory and Language, 33,* 332–356.

Wijnen, F. (1990). The development of sentence planning. *Journal of Child Language, 17,* 651–675.

Wijnen, F. (1992). Incidental word and sound errors in young speakers. *Journal of Memory and Language, 31,* 734–755.

Wright, C. E. (1979). Duration differences between rare and common words and their implications for the interpretation of word frequency effects. *Memory & Cognition, 7,* 411–419.

Zhang, G., & Simon, H. A. (1985). STM capacity for Chinese words and idioms: Chunking and the acoustical loop hypothesis. *Memory & Cognition, 13,* 193–201.

CHAPTER 7

Sentence Comprehension

Michael K. Tanenhaus
John C. Trueswell

I. INTRODUCTION

The goal of research in sentence comprehension is to understand the representations that are formed as people understand a sentence and the processes involved in developing these representations. This involves recognizing the words in the sentence, determining the syntactic and semantic relationships among the words and phrases, and interpreting contextually dependent expressions. These processes draw upon specifically linguistic knowledge as well as knowledge about the world and the specific context of a sentence or utterance (see Frazier, Chapter 1, this volume).

Given space limits, we have not attempted a comprehensive review. Rather, we have tried to provide the reader with an understanding of some of the central theoretical perspectives and empirical questions that are guiding current research, and some historical perspective on how the field has developed. In doing so, we have chosen to focus primarily on the problem of how readers and listeners determine grammatical relationships as they are processing a sentence. As a result, we do not address several important topics, including how word meanings are combined during sentence processing (see Schwanenflugel, 1991, for a representative collection of current papers) and the processing of figurative language, in particular idioms and metaphor (see Cacciari & Tabossi, 1993). We also have relatively little to say

Speech, Language, and Communication

about lexical processing, except as it is directly related to syntactic processing, because that topic is covered in Chapter 4 by Cutler and Chapter 5 by Seidenberg in this volume.

The organization of the chapter is as follows. Section II previews the territory covered and introduces an example sentence that is used throughout. Section III, which forms the core of the chapter, examines how words and phrases are combined during sentence processing and how linguistic expressions whose interpretation depends on information provided by the context of a sentence or utterance are processed. The section begins with a short historical review. We then outline more recent models and use these models to guide brief reviews of some central empirical issues. Section IV concludes with a summary and a discussion about emerging issues and trends.

II. AN EXAMPLE AND SOME PRELIMINARIES

During comprehension, readers and listeners construct a *mental model* or *discourse model* (Garnham, 1981; Gernsbacher, 1991; Johnson-Laird, 1983; Marslen-Wilson & Tyler, 1987; Morrow & Bower, 1989; Webber, 1979). In order to build the model the comprehender must recognize each of the words in the sentence and determine the syntactic (and semantic) relationship among them, as defined by the grammar of the language. The process of assigning syntactic relationships is generally referred to as *parsing,* though this term is sometimes used to include both the assignment of syntactic relationships and interpretation (Altmann, 1989). As a result of parsing the sentence, the comprehender can determine the propositional content or "message" expressed by the sentence, that is, who did what to whom.

As the propositional content of the sentence is extracted, new events and entities are introduced into the model and reference is made to those that have already been introduced. Referring expressions known as *anaphors* and other contextually dependent expressions play a primary role in this process. In addition, readers and listeners may routinely incorporate some inferences that are triggered by information in the sentence, the context of the sentence or utterance, and general world knowledge.

In order to make our discussion more concrete, it will be helpful to introduce a specific example that can then be used as a touchstone throughout the chapter. Consider the sentence in (1).

(1)   *The pupil spotted by the proctor was expelled.*

Syntactically, *pupil* is the head noun in the noun phrase *the pupil spotted by the proctor,* which is the subject noun phrase for the verb phrase *was expelled. The pupil* is modified by a relative clause (*spotted by the proctor*). Both the main clause and the embedded clause are in the passive voice and both are in the past tense.

Semantically, the sentence describes two events: a spotting event and an expelling event, each of which takes place in the past. The proctor and the pupil are *discourse entities* that each participate in the spotting event in different ways or modes, commonly referred to as *thematic roles*. The proctor is the Agent of the spotting event, the one doing the spotting, and the pupil is the Theme or Patient, what is being spotted. The pupil is also the Theme or Patient of the expelling event. Thematic roles are closely linked to the syntactic relationships among verbs (and other relational words) and their syntactic *complements* or *arguments*.

The syntactic and semantic relationships in a sentence are in large part determined by constraints defined by the grammar of a language. However, the way that they are recovered in sentence processing is strongly influenced by the sequential nature of the input. The input is sequential in spoken language because of the nature of auditory stimuli. It is sequential in written language because readers typically fixate successively on each word in a sentence, processing only a limited amount of information from the periphery (Rayner, McConkie, & Zola, 1980; Rayner & Pollatsek, 1987).

Many aspects of sentence comprehension take place on-line as soon as the relevant input is encountered (cf. Marslen-Wilson, 1975; Marslen-Wilson & Tyler, 1987). For example, spoken words are recognized shortly after enough phonetic input is received to distinguish the input from other likely alternatives, often well before the end of the word (Marslen-Wilson, 1987). Lexical, syntactic, and contextual information all determine the likelihood that close shadowers (people who can repeat back a message at a lag of about one syllable) will fluently restore a distorted word in running speech (e.g., Marslen-Wilson, 1973; Marslen-Wilson & Welsh, 1978). The disambiguation of a word with multiple meanings using information from the preceding context takes place within 200 ms in spoken language processing (Seidenberg, Tanenhaus, Leiman, & Bienkowski, 1982; Swinney, 1979; Tanenhaus, Leiman, & Seidenberg, 1979), and it begins on the initial fixation to the ambiguous word in reading (Frazier & Rayner, 1987). When a syntactically ambiguous sentence fragment is disambiguated in favor of its less preferred alternative, processing consequences can be seen on the initial fixations to the disambiguating information (Frazier & Rayner, 1982; Rayner, Carlson, & Frazier, 1983). Numerous studies investigating syntactically anomalous sentences find clear processing effects on or immediately after the word where the anomaly occurs (Boland, Tanenhaus, & Garnsey, 1990; Hagoort, Brown, & Groothusen, 1993; Marslen-Wilson, Brown, & Tyler, 1988; Osterhout & Holcomb, 1992; West & Stanovich, 1986; Wright & Garrett, 1984). And, under at least some circumstances, the interpretation of a referential expression begins almost immediately using information from the discourse context (S. B. Greene, McKoon, & Ratcliff, 1992; Marslen-Wilson & Tyler, 1987; Sanford & Garrod, 1989) and it can rapidly influence syntactic ambiguity resolution (Altmann & Steedman, 1988).

Evidence for on-line comprehension has led researchers to focus on ex- perimental measures that are closely time locked to the input (see Cutler, Chapter 4, this volume). The most widely used methodologies include: (1) *monitoring* tasks in which the subject is timed while monitoring the incom- ing linguistic input for various units, for example, phonemes, words, cate- gory members, and rhymes (Cutler & Norris, 1979); (2) *probing* and *priming* tasks in which the developing representation is probed by examining re- sponse times to targets that occurred in the sentence or are related to a word or a phrase in the sentence (McKoon & Ratcliff, 1979; Swinney, Onifer, Prather, & Hirshkowitz, 1978); (3) subject controlled or *self-paced* reading in which reading times are measured while subjects read text in presentation "windows" of various sizes, often while performing a secondary task, such as answering a question or monitoring the sentence for grammaticalness or sensibility (e.g., Just, Carpenter, & Woolley, 1982); (4) *eye-movement* record- ing in which fixation patterns and durations are measured as the subject reads a sentence (Rayner, Sereno, Morris, Schmauder, & Clifton, 1989); and (5) monitoring *event-related potentials* (ERPs) as subjects read or listen to sentences (Garnsey, 1993).

When viewed from the perspective of an on-line processing system, nearly all sentences contain numerous temporary ambiguities. While ambi- guity exists at all levels of language comprehension, from categorizing a phoneme to recognizing a speaker's intentions, researchers in sentence com- prehension have been primarily concerned with how comprehenders re- solve the structural ambiguity that arises in assigning grammatical relation- ships to words and phrases as a sentence unfolds. Structural ambiguity arises because of several characteristics of natural language. Linguistic forms such as words and morphemes are frequently ambiguous with respect to their syntactic category. In our example, the word *spotted* is ambiguous with respect to syntactic category; it could be either an adjective or a verb. It is also ambiguous as to the tense and voice of the clause it occurs in because the morpheme *ed* can be used for both the simple past and for the passive participle.

Syntactic structure is hierarchical and, at least partially, recursive. This results in frequent grammatical dependencies between nonadjacent words and phrases. For example, the noun phrase *the pupil spotted by the proctor* contains a sentence embedded within a noun phrase. Consequently, *the pupil* is the subject of the verb *expelled* even though several words intervene, including another noun phrase, *the proctor*. Similarly, the verb *was* agrees in number with the noun *pupil,* and not the most local noun *proctor*.

Ambiguous forms and nonadjacent grammatical dependencies often combine to result in fragments that are temporarily ambiguous among multiple syntactic structures. For example, *the pupil spotted . . .* is ambiguous between a past-tense main clause in the active voice (e.g., *The pupil spotted the proctor*) and a relative clause (e.g., *the pupil spotted by the proctor. . .*).

The alternative syntactic structures for a temporarily ambiguous fragment typically have different semantic and discourse consequences. As a result, information at these higher levels could provide constraints that are relevant to resolving ambiguities at lower levels. We can illustrate how these correlated constraints might be used in ambiguity resolution by considering how thematic information is relevant to resolving the main clause/relative clause ambiguity in the fragment *the pupil spotted. . ..*

In a main clause, *the pupil* would be assigned the Agent thematic role (i.e., the Agent of the spotting event), whereas it would be assigned the Theme role in a relative clause. Therefore, the thematic fit of the noun phrase to each of these potential roles could be useful in resolving the syntactic ambiguity. *Pupil* is both a good Agent and a good Theme for a spotting event; however another noun such as *crib sheet* is a good Theme but a poor Agent. Thus, thematic fit might be used to help disambiguate a fragment such as *the crib sheet spotted. . .* in favor of a relative clause at the verb.

A past-tense main clause and a (restrictive) relative clause also differ with respect to how they would be integrated into the discourse model. A main clause is used to introduce a new event into the model, whereas a restrictive relative clause can be used to refer to an already established event. Thus the felicity with which each type of event could be incorporated into the model in specific discourse contexts is another potential source of constraint.

How and when the processing system exploits correlated constraints across different levels of representation have emerged as central questions in sentence processing. Two broad classes of approaches to these questions have been explored, each of which explains the speed and efficiency of sentence processing differently. One approach, which has its roots in Marslen-Wilson's early work (1973, 1975), assumes that the processing system is able to rapidly and optimally integrate different types of information by taking advantage of correlated constraints to evaluate the evidence for multiple alternatives. In these *constraint-based* or *interactive* approaches, use of correlated constraints is what underlies the speed and efficiency of on-line comprehension. As a consequence, processing at different levels is closely intertwined. For example, lexical and syntactic processing are interleaved with interpretation and the construction of a discourse model (e.g., Marslen-Wilson & Tyler, 1987).

A second approach is to have informationally encapsulated subsystems or modules that are each responsible for processing distinct types of representations. In modular models, the speed and efficiency of on-line comprehension arises, in part, because certain processes are insulated from others.

Thus correlated constraints are ignored in initial processing. Fast mandatory processes are often viewed as restricted to recovering the syntactic and perhaps semantic relationships defined by the grammatical structure of the sentence. These processes are insulated from higher-level interpretative and inferential processes that relate a sentence to its context (J. A. Fodor, 1983).

These contrasting perspectives lie at the center of the *modularity* debate that has played a prominent theoretical role in sentence processing research, especially research on parsing (J. A. Fodor, 1983; Garfield, 1987; Frazier, Chapter 1, this volume). The modularity issue is closely intertwined with questions about the nature of linguistic representation and how grammatical knowledge is accessed and used in processing. Together these issues have played a primary role in sentence comprehension research.

In order to appreciate how these issues have evolved, we begin with a brief historical overview of early research on sentence comprehension, focusing on syntactic processing. We then turn to more contemporary models and some current theoretical and empirical issues.

III. SENTENCE PROCESSING

A. Historical Perspective

Much current research on sentence processing has it roots in a research program initiated by George Miller in the 1960s that was directly inspired by Noam Chomsky's theory of transformational grammar. Miller's work placed syntactic processing at the core of sentence processing. It also established what Clark (1992) has labeled the "language-as-product" tradition in which recovering the linguistic structure of a sentence or utterance was viewed as the primary goal of sentence processing.

Miller proposed that the language processing system directly incorporated a transformational grammar (for review, see Bever, 1988; J. A. Fodor, Bever, & Garrett, 1974). The view of grammar that guided this research was initially developed in Chomsky (1957) and then expanded and modified in Chomsky (1965). Both theories of grammar were rule based and derivational. The underlying structure of a sentence was generated by recursive phrase structure rules defined in terms of syntactic categories (e.g., S $\rightarrow$ NP + VP; NP $\rightarrow$ DET + N). Transformational rules mapped the underlying structure of a sentence onto a surface structure. Chomsky's (1965) "Aspects" theory introduced a semantic component of grammar and identified deep structure as a syntactic level at which terminal syntactic categories (e.g., N, V) were replaced by words (lexical insertion) and semantic interpretation took place.

The specific hypothesis explored by Miller and his students was that listeners compute the surface structure of a sentence and then use transformations to map the surface structure onto its deep structure (e.g., Miller, 1962; Miller & Isard, 1963). The representation of a sentence in memory was its deep structure and a list of transformational tags (e.g., Clifton, Kurcz, & Jenkins, 1965; Mehler, 1963; Miller, 1962). The perceptual complexity of a sentence was hypothesized to be a function of the complexity of its derivation, determined largely by the number of transformations that applied, an hypothesis that was later dubbed the Derivational Theory of Complexity (DTC).

Miller also assumed that sentence processing operated under performance constraints imposed by a limited capacity information processing system, in particular a limited working memory. For example, sentences with multiple center embeddings such as *The pupil the proctor spotted cheated* were hypothesized to be difficult because *the pupil* has to be held in working memory while the embedded constituent *the proctor spotted* is processed. It then must simultaneously be assigned the grammatical roles of object of *spotted* and subject of *cheated* (Bever, 1970; Miller & Chomsky, 1963). The idea that limited working memory shapes syntactic processing continues to play an important role in current models.

The hypothesis that the deep structure of a sentence is retained in memory remained viable throughout the 1960s. Sachs (1967) found that people remember the gist of a sentence but not its syntactic structure. This was inconsistent with Miller's initial formulation of the deep structure hypothesis, but broadly consistent with a revised version based on Chomsky's (1965) theory. The most compelling support came from ingenious experiments by Blumenthal (1967) and Wanner (1974). In these experiments, the effectiveness of a probe word as a recall cue for a memorized sentence was correlated with the number of times it appeared in its deep structure. In our example, *pupil* would be a better recall cue that *proctor* because *pupil* is the object of both *spotted* and *expelled* in deep structure, whereas *proctor* is only the subject of *spotted*. However, as Wanner himself later argued, these results are compatible with the more general claim that comprehenders extract the propositional content of a sentence (Wanner, 1977). Subsequent research aimed at establishing the "psychological reality" of specific syntactic frameworks has run into a similar problem. Ruling out alternative explanations in terms of other levels of representation is challenging and few attempts have been convincing.

In the early 1970s, important studies by Johnson-Laird and Stevenson (1970) and by Bransford and Franks and their colleagues (e.g., Bransford, Barclay, & Franks, 1972; Bransford & Franks, 1971) showed that memory representations do not preserve the deep structures of sentences. Rather, people remember the general content of a sentence that is relevant to the particular context or situation in which the sentence appears. These results played a central role in the development of the currently influential mental models approach to anaphora and discourse (e.g., Garnham, 1981; Johnson-Laird 1984). They also marked the start of separation between the community of researchers studying sentence processing, which retained strong ties to theoretical linguistics, and the much larger community of researchers studying text processing and lexical processing, which did not.

The brief history of the DTC is well known (for detailed accounts, see Bever, 1988, and J. A. Fodor et al., 1974). After initially promising results, attempts to relate the processing complexity of a sentence to its derivational history were largely abandoned (but cf. Berwick & Weinberg, 1984). The DTC faced empirical difficulties in the form of clear counterexamples. Rapid changes in syntactic theory made experimental results difficult to interpret. And, many effects initially attributed to derivational complexity had plausible alternative accounts which did not involve transformations or even syntactic structure. For example, whether or not a passive sentence such as *The pupil was spotted by the proctor* is more difficult to comprehend than an active sentence such as *The proctor spotted the student* depends on the prior linguistic context (J. M. Greene, 1970) as well as on the semantic properties of the noun phrases (Slobin, 1966). This makes it difficult to attribute complexity differences to syntactic factors per se (but cf. Forster & Olbrei, 1973).

By the late 1960s, little evidence remained in support of the hypothesis that transformations corresponded to mental operations in sentence comprehension. However, a growing body of empirical studies suggested that syntactic structure, especially surface constituent structure, played an important role in sentence processing (for reviews, see J. A. Fodor et al., 1974; Levelt, 1978). In addition, the evidence at the time still supported the deep structure hypothesis. This raised the question of how comprehenders map surface structure onto deep structures without using transformations. J. A. Fodor and Garrett (1966) and Bever (1970) proposed that listeners make use of perceptual strategies that map surface features onto deep structures. The first detailed formulation of these parsing strategies is presented in Bever (1970). For example, the NVN strategy proposed that a Noun Verb (NP) sequence is interpreted as the Subject Verb (Object) of a deep structure sentence (e.g., J. A. Fodor et al., 1974). This straegy accounts for why the temporarily ambiguous fragment in (2) is initially misparsed as a main clause, thus leading the comprehender down the "garden path."

(2)   The horse raced past the barn *fell*.

Perceptual strategies, especially as formulated by Bever (1970), marked the beginning of the transition from the transformational era to current investigations of syntactic processing. The goal of explaining the perceptual complexity of a sentence by its derivational history was largely abandoned. Instead, attention shifted to how grammatical relationships are recovered as a sentence unfolds. As a result, local ambiguity emerged as an important theoretical and empirical domain. While there were a number of prior studies of ambiguity (cf. Levelt, 1978, for a partial review), the focus had been on the much rarer phenomenon of global ambiguity in which a complete sentence is ambiguous (e.g., *Visiting relatives can be boring*). Perceptual strategies were also a precursor to current constraint-based models because the strategies were frequency sensitive and they made use of both syntactic and semantic constraints.

The strategies were embedded in a *clausal processing* model in which deep structure clauses were taken to be the primary perceptual units of sentence processing. The need for perceptual units was motivated by Miller's (1956) view of short-term memory as a limited capacity system that could be extended by recoding the input into higher-order structures (e.g., Carroll, Tanenhaus, & Bever, 1978). This led to a view of comprehension as a "catch-up" game in which the comprehender had to recode the linguistic input at linguistically defined boundaries in order to free working memory for further processing (Bever & Hurtig, 1975).

Evidence for clauses as units came from a series of experiments by Bever and colleagues and others, summarized in J. A. Fodor et al. (1974), Carroll and Bever (1978), and Levelt (1978). Among the central results were the following: (1) clicks within words migrated toward clause boundaries during recall; (2) reaction times to a tone were slow at the end of a clause and faster at the beginning of a clause; (3) multiple readings for ambiguous structures were more available within a clause than after a clause boundary; and (4) memory for surface form declined after clause boundaries.

Important processes clearly take place at clause boundaries, including integrative processes, which Just and Carpenter (1980) have labeled "sentence wrap-up" effects. Although, the clausal model has also continued to generate some interesting results, especially on different types of interclausal relationships (Townsend & Bever, 1978), the influence of the model has declined. More on-line investigations demonstrated that extensive processing occurs prior to clause boundaries (e.g., Marslen-Wilson, 1973, 1975). Moreover, the degree to which processing changes are seen across clause boundaries depends on the information within the clause and the discourse context (Carroll et al., 1978; Marslen-Wilson, Tyler, & Seidenberg, 1978; Tanenhaus & Seidenberg, 1981). Thus the clause boundary in particular, and linguistically defined units in general, lost their special status.

By the middle 1970s, there was an emerging consensus that the linguistic representations incorporated into the transformational grammars of the time were poorly suited for use in on-line comprehension (cf. Bresnan, 1978; Marslen-Wilson, 1975). The problem was that much of syntactic knowledge was incorporated into ordered rules in a derivation. Moreover, the rules were defined over clause-length sequences. Thus the only natural way to incorporate a transformational grammar into a real-time processing model was either to posit that processing was delayed until the end of linguistic units like clauses, which was incompatible with the emerging evidence for on-line comprehension (cf. Marslen-Wilson, 1975), or to propose that grammatical relatioships are recovered using procedure that did not make direct use of grammatical knowledge (e.g., Bever, 1970; J. A. Fodor et al., 1974).

Throughout the 1980s and early 1990s, there has been renewed optimism that grammatical representations can be directly incorporated into on-line comprehension models, as suggested by Bresnan's *strong competence* hypothesis (Bresnan, 1978). This is largely because of two developments in syntactic theory. First, more syntax is incorporated into lexical representations, a trend that began with Chomsky (1970) and especially Bresnan and Kaplan (1982). Second, syntactic structure is increasingly viewed as a set of intersecting but unordered local constraints, rather than as a set of more global ordered rules that apply during a derivation. An important consequence of a constraint-based view of grammar is that, in principle, constraints can be satisfied as they become relevant (Pollard & Sag, 1993), making it is easier to interleave different types of constraints.

B. Current Issues

We now turn to a survey of some current issues in sentence processing, focusing primarily on how readers and listeners determine the syntactic and semantic relationships among words and phrases. Ambiguity resolution will be a unifying theme throughout most of this section. We begin with syntactic category ambiguity and then turn to attachment ambiguity, which has dominated much of the literature since Bever (1970). Our discussion of attachment ambiguity introduces the models and perspectives that are currently most influential in the literature. We conclude our discussion of syntactic processing with a section on empty categories and then briefly discuss anaphors and other contextually dependent expressions.

1. Syntactic Category Ambiguity

Determining the grammatical relationships among words and phrases in a sentence requires the comprehender to determine the syntactic category of each word. As we illustrated in our example, words are often temporarily ambiguous among two or more syntactic categories. Syntactic category ambiguities are frequently strongly disambiguated by prior syntactic context. In some cases, however, multiple possibilities remain for several words or even phrases (e.g., *Cast iron sinks quickly*).

Studies investigating syntactic category ambiguities (e.g., *rose, watch, patient, that*) using cross-modal priming paradigms generally find that senses of words from both contextually appropriate and inappropriate syntactic categories are initially activated even in constraining syntactic contexts (Seidenberg et al., 1982; Tanenhaus & Donnenwerth-Nolan, 1984; Tanenhaus et al., 1979). This is consistent with results from the more extensive literature on within-category sense ambiguities (Simpson, 1984). This *multiple access* pattern might arise because the lexical access system is an encapsulated processing module (J. A. Fodor, 1983; Swinney, 1991) or because syntactic context is only weakly constraining until the set of alternatives consistent with the sensory input has become activated (Kawamoto, 1993; MacDonald, Pearlmutter, & Seidenberg, 1994b; Tanenhaus, Dell, & Carlson, 1987). Under conditions where syntactic context places strong constraints on a limited set of alternatives, only the biased sense shows priming (Shillcock & Bard, 1993). This situation arises in spoken language when there is an ambiguity involving a function word and a content word (e.g., *would* vs. *wood*) and the syntactic context is consistent with only the function word.

The relative frequency of the alternatives in a syntactic category ambiguity often changes dramatically with the preceding context. These "contingent" frequencies and how they interact with simple frequencies are just beginning to be explored in the literature.

Juliano and Tanenhaus (1993) investigated the effects of context on reader's initial preferences to interpret the word *that* as a demonstrative (. . . *that cheap hotel*. . .) or as a complementizer (. . . *that cheap hotels*. . .). Biases were predicted by the frequency with which each form occurs in different syntactic environments as determined by corpus analyses and not by simple lexical frequency.

Frazier and Rayner (1987) investigated category ambiguity resolution in sentences beginning with phrases such as *warehouse fires*, in which *warehouse* could either be the head of a noun phrase (*The warehouse fires employees over sixty*) or part of a noun compound (*The warehouse fires were set by an arsonist*). Fixation durations to disambiguated phrases such as *these warehouse fires* were contrasted with ambiguous phrases such as *the warehouse fires*. They concluded that the parser delays interpretation of category ambiguities on the basis of (1) faster fixation durations for the ambiguous fragments compared to the controls at the noun phrase (e.g., *the warehouse fires*), and (2) slower fixation durations to the ambiguous fragments compared to controls in the disambiguating region.

However, MacDonald (1993) has recently shown that the same data pattern arises with unambiguous phrases because the use of the demonstrative *these* is pragmatically odd when it is not preceded by a referential context. In cross-modal naming and self-paced reading studies, she found that the resolution of noun compound/noun–verb ambiguities depends both on biasing context and on the frequency with which the noun occurs as the head of a phrase, as determined by corpus analyses.

Finally, *visiting relatives* constructions are a well-known example of a syntactic category ambiguity that has played an important historical role in investigations of modularity issues. The verb + *ing* form could either be an adjective (e.g., *laughing relatives*) or a gerund (e.g., *bothering relatives*). On the basis of fragment completion times, Bever, Garrett, and Hurtig (1973) concluded that both alternatives were computed and maintained until a clause boundary. Tyler and Marslen-Wilson (1977) demonstrated rapid effects of semantic context on the resolution of the verb + *ing* noun ambiguity. Subjects named the target *is* or *are* when it was presented visually after a fragment such as *You should avoid going on a runway because landing planes. . ..* Naming times were faster when the target was congruent with the contextually biased interpretation. The materials in this study have been criticized by Townsend and Bever (1982), who argued that morphological factors could underlie the effects, and by Cowart and Cairns (1987), who demonstrated that the Tyler and Marslen-Wilson results could have been due to biases introduced by using the pronoun *they* in the gerundive contexts rather than to semantic effects from the context. Recently, Farrar and Kawamoto (1993) have replicated the Tyler and Marslen-Wilson (1977) findings using materials that avoid these problems.

The picture that emerges from studies of syntactic category ambiguities is that multiple syntactic categories are initially accessed, with rapid evaluation based on syntactic and semantic context. The system also appears to be sensitive to contingent frequencies.

2. Attachment Ambiguity

Table 1 presents some of the ambiguous structures that have played a prominent role in the literature. For each structure, ambiguity arises because the underlined word or phrase could be incorporated or "attached" in more than one way into the constituent structure of the fragment of the sentence that has already been parsed.

Three interrelated questions arise with these (and other) ambiguities: (1) what alternatives are available at the point of the ambiguity?; (2) what degree of commitment is made to one or more alternatives?; and (3) what information is used to guide these commitments?

These issues have been addressed in a number of theoretical parsing models that combine detailed grammatical assumptions with decision principles for resolving attachment ambiguity. The assumption common to these models is that syntactic analysis is accomplished by a special computational device that makes direct use of grammatical information. Difficulties

TABLE 1   Some Important Attachment Ambiguities

Ambiguous fragment	Alternative completions
The student spotted[a]	the proctor and hid his crib sheet. (main clause)
	by the proctor was expelled. (reduced relative clause)
The spy saw the cop with . . .	the telescope. (preposition attached to the verb phrase)
	the revolver. (preposition attached to the noun phrase)
John remembered the answer . . .	from an earlier class. [noun phrase (object) complement]
	was in the book. (sentence complement)
Bill told the woman that. . .	he liked her. (sentence complement)
	he was engaged to a story. (relative clause)
After the patient visited the doctor . . .	he developed a cough. (object complement)
	became worried. (subject of main clause)

[a]The attachment of the underlined word or words in each fragment is ambiguous. The continuations disambiguate the fragment in favor of the structure in parentheses. The preferred attachment is presented above the less preferred attachment.

in processing, including garden paths, arise from the architecture of the parser in conjunction with how it applies grammatical rules or principles. (See Pritchett, 1992, and Gibson, 1991, for recent reviews of parsing models and Allen, 1994, for an introduction to computational techniques for ambiguity resolution.)

Almost all of the possible answers to the three questions introduced above have been proposed in the parsing literature including: (1) delaying commitments until enough information accrues to make an informed decision (e.g., Marcus, 1980); (2) making partial syntactic commitments that are consistent with the upcoming syntactic alternatives (Marcus, Hindle, & Fleck, 1983; Weinberg, in press); (3) making an initial commitment to a single analysis using only syntactic category information (Frazier & Fodor, 1978; Kimball, 1973; (4) making a single commitment guided by lexical representations (Ford, Bresnan, & Kaplan, 1982); and (5) developing multiple analyses in parallel (Gorrell, 1989; Kurtzman, 1985) with selection based on maximally satisfying grammatical principles (Pritchett, 1992), pragmatic fit to the discourse model (Altmann & Steedman, 1988; Crain & Steedman, 1985), or multiple constraints, including memory demands (Gibson, 1991).

a. Models of Attachment Ambiguity Resolution

Experimental research on attachment ambiguity has been guided by three broad frameworks. The first is the *garden-path* model, which maintains that there is an initial syntactically defined stage in parsing that is embedded within a modular architecture. The second is *referential theory,* which proposes that ambiguity resolution is based on selecting the structure that best fits the discourse model. The third is a set of *constraint-based* approaches, which emphasize rich lexical representations, an evidential approach to ambiguity resolution, and rapid use of correlated constraints.

  i. The garden-path model. Kimball (1973) showed that parsing preferences for a wide range of locally ambiguous sentences, including those sentences that Bever had used to argue for perceptual strategies, could be modeled by assuming that comprehenders directly used phrase structure rules defined over syntactic categories (e.g., NP → Determiner + Noun) to build a surface constituent structure. When more than one attachment was consistent with the phrase structure rules, a single parse was chosen using decision principles that made reference only to the character of the rules themselves and the syntactic tree being constructed (e.g., avoid adding new nodes).

  Frazier and Fodor (1978) argued that all of Kimball's principles could be unified by the single principle of Minimal Attachment (build the simplest structure consistent with the rules of the grammar). In response to criticisms from Wanner (1980), who defended an Augmented Transition Network account for the same data, Fodor and Frazier added Late Closure, a variant of Kimball's principle of Right Association. Late Closure states that the parser prefers to make an attachment into the phrase that is currently being processed as long as the alternative attachments are equally simple. Thus, the processing system has a general preference for a recent attachment site over an attachment site that occurred earlier in the sentence. For example, in a sentence such as *John said he will leave this morning,* people prefer to interpret the adverbial phrase *this morning* as modifying the most recent verb phrase *leave* rather than the more distant verb phrase *said.*

  Minimal Attachment and Late Closure provide a unified account for a wide range of attachment ambiguities, including all of those illustrated in Table 1. These parsing principles have been embedded in the garden-path model of sentence processing, which has played an influential role in guiding experimental studies throughout the last decade (Clifton & Frazier, 1989; Clifton, Speer, & Abney, 1991; Frazier, 1987, 1989; Frazier & Rayner, 1982; Rayner et al., 1983).

  In the garden-path model, the sentence processing system is organized into informationally encapsulated processing modules, each of which computes a distinct type of representation. Modules may differ in their computational properties. Thus the model has focused attention on potential differences in how and when different classes of grammatical and nongrammatical information are used in comprehension. The input is initially structured by a serial "first-stage" parser or constituent-building module, which builds a syntactic structure by attaching each incoming work in accordance with the Minimal Attachment and Late Closure principles (cf. Clifton & Ferreira, 1989; Frazier, 1987, 1989). As a result, the input can be rapidly structured using a restricted domain of information, thus minimizing working memory load. However, the initial structure will frequently be incorrect, resulting in local garden paths whenever the subsequent input is incompatible with the initial structure or when the initial structure is incompatible with information that is not used in the first stage of parsing. The garden–path and revision process results in temporary increases in processing difficulty. Revisions are guided by a "thematic processor" that makes use of discourse context and semantic/thematic information to evaluate the first-stage parse and, if necessary, direct revisions (Frazier, 1987; Rayner et al., 1983). The revision process has received relatively little attention (but cf. Ferreira & Henderson, 1991).

In order to see how the garden–path model works, we return to the example *The pupil spotted by the proctor was expelled.* The fragment *the pupil spotted. . .* is temporarily ambiguous between a past-tense active verb and a passive participle. When the parser encountered the word *spotted* it would attach it as a main verb because that attachment requires fewer nodes than attachment into a relative clause. The word *by* would successfully be attached into the structure because a verb in a main clause can be used intransitively with a prepositional phrase (e.g., *The pupil cheated by using a crib sheet*). At some point in the prepositional phrase, the parser would receive an error signal because the verb *spotted* requires an object complement when it occurs in a main clause. This revision would come about as a result of the parser using lexical information to evaluate and filter the structure built during the first-stage parse.

Alternatives to the garden–path approach have generally assumed that there is some degree of initial parallelism in the system. The parallelism allows the system to avoid making complete commitments and thus to take advantage of correlated constraints from the preceding context as well as subsequent information as the sentence unfolds (e.g., Altmann & Steedman, 1988; Carlson & Tanenhaus, 1988; Gorrell, 1989; Kurtzman, 1985; MacDonald, Just, & Carpenter, 1992).

ii. Referential theory.   Crain and Steedman (1985) proposed that attachment preferences in "null" contexts arise because comprehenders are making the minimal presuppositions necessary to interpret the input with respect to a discourse model (also see Altmann & Steedman, 1988; Ni & Crain, 1990; Trueswell & Tanenhaus, 1991). The parser computes structures in parallel and the structure that best fits the pragmatic constraints provided by the discourse model is incorporated into the model. If readers and listeners are processing incrementally, the discourse model will be frequently consulted and updated as a sentence is processed (Ades & Steedman, 1982; Marslen-Wilson & Tyler, 1987). Information about the fit between a possible parse and the model could then be available to evaluate the alternatives. The use of context in referential theory is similar to that in two–stage models of lexical ambiguity resolution (e.g., Swinney, 1979; Tanenhaus et al., 1979) in which multiple senses are accessed in a first stage of processing and then context is used to select a single sense. This approach has been labeled as "weakly interactive" in the parsing literature (e.g., Crain & Steedman, 1985), though it is fully consistent with the modular "propose and filter" architecture argued for by Forster (1979) in which lower-level systems pass on ambiguous outputs to higher-level systems. The different terminologies arise because the term interactive is used in the parsing literature to refer to any model in which syntactic decisions are informed by correlated nonsyntactic constraints, regardless of whether or not there is top-down feedback in the system. In contrast, feedback is the defining characteristic of interactive models in the word recognition literature (see Cutler, Chapter 4, this volume).

The Crain and Steedman (1985) proposal has become known as the referential theory because many of the crucial predictions hinge on what presuppositions are necessary to find or create a referent for definite noun phrases and other referring expressions. Presuppositional complexity is correlated with syntactic simplicity for those attachment ambiguities for which the less preferred structure involves noun phrase modification. The reduced relative ambiguity, many prepositional phrase attachment ambiguities, and the sentence complement/relative clause ambiguity all fall into this category. The referential theory predicts that discourse context can shift parsing preferences, eliminating garden paths that occur in "null" contexts, and inducing garden paths in normally preferred structures.

Consider our example again. In a relative clause the phrase *the pupil spotted* refers to a discourse entity that plays the theme of some spotting event. Because the relative clause modifies the noun phrase *the pupil*, Crain and Steedman (1985) argue that a set of possible discourse referents (i.e., a set of pupils) needs to be in discourse focus. The modifying relative clause then distinguishes a unique referent. In a null context, inferring a set of pupils would be a more complex presupposition than inferring a single pupil, leading to the main clause bias. However, in a context that established the appropriate discourse conditions (e.g., *Two pupils were cheating on an exam. The proctor spotted one pupil cheating, but not the other*), readers would correctly treat *the pupil spotted* as the beginning of a relative clause, because the discourse model does not contain a unique referent for *the pupil*.

iii. Constraint-based models. Constraint-based models have typically assumed some degree of parallelism and an evidentially based ambiguity resolution process in which multiple sources of constraint provide evidence in support of the most likely syntactic alternatives (e.g., Bates & MacWhinney, 1989; Marslen-Wilson, 1973; Oden, 1978; Taraban & McClelland, 1988). Ambiguity resolution is viewed as a constraint-satisfaction process, involving competition among incompatible alternatives. As a sentence unfolds, the alternatives are evaluated using evidence provided by the local input as well as the preceding and following ("right") context (MacDonald, 1994). Processing difficulty occurs when information is inconsistent (e.g., incompatible alternatives are equally supported) and when input is encountered that is inconsistent with the previously biased alternative. Conscious garden paths represent the end of a continuum in which the correct structure is no longer activated when the disambiguating input is encountered. In contrast to serial models like the garden-path model, constraint-based models do not sharply distinguish between a first stage of structure building and a second stage of evaluation and revision.

Constraint-based models have generally suffered from underspecification, leaving them open to the criticism that they do not make clear predictions beyond the general claim that context matters. For example, constraint-based models have typically not incorporated detailed assumptions about grammatical representations. This is problematic because linguistic representations play a central role in defining which constraints are relevant for sentence processing. In addition, claims about frequency, which are central to constraint-based systems, have been difficult to test until recently because large-scale parsed corpora are only now becoming available (e.g., Marcus, Santorini, & Marcinkiewicz, 1993).

Some of these concerns are beginning to be addressed in recent *constraint-based lexicalist* models. This framework emphasizes that the combinatory information that is part of lexical representation plays a central role in making available multiple syntactic alternatives and defining syntactic, semantic, and discourse constraints that are relevant to evaluating those alternatives (e.g., Carlson & Tanenhaus, 1988; Tanenhaus & Carlson, 1989).

In the constraint-based lexicalist framework, attachment ambiguities arise out of the intersection of several types of ambiguities (e.g., MacDonald et al., 1994a, 1994b), including argument structure ambiguities, syntactic category ambiguities, and morphological ambiguities of various kinds. Access to lexical representations is assumed to be frequency weighted (MacDonald, 1994; Tabossi, Spivey-Knowlton, McRae, & Tanenhaus, 1994; Trueswell & Tanenhaus, 1994; Trueswell, Tanenhaus, & Garnsey, 1994). Contextual effects are hypothesized to be mediated by lexical representations. When these factors are quantified and combined, it is claimed that there is no need for either an initial category-based parsing stage or a separate revision stage.

In order to make these ideas more concrete, we briefly consider an example using *donate,* a verb with multiple argument structures. Like all English verbs, *donate* requires a subject noun phrase when it appears as the matrix verb in a sentence. It also licenses, or subcategorizes for, two additional types of internal syntactic complements, a noun phrase and a prepositional phrase. *Donate* can be used with both of these complements together, as in (3a), or with each alone as in (3b) and (3c).

(3) a. *John donated a gift to the charity.*
    b. *John donated a gift.*
    c. *John donated to the charity.*

The semantic component of argument structure specifies the "thematic" role or mode of participation that each of the subcategorized complements plays in the event denoted by the verb. The combination of subcategorization frames and thematic roles results in three distinct argument structures for the verb *donate,* shown in:

(4) a. NP <Agent> NP <Theme> PP <Recipient>
    b. NP <Agent> NP <Theme>
    c. NP < Agent > PP <Recipient>

These argument structures are realized in sentences (3a) to 3(c), respectively.

Now assume that a reader or listener encounters *John donated.* At this point, the likely set of syntactic possibilities and their associated thematic roles would be available. The usefulness of this information is highlighted if we have a question such as *which charity did Bill donate . . .* Access to the argument structures and their thematic properties would allow the reader or listener to provisionally interpret *which charity* as the Recipient of the donation since a charity is a good *donate* recipient and a poor *donate* theme. The argument structures would also make available syntactic constraints that are relevant to this assignment. In contrast, a painting would be a good *donate* theme and a poor *donate* agent. Similarly, in a fragment such as *the painting donated. . .,* the fact that paintings are poor *donate* agents would provide evidence against any of the argument structures in (4), which define the possible set if the verb is in the active voice. However, if *donate* is a passive, then the subject NP becomes the Theme (e.g., NP <Theme> PP <Recipient>; NP <Theme>; Np<Theme>PP<Agent>). Thus thematic fit would provide evidence that *donated* was a passive voice and therefore that *the painting donated. . .* was the start of an object relative clause.

In the most detailed presentation of the constraint-based lexicalist framework, MacDonald et al. (1994b) analyze the reduced relative/main clause ambiguity as arising from several intersecting lexical ambiguities, including tense, voice (active or passive), and argument structure, adopting the interactive activation framework of McClelland and Rumelhart (1981). The constraint-based lexicalist framework makes similar predictions as the garden-path model when local constraints initially favor the main clause analysis (e.g., in our example *the pupil spotted. . .*), though the mechanisms differ. However, the predictions diverge as lexical frequencies and contextual constraints vary. For example, *The horse raced past the barn fell* is predicted to be especially difficult because *raced* is typically used as an active intransitive and *horse* is a good Agent for *raced.* In contrast, a sentence with the same syntactic structure (e.g., *The land mine buried in the sand exploded*) is predicted to cause little or no difficulty compared to an unambiguous control (e.g., *The land mine hidden in the sand exploded*) because *buried* is typically used transitively, it is frequently used as a participle in the passive voice and *land mine* is a poor *bury* agent.

b. Empirical Studies of Attachment Ambiguity

i. Structural preferences. The Minimal Attachment and Late Closure principles received striking support from a series of important eye-movement experiments initiated by Frazier and Rayner (1982), which showed that readers experience processing difficulty as soon as they encounter evidence that disambiguates a sentence in favor of the nonminimally attached alternative. In a typical study a locally ambiguous sentence is contrasted with an unambiguous control sentence with similar lexical content. For example, a reduced relative clause such as *The pupil spotted by the proctor was expelled* would be compared with an unambiguous full relative, *The pupil who was spotted by the proctor was expelled* (Ferreira & Clifton, 1986), or with an unambiguous reduced relative clause, *The pupil seen by the proctor was expelled* (Trueswell et al., 1994). The standard pattern of results is that fixation durations increase when the eye first enters the "disambiguating region" of the sentence (the prepositional phrase *by the proctor*). Readers are also more likely to make a regressive eye movement to reread earlier parts of the sentence, resulting in longer "second-pass" reading times. Similar results have been found for a variety of minimal attachment ambiguities, including the sentence complement ambiguity, prepositional phrase attachment ambiguities, and the relative clause/sentence complement ambiguity (cf. Clifton & Ferreira, 1989; Clifton et al., 1991; Frazier, 1987; Rayner & Frazier, 1987).

In most of these studies, comparisons of sentences that were disambiguated in favor of the minimally attached structure with unambiguous controls showed no systematic processing differences. On the assumption that computing parallel structures increases processing difficulty, this result provides strong support for the claim that the parser initially pursues a single analysis. Thus syntactic ambiguity resolution appeared to be strikingly different than lexical ambiguity resolution, where a variety of evidence from spoken language processing and from reading converges on the conclusion that initial contact with the input activates multiple candidates (e.g., Duffy, Morris, & Rayner, 1988; Kawamoto, 1993; Marslen-Wilson, 1989; Simpson, 1984). Rayner and Morris (1991) argue that these differences arise because lexical processing involves accessing stored forms, whereas syntactic processing uses rules to build novel structures.

Several important studies suggested that initial attachments might be unaffected by lexically specific syntactic information, local semantic context, and discourse context (e.g., Ferreira & Clifton, 1986; Ferreira & Henderson, 1990; Mitchell, 1987; Rayner et al., 1983), though more recent work has strongly qualified this conclusion.

Finally, although Minimal Attachment has received support in cross-linguistic studies, important exceptions to Late Closure have been identified, beginning with Cuetos and Mitchell's (1988) work in Spanish (also see Carreiras & Clifton, in press). Mitchell and Cuetos (1991) argue that attachment preferences differ across languages because they are tuned to be frequency sensitive. Gibson, Pearlmutter, Canseco-Gonzalez, and Hickock (in press) offer an account within the framework of Gibson's parser in which languages assign different weights to two parameters: *recency* and *preference* to attach a phrase to an argument of a verb. Finally, Frazier and Clifton (1994) develop the hypothesis that multiple attachment sites are evaluated in parallel for phrases that are not potential arguments, whereas primary grammatical relations are initially assigned serially according to Minimal Attachment and Late Closure.

ii. Verb information. A number of studies have focused on the time course with which verb-specific information becomes available, typically by examining congruity effects with syntactic or semantic/thematic anomalies (Boland, 1993; Gorrell, 1989; Marslen-Wilson et al., 1988; McElree, 1993; McElree & Griffith, in press; Osterhout & Holcomb, 1992; Tanenhaus, Garnsey, & Boland, 1991; Trueswell, Tanenhaus, & Kello, 1993). The conclusion that arises from all of these studies is that both subcategorization and thematic information become available when a verb is encountered.

Shapiro and colleagues show that multiple argument structures temporarily increase processing complexity, as initially suggested by J. A. Fodor et al. (1974). These experiments use lexical decision times in a cross-modal task as a measure of local processing difficulty (Shapiro, Zurif, & Grimshaw, 1989, but cf. Schmauder, Kennison, & Clifton, 1991). Processing complexity also increases when a less preferred argument structure is used (Clifton, Frazier, & Connine, 1984), with effects emerging most clearly when preferences are independently established for individual subjects (Shapiro, Nagel, & Levine, 1993).

The finest-grained temporal information comes from recent work by McElree (1993) and McElree and Griffith (in press) using Speed Accuracy Trade-off functions to examine retrieval processes. Category and subcategory information are activated equally quickly in memory, with less frequent subcategorizations accessed as rapidly (but perhaps not as strongly) as more frequent ones, indicating that lexically based syntactic alternatives are available in parallel. Access to thematic information may be delayed relative to subcategorization information.

The rapid access of argument structure information supports the constraint-based lexicalist assumptions. However, it is important to separate the question of when information becomes available from the question of how it is used. One possibility consistent with the garden-path frame-work is that verb-specific information is used as a "filter" to evaluate and, if necessary, revise the initial analysis posited on the basis of category informa-tion (Clifton, 1993; Clifton et al., 1991; Ferreira & Henderson, 1990, 1991; Frazier, 1987, 1989; Mitchell, 1987, 1989).

The sentence complement ambiguity has served as an important empiri-cal arena for studies investigating what happens when verb preferences and Minimal Attachment make different predictions (e.g., Ferreira & Hender-son, 1990, 1991; Garnsey, Lotocky, & McConkie, 1992; Holmes, Stowe, & Cupples, 1989; Juliano & Tanenhaus, 1993; Mitchell & Holmes, 1985; True-swell et al., 1993). Many of these studies were motivated by Ford et al.'s (1982) hypothesis that verb attachments are determined by the verb's most frequent subcategorization frame.

According to the lexical filtering hypothesis, readers and listeners should experience temporary difficulty in processing ambiguous sentences in which lexically specific constraints conflict with category-based attachment principles. Clear examples of this occur with the subject/object ambiguities that arise in the sentence complement ambiguity and the subordinate/main clause ambiguity. When a noun phrase follows a verb, readers have a strong preference to parse it as an object complement rather than as the subject of a main clause or a sentence complement, resulting in increased reading times at the underlined verbs for examples like those in (5).

(5) a.   *After the child visited the doctor <u>prescribed</u> a course of injections.*
    b.   *The student forgot the solution <u>was</u> in the back of the book.*

Mitchell (1987) demonstrated that processing difficulty is still found when the verb in the main clause does not permit an object; however, the diffi-culty then begins at the preceding noun as is illustrated in the examples in (6).

(6) a.   *After the child sneezed <u>the doctor</u> prescribed a course of injections.*
    b.   *The student hoped <u>the solution</u> was in the back of the book.*

Within a lexical filtering framework, these effects suggest an initial category-based NP attachment followed by rapid lexical filtering. However, these effects also emerge naturally in constraint-based lexicalist systems whenever the category-based generalization corresponds to the most fre-quent attachment across the set of individual lexical items. For example, corpus analyses show that a noun phrase following a verb is typically its object. Thus a constraint-based system will have a residual bias for the regular (e.g., more frequent) pattern in the language, even when that pat-tern is not independently represented, but rather arises because of shared features among specific items. This is analogous to the explanation for spelling-sound regularity effects in pronunciation developed by Seidenberg and McClelland (1989). On this view, there will be some processing difficulty for verbs that do not conform to the regular attachment pattern. However, the magnitude of the difficulty should be correlated with the frequency of that verb, with little or no processing difficulty for the highest-frequency verbs. Recent experimental studies using regression analyses (e.g., Juliano & Tanenhaus, 1993; Trueswell et al., 1993) and simulations with connectionist models that learn the mappings between individual verbs and complement types from a corpus (Juliano & Tanenhaus, 1994) have confirmed these predictions.

   iii. Thematic fit and argument assignment.   How and when the thematic fit between a noun phrase and a potential thematic role influences syntactic processing has received extensive attention in the recent literature, including studies using the subject/object ambiguity (Stowe, 1989; also Clifton, 1993), filler-gap dependencies (Tanenhaus, Boland, Mauner, & Carlson, 1993; Tanenhaus et al., 1991), and especially the relative clause ambiguity.

   In an important study, Ferreira and Clifton (1986) varied the animacy of the subject noun phrase in reduced and unreduced relative clauses (e.g., *The evidence/defendant examined by the lawyer turned out to be unreliable*). Inanimate nouns are poor Agents and thus provide a thematic constraint that supports the reduced relative. The results provided striking support for the independence of initial parsing decisions. First- and second-pass reading times were unaffected by the animacy manipulation. In addition, fixation times at the verb were longer for the inanimate nouns. Ferreira and Clifton (1986) argued that readers were aware of the implausibility of the inanimate Agent, but that still did not influence their initial attachment.

   However, subsequent studies have provided a different perspective on these results. For example, Trueswell et al. (1994) found clear effects of animateness at the disambiguating prepositional phrase, using more strongly constraining materials. In addition, correlations with typicality norms that quantified goodness of fit showed that the Ferreira and Clifton (1986) pattern occurs for weakly constraining nouns. For the most strongly constraining items, Trueswell et al. (1994) found no hint of processing difficulty for reduced relatives compared to unambiguous controls. Finally, the effects that Ferreira and Clifton (1986) found at the verb are similar to effects that are found for "sense" ambiguities when context biases a low-frequency sense (e.g., when context would bias the *eye* sense of the ambiguous noun *pupil*).

   There are now a number of studies that have found thematic effects with reduced relative clauses, including effects with animate nouns that are poor Agents and good Themes (for review, see MacDonald et al., 1994). Thematic constraints interact with argument structure and with postambiguity constraints (MacDonald, 1994). They also interact with the availability of the syntactic alternatives, as manipulated by parafoveal information that biases a passive participle (Burgess, 1991; Spivey-Knowlton, Trueswell, & Tanenhaus, 1993), and as determined by lexical frequency. A metanalysis of all of the context studies in the literature by MacDonald et al. (1994) shows that thematic effects are strongest for verbs that frequently are used in passive participle constructions and weakest for verbs that are typically used in the simple past tense.

iv. Referential context. Most research on how discourse context affects ambiguity resolution has been guided by the referential theory. The focus has been on how contexts that set up expectations for noun modification affect ambiguity resolution when the normally less preferred structure requires noun phrase modification. Three types of ambiguities have featured most prominently in the literature: (1) the prepositional phrase attachment ambiguity (Altmann & Steedman, 1988; Britt, Perfetti, Garrod, & Rayner, 1992; Ferreira & Clifton, 1986; Rayner, Garrod, & Perfetti, 1992; Spivey-Knowlton & Sedivy, in press); (2) the sentence complement/relative clause ambiguity (Altmann, 1989; Altmann, Garnham, & Dennis, 1992; Mitchell, Corley, & Garnham, 1992); and (3) the main clause/relative clause ambiguity (Britt et al., 1992; Ferreira & Clifton, 1986; Murray & Liversedge, 1994; Ni & Crain, 1990; Rayner et al., 1992; Spivey-Knowlton & Tanenhaus, 1994; Spivey-Knowlton et al., 1993).

The empirical support for referential effects is mixed (for a recent review, see Spivey-Knowlton & Tanenhaus, 1994). Some studies find immediate effects of referential context, with context reducing or eliminating processing difficulty for the less preferred structure (e.g., Altmann, 1989; Altmann et al., 1992; Altmann & Steedman, 1988; Ni & Crain, 1990; Spivey-Knowlton & Tanenhaus, 1994; Spivey-Knowlton et al., 1993). Other studies have found only weak or delayed effects of referential context (Britt et al., 1992; Ferreira & Clifton, 1986; Mitchell et al., 1992; Murray & Liversedge, 1994; Rayner et al., 1992).

However, generalizations are beginning to emerge in the literature from recent experiments in which referential effects are manipulated within the same experiment and with the same response measures (e.g., Britt, 1994; Britt et al., 1992; Spivey-Knowlton & Sedivy, in press; Spivey-Knowlton et al., 1993). Referential effects are found most consistently with prepositional phrase attachment, the ambiguity for which the alternative attachments are most similar in frequency. In contrast, the weakest effects come from studies with reduced relative clauses where there is a large frequency asymmetry. In addition, changing the availability of the normally less preferred structure controls the effectiveness of referential manipulations (Spivey-Knowlton et al., 1993), and they interact with local semantic constraints (Spivey-Knowlton & Tanenhaus, 1994).

The most compelling evidence for the availability hypothesis comes from recent studies by Britt (1994) and by Spivey-Knowlton and Sedivy (in press) using prepositional phrase attachment. Both of these studies demonstrate that the effectiveness of a referential context interacts with the strength of verb preferences. Britt showed that referential context shifted the preferred attachment for a prepositional phrase from VP modification to NP modification (e.g., *put away the book on the top shelf/the Civil War*) for verbs that optionally take a locative argument, but not for verbs that require one. Thus referential context was ineffective when it biased an attachment that was inconsistent with a strong local verb preference.

Spivey-Knowlton and Sedivy manipulated presuppositional complexity by varying the definiteness of the article in materials modified from those used by Altmann and Steedman (1988). Definite articles presuppose a unique discourse referent, whereas indefinites do not (e.g., *the thief blew up the/a safe with. . .*). The effect of the referential manipulation was weak for *action* verbs, which have a strong verb phrase attachment preference as determined by corpus analysis, and strong for *psych* and *perception* verbs, which have a slight NP preference attachment.

There are also individual differences in how context is used in processing temporarily ambiguous sentences. Just and Carpenter and their colleagues propose that readers with high memory span are better able to maintain multiple possibilities in parallel. Thus, high-span readers have less difficulty than low-span readers when the reading of an ambiguous word initially biased by context turns out to be incorrect (Just & Carpenter, 1992). High-span readers are also more sensitive to the less preferred reading of a structural ambiguity (MacDonald et al., 1992), and, are better able to use biasing contextual information to resolve local syntactic ambiguities (Just & Carpenter, 1992; King & Just, 1991). One possibility is that high-span readers have larger or more efficient working memories and therefore are better able to maintain alternative meanings, parallel structures, and contextual information. Alternatively, high-span readers may be more familiar with lower-frequency forms than low-span readers and thus they are better able to make use of correlated constraints (MacDonald et al., 1994b).

In conclusion, the referential context of an utterance can clearly provide constraints that are rapidly used in ambiguity resolution. However, the claim that parsing preferences can be reduced to discourse factors is almost certainly incorrect. Rather, the effects of discourse context are strongly modulated by within-sentence factors that govern the availability of the syntactic alternatives.

The overall generalization that emerges from the literature on thematic and discourse context effects on attachment ambiguity resolution is that context has immediate effects when it is strongly correlated with a syntactic alternative and when that alternative is available. Availability is strongly modulated by lexical factors, including the frequency of the lexical candidates. This is the case for syntactic category ambiguities as well as sense ambiguities, suggesting that uniform mechanisms may be involved (Mac-

Donald, 1993; Tabossi et al., 1994; Trueswell et al., 1994). MacDonald et al. (in press) argue that lexical and syntactic ambiguity resolution follow similar principles because syntactic ambiguity resolution is a variant of lexical ambiguity resolution.

The referential effects in parsing that we have reviewed demonstrate that readers incrementally update their discourse models to relate anaphoric expressions to entities in their model. Trueswell and Tanenhaus (1991, 1992) showed that readers also incrementally update events. They presented sentences such as *The student spotted by the proctor was later expelled* in future and past contexts such as those in (7):

(7) *Several students will take (took) an exam tomorrow (yesterday).*
     A proctor will notice (noticed) one of the students cheating.

The reduced relative ambiguity involves an ambiguity of tense, and tense is a contextually dependent expression with anaphorlike characteristics (Webber, 1988). Introducing a new past event in a future context is generally infelicitous. However, it is felicitous to use a relative clause to refer back to an event that will take place in the future as long as the event has already been introduced into the discourse model. Trueswell and Tanenhaus found that fragments such as *the student spotted. . .* were typically completed as main clauses in past contexts and as relative clauses in future contexts. Future contexts also sharply reduced difficulties for reduced relative clauses compared to unambiguous base line sentences in self-paced reading and eye-monitoring experiments.

v. Intonation and prosody.   Most recent research on attachment ambiguity resolution has examined reading for primarily methodological reasons. Visual stimuli are easy to control using microcomputers. In addition, experimental techniques such as eye tracking and self-paced reading permit experimenters to obtain continuous and relatively natural measures that are time locked to the input. However, prosodic and intonational variables are likely to play an important role in spoken language comprehension. Moreover, their presence in spoken language, and absence in printed language, may result in differences in how language in each modality is processed.

Several recent studies suggest that prosody can have clear effects on syntactic ambiguity resolution. For example, the duration of a segment tends to increase and the pitch (F0) tends to decrease at major syntactic boundaries (e.g., Cooper & Paccia-Cooper, 1980). Listeners are sensitive to this pattern in English and can use it in resolving phrase boundary ambiguities (Price, Ostendorf, Shattuck-Hufnagel, & Fong, 1991).

Consider the subject/object clause boundary examples in (8) taken from Speer and Kjelgaard-Bernstein (1992).

(8) a. *Whenever the guard checks the door, it's locked.*
    b. *Whenever the guard checks, the door is locked.*

In (8a) *checks* is not followed by a major phrase boundary since the following NP is the object of the verb, whereas in (8b) it is followed by an S (Major clause) boundary. Speer and Kjelgaard-Bernstein found that speeded comprehension judgments were fastest when the intonation was consistent with the correct parse of the sentence. Moreover, there was not a late closure advantage for sentences with early closure prosody, suggesting that prosody can eliminate the usual late closure preference.

Beach (1991) found that duration and F0 determined the preferred continuation of fragments ending in a noun phrase that could either be the object of the preceding verb or the subject of a sentence complement. Marslen-Wilson, Tyler, Warren, Grenier, and Lee (1992) found similar effects using a cross-modal integration task. Subjects listened to ambiguous fragments like those in (9a) in which the underlined phrase could either be the object of the verb or the subject of a sentence complement, and then named aloud a visual target (e.g., *was*) that continued the fragment as a sentence complement.

(9) a.   *The workers considered the offer from management.* . .
    b.   *The workers considered that the offer from management.* . .

Naming times to *was* were longer compared to an unambiguous control condition (9b) when prosody was consistent with an object continuation, but not when it was consistent with a sentence complement.

Finally, it is important to note that many of the prosodic cues provided by speakers are likely to be related to interpretive and referential processes (cf. Speer, Crowder, & Thomas, 1993). A clear example is contrastive focus (e.g., *Touch the LARGE red triangle*), which focuses attention on both the referent in the asserted proposition, and the entities or propositions to which it is being contrasted (e.g., Sedivy, Carlson, Tanenhaus, Spivey-Knowlton, & Eberhard, in press; Tanenhaus, Spivey-Knowlton, Eberhard, & Sedivy, in press). Pierrehumbert and Hirschberg (1990) outline an approach for exploring how prosody maps onto discourse representations that is likely to play an important role in future research.

3. Empty Categories

Sentences with *empty categories* have been studied extensively in the sentence processing literature, especially by researchers with a linguistic orientation. Several factors have contributed to the interest in these constructions. First, they have been important in the development of transformational grammar, with their properties having been used to motivate novel and often controversial syntactic proposals. In particular, the notion of a phonetically unrealized syntactic category clearly emerged within Chomsky's (1981) Government and Binding (GB) theory where it plays a central role. Second, competing syntactic frameworks typically differ in how these constructions are explained. Theories that make use of multiple levels of syntactic representation and movement rules (transformations) rely heavily on empty categories, whereas other theories with a more surface-oriented syntax make limited use of empty categories or do without them completely. These differences have motivated experiments to find evidence for the "psychological reality" of empty categories. Finally, certain types of empty category constructions, especially those with *long-distance dependencies,* are useful for studying how different types of linguistic and nonlinguistic information are coordinated in on-line comprehension.

The sentence in example (10) contains a long-distance dependency between the noun phrase *which car* and the verb *put.*

(10) *I wonder which car$_i$ Tom put _____$_i$ in the garage.*

The verb *put* normally requires two internal arguments: a noun phrase complement that immediately follows the verb and plays the role of Theme; and a second complement, usually a prepositional phrase, that plays the role of Location. Leaving out either of these arguments results in an anomalous sentence (e.g., **Tom put the car* or **Tom put in the garage*). However, the example sentence is perfectly comprehensible even though *put* seems to be missing its noun phrase complement, resulting in the normally anomalous sequence *put in the garage.* The sentence is grammatical because *which car* functions as the missing argument. Following terminology introduced by J. D. Fodor (1978), the "missing" syntactic argument after the verb will be referred to as a *gap* and the phrase that functions as the argument in the interpretation of the sentence as a *filler.* Gap locations are marked with an underline and subscripts are used to "co-index" the gap and the filler.

In a long-distance dependency, the interpretation of the filler depends, in part, on identifying the gap, which itself is temporarily ambiguous, as is illustrated by the examples in (11).

(11) a. *I wonder which book$_i$ Tom read_____$_i$ to us?*
     b. *I wonder which book$_i$ Tom read about_____$_i$?*

In (11a) *which book* is the object of the verb *read,* that is, what Tom is reading, whereas in (11b) *read* is being used intransitively and *which book* is the object of the preposition *about,* that is, what is being read about.

In an important early study, Wanner and Maratsos (1978) proposed that a filler is held in temporary storage until the gap is encountered. Using a concurrent memory load task, they found that memory load increases after a filler is encountered and then returns to a normal base line after the gap location. Kleunder and Kutas (1993) present ERP data implicating phonological working memory in processing long-distance dependencies.

Readers have a strong tendency to propose and fill a gap as soon as a verb is encountered. The most striking evidence comes from a study by Stowe (1986), which used sentence pairs similar to those illustrated in (12).

(12) a.   *I wonder which guest$_i$ the hostess invited us to meet____$_i$at the party.*
     b.   *I wonder if the hostess invited us to meet the guest at the party.*

Reading times to *us* were longer in the *wh* conditions (12), where there was a possible gap after the verb, than in the *if* control sentence (12b), where there was not a possible gap. This demonstrates that readers initially interpreted the filler, *which guest* as the object of the verb *invite* and then had to revise the gap analysis at *us,* resulting in longer reading times (cf. Clifton & Frazier, 1989; Crain & Fodor, 1985). Stowe also showed that readers do not postulate gaps in environments where they would be ruled out by other syntactic constraints (also Kleunder & Kutas, 1993).

As in the attachment ambiguity literature, lexical variables have played an important role with some models assigning a primary role to lexical factors (e.g., J. D. Fodor, 1978), whereas other models assume that gap filling is initially determined by category-based principles (Clifton & DeVincenzi, 1990; Clifton & Frazier, 1989). Several studies have examined whether the early filling bias is eliminated when a verb is typically used intransitively (Clifton & Frazier, 1989; Clifton et al., 1984; Stowe, Tanenhaus, & Carlson, 1991). The results have been somewhat inconclusive, perhaps because lexical effects depend on aspects of argument structure that are only partially correlated with transitivity. Boland, Garnsey, and Tanenhaus (in various combinations) and their colleagues have manipulated argument structure in experiments in which the plausibility of a *wh* phrase is manipulated with respect to a potential gap after the verb. For example, in a study measuring event-related potentials, Garnsey, Tanenhaus, and Chapman (1989) contrasted sentences like those illustrated in (13).

(13) a.   *I wondered which book$_i$ the boy read____$_i$in class yesterday.*
     b.   *I wondered which food$_i$the boy read____$_i$in class yesterday.*

Garnsey et al. (1989) found that the N400 component of the ERP wave form to the verb was larger when the filler was implausible, indicating that readers had immediately attempted to relate the filler to the verb, resulting in an incongruous interpretation. Subsequent work has shown that these anomaly effects are mediated by argument structure. Readers take thematic fit into account in gap assignment as long as the verb's argument structure provides multiple gap sites (e.g., Tanenhaus et al., 1991, 1993), confirming the generalization we drew earlier about the conditions under which context affects syntactic processing.

In the GB framework, empty categories are treated as a type of referential dependency, in effect, a type of unexpressed or implicit pronoun with the filler as its antecedent. Since pronouns facilitate recognition of their antecedents in probe recognition and lexical priming paradigms (e.g., Dell, McKoon, & Ratcliff, 1983), similar "priming" effects are expected for empty categories. A number of studies have confirmed this prediction, beginning with Bever and McElree (1988; for review, see J. D. Fodor, 1989; Nicol & Swinney, 1989).

Swinney, Ford, Frauenfelder, and Bresnan (1989) used sentences similar to the example in (14).

(14)   *That's the actress$_i$ that the doctor from the new medical center invited____$_i$to the party.*

Lexical decisions and naming times were faster to an associate of the word *actress* than to an unrelated control word when the target was presented after *invite*. Nicol (1993) has reported priming at the verb, even when the gap occurred several words after the verb, suggesting that argument structure information was mediating gap filling. This is consistent with the conclusions of the anomaly studies that we reviewed earlier. It is also consistent with evidence from intuitions presented in Pickering and Barry (1991) who used these, and other, data to argue against empty categories (but cf. Gibson & Hickock, 1993).

However, the interpretation of cross-modal priming effects as reflecting gap filling has recently been called into question by McKoon and colleagues who argue that the effects are due to general congruence between the target and local context rather than true lexical priming (McKoon & Ratcliff, in press; McKoon, Ratcliff, & Ward, in press; but cf. Nicol, Fodor, & Swinney, in press).

GB theory also makes use of several types of empty categories and it uses them in places where other grammatical frameworks do not. For example, GB posits an empty category (NP-trace) following a verbal passive such as (15) to account for why the surface subject of verb in the passive is assigned the thematic role that is canonically assigned to its object, and it posits a null pronominal (PRO) in infinitive clauses such as (16) to account for the fact that the infinitives have an "understood" subject. Other grammatical theories such as Lexical Functional Grammar (Bresnan & Kaplan, 1982), Generalized Phrase Structure Grammar (Gazdar, Klein, Pullum, & Sag, 1985), and its descendent, Head-Driven Phrase Structure Grammar (Pollard & Sag, 1993) account for these phenomena in the semantics or by using lexical rules.

(15)   *The mayor$_i$ on the podium was shot____$_i$.*

(16)   *Which friend$_i$ did Bill invite____$_i$PRO____$_i$to go to the party?*

Several studies using probe recognition paradigms, beginning with Bever and McElree (1988), have found priming to the filler in constructions in which only GB theory posits an empty category. For example, MacDonald (1989) found speeded probe recognition to the target *mayor* following sentences with verbal passives such as (15) compared to adjectival passives such as *The mayor on the podium was furious,* which, according to GB theory, do not contain an NP-trace. Bever and McElree (1988) and McElree and Bever (1989) found speeded recognition to adjective probes in a variety of syntactic constructions in which GB theory posits an empty category compared to control conditions with similar lexical content. While these results are consistent with predictions generated from GB theory, it remains to be seen whether explanations couched in terms of other levels of representation can be ruled out (cf. J. D. Fodor, 1989).

4. Sentence Memory

Relatively little recent research on sentence processing has made use of memory paradigms. However, the nature of people's immediate memory for surface form remains an important issue. Studies conducted in the 1970s, including Jarvella (1971) and Wanner (1974), found that people have verbatim memory for the clause they are processing and perhaps one additional clause. These studies used recognition paradigms in which subjects judged whether a probe sentence was "new" or "old." Gernsbacher (1985) showed that the loss of surface memory is tied to integration processes (also see Murphy & Shapiro, 1994). However, more recent work by Potter and Lombardi (1990) challenges the idea that there is verbatim memory for even the most recent clause. Their results suggest that what appears to be verbatim recall is actually reconstructed from lexical representations and their argument structures.

Finally, although studies using explicit memory paradigms find little evidence that memory for linguistic structure is preserved, structural processing does have long-term consequences. In a classic study, Carey, Mehler, and Bever (1970) demonstrated that processing sentences with similar structures biases the interpretation of an ambiguous sentence. Interest in the mechanisms underlying these "priming" effects is re-emerging, sparked by Bock's (1986) striking evidence for structural priming in language production. Research on this issue is beginning to focus on whether or not similar effects occur in sentence comprehension and, if so, what is the nature of the priming (e.g., are syntactic constructions primed, or is priming restricted to lexical/syntactic features?). The syntactic structure used to introduce a phrase also has clear effects on its salience or accessibility in memory (McKoon, Ratcliff, Ward, & Sproat, 1993).

5. Context and Anaphora

There is now a substantial literature demonstrating that there is not a separate stage in processing during which sentence meaning (i.e., a literal or a context-independent meaning) is constructed (e.g., Gibbs, 1984). Rather, the interpretation of a sentence takes place against the contextual backdrop established by the comprehender's discourse model, which is updated incrementally as the sentence unfolds. The importance of context can be illustrated by comparing the interpretation of our example sentence when it occurs in isolation and when it is preceded by the following context:

(17)　　*A math exam was being held to screen applicants for admission to a special high school. Two pupils were cheating with a crib sheet. The assistant principal, who was proctoring the exam, noticed one of the students cheating, but not the other. The pupil spotted by the proctor was expelled.*

When the sentence is presented in a null context, the reader (or listener) knows that the proctor spotted the pupil (doing something) and that the student was expelled (by someone). When presented in the context of (17), the reader can establish more specific information about the content of the sentence. For example, the reader knows that the student was cheating on an exam with a crib sheet and it is likely that he was expelled from the exam. The context also provides more specific information about the student and about the proctor.

Many of the explicit links between a sentence and its context occur through referential expressions, or *anaphors,* whose interpretation depends on entities and events that have already been introduced into the model (Haviland & Clark, 1974). In our example, *the pupil* and *the proctor* are each anaphoric expressions that refer to entities previously established in the discourse model and *spotted* refers to the event in which the proctor noticed one of the pupils cheating (Webber, 1988). The linguistic expression that initially introduces the discourse entity is the *antecedent,* though this term is often used more loosely to refer to either the antecedent or the discourse entity. *The assistant principal, who was proctoring the exam,* is the linguistic antecedent for *the proctor* in the last sentence, and *two pupils* is the antecedent for the anaphoric expression *one of the students.*

Natural languages make use of a rich variety of anaphoric devices, a small subset of which are illustrated in Table 2. In addition to anaphors that are explicitly expressed (pronouns, definite noun phrases, *one* anaphora, *do so* and *do it* anaphora, etc.), there are many kinds of anaphors that are unexpressed or implicit, typically because an optional argument of a verb has been omitted in context. Research on anaphora has focused on four general questions: (1) what is the nature of the representations that different types of anaphors access?; (2) what factors influence the processes by which anaphors find their antecedents?; (3) what is the time course with which anaphors are assigned interpretations?; and (4) what is the discourse function of different anaphors?

Hankamer and Sag (1976) proposed that anaphors could be grouped into

TABLE 2   Some Types of Anaphoras[a]

Definite pronouns:	*He gave it to her.*
Reflexive pronouns:	*Julie defended herself.*
Demonstrative pronouns:	*Please hand me that cup.*
Repeated noun anaphora:	*David called up Gail, but Gail wasn't home.*
Definite noun phrase anaphora:	*A tall man walked into the room. The man took off his coat.*
One anaphora:	*Cornell bought a used bicycle and Kathy bought a new one.*
Do it anaphora:	*Michael asked Sheryl to take out the garbage, but she refused to do it.*
Do so anaphora:	*Michael asked Sheryl to take out the garbage, but she refused to do so.*
Verb phrase ellipsis:	*Michael asked Sheryl to take out the garbage, but she refused to ____.*
Null complement anaphora:	*Michael asked Sheryl to take out the garbage, but she refused ____.*
Gapping:	*Kenzo ordered steak and Josh ____ chicken.*
Null pronominal anaphora:	*____ Noticing the fallen man, Joy came to his rescue.*

[a]The anaphoric expression is underlined. For expressions that are anaphoric because they have an unexpressed constituent, both the omitted constituent and its antecedent are underlined.

two categories, which they labeled *deep* and *surface* anaphora. Sag and Hankamer (1984) later hypothesized that deep anaphors access a conceptual level of representation in a discourse or mental model, whereas surface anaphors initially access a linguistic level of representation. The distinction is motivated by the observation that surface anaphors (e.g., verb phrase ellipsis and *do so* anaphora), but not deep anaphors (e.g., pronouns, null complement anaphora and *do it* anaphora) require their antecedents to be introduced linguistically and place structural constraints on the linguistic form of their antecedent.

Experimental tests of the deep–surface distinction have failed to support the strong form of the Sag and Hankamer (1984) hypothesis. Some studies have found that the structural characteristics of a linguistic antecedent affect surface anaphors more than deep anaphors (Mauner, Tanenhaus, & Carlson, in press-b; Tanenhaus & Carlson, 1990), whereas others have not (e.g., Murphy, 1985). Mauner et al. (in press-b) suggest that clear differences emerge when pragmatic effects are controlled for, whereas Murphy (1990) argues that differences are seen only when subjects are asked to make explicit judgments about the target sentences. Garnham and Oakhill (1987) show that pragmatic context can influence the interpretation of surface anaphors.

The claim that deep anaphors are interpreted using conceptual or mental model representations has received strong support in the literature (e.g., Cloitre & Bever, 1988; Garnham, 1981; Gernsbacher, 1991; Lucas, Tanenhaus, & Carlson, 1990; McKoon et al., 1993). Garnham and Oakhill (1992) present a useful overview of the mental models approach to anaphora. Particularly striking evidence for conceptual effects on deep anaphors comes from work by Gernsbacher and colleagues (e.g., Carreiras & Gernsbacher, 1992; Gernsbacher, 1991; Oakhill, Garnham, Gernsbacher, & Cain, 1992), which shows that notional number rather than grammatical number is relevant for interpreting deep anaphoras in discourse context. For example, in (18) the plural pronoun *them* is used to refer to the conceptual entities knives, though the linguistic antecedent *knife* is singular.

(18)   *I need a knife. Where do you keep them?*

The time course with which anaphors are interpreted in context has been the subject of numerous experiments. Most of this literature has examined the processing of pronouns and definite noun phrases, using either reading time measures or priming paradigms. A review of this literature goes well beyond the scope of this chapter. In general, the literature shows that people begin to interpret anaphoric expressions immediately. Factors such as grammatical position, verb semantics, the distance between the antecedent and the anaphor, and local and global focus in the discourse model, determine the speed with which an anaphor will be interpreted. These factors also affect which of several possible antecedents is most likely to be assigned when the anaphor is ambiguous (for reviews, see Gernsbacher, 1989; S. B. Greene et al., 1992; MacDonald & MacWhinney, 1991; Sanford & Garrod, 1989).

Although most research has focused on the salience of the antecedent, anaphors themselves are likely to play an important role in helping listeners manage attentional resources (Brennan, in press) as they integrate the sentence into the discourse model as it unfolds. This idea has been developed in some detail within the *centering* framework, initially proposed by Grosz, Joshi, and Weinstein (1983). Preliminary empirical support comes from work by Brennan (in press), Gordon, Grosz, and Gilliom (1993), and Hudson-D'Zmura and Tanenhaus (in press).

Implicit anaphors have generally received less attention than explicit anaphors. Tyler and Marslen-Wilson (1982) show that null pronominal anaphoras are interpreted as rapidly as noun anaphors and explicit pronouns. Some arguments of verbs are omitted only when context specifies their content. Several recent studies have found that these unexpressed arguments are "filled in" using information from context (Halpern, Mauner, & Tanenhaus, 1993; McKoon & Ratcliff, 1992). Other classes of unexpressed arguments may be represented semantically as unspecified or partially specified entities, even in the absence of specific contextual information (Mauner, Tanenhaus, & Carlson, in press-a. For example, the interpretation of *The pupil spotted by the proctor was expelled* out of context might be something like: The pupil spotted by the proctor (doing something) was expelled (by someone) (from someplace).

In conclusion, research on the processing of anaphors and on referential effects on syntactic processing each demonstrate that anaphoric and other contextually dependent expressions provide important links between the discourse model and the sentence. Readers and listeners exploit these links to develop incremental interpretations as the sentence unfolds over time.

IV. SUMMARY AND FUTURE DIRECTIONS

The goal of this chapter has been to provide the reader with an overview of some of the central theoretical and empirical issues in sentence comprehension, including some historical perspective on how the field has developed. In doing so, we have necessarily focused on only a subset of issues. However, we have tried to provide enough detail for a reader to be able to reconstruct how our example sentence would be comprehended, from the perspective of what we currently know about sentence processing. We conclude with a brief discussion of some trends that are emerging in the recent literature and how we expect they will shape the field during the next few years.

Although most research in sentence processing is still conducted primarily in English, recent years have seen an increase in research across a spectrum of languages. This is important because focus on a single language can result in a distorted picture of which aspects of language processing are adaptations to a particular language and which reflect basic processing principles. Cross-linguistic research has already begun to have an important theoretical impact, especially on models of syntactic processing, and this trend is likely to continue.

During the next few years, the field is likely to show more emphasis on statistical and computational models that generate quantitative predictions about behavioral data. As a result, there should be more focus on mechanisms and explicit links to related areas in perception and cognition, including work in learning, attention, and categorization. We expect that the problem of ambiguity resolution will increasingly be viewed within the broader context of models of perceptual indeterminacy and of information integration. The development of learning models, and an increased focus on lexical representation, should also lead to more productive interaction between researchers investigating sentence processing in adults, and researchers who are studying related issues in language development.

The ability to make use of data from corpora is likely to be crucial to any modeling efforts because it allows researchers to quantify and test claims about frequency, co-occurence, and strength of correlation among constraints. Corpus analyses can also be used to evaluate potential biases in experimenter-constructed materials, and to test hypotheses derived from a variety of models.

While research on reading will continue to be important, there will be an increased focus on spoken language, including prosodic information that is correlated with structure and with interpretation. As work in both modalities develops, there will be increased awareness of different modes of language use. For example, reading sentences in a narrative text may represent a very different mode of language processing from understanding an utterance in a cooperative task with visually accessible referents. Focus on different modes of language processing may help to clarify which aspects of processing reflect architectural properties of the system, and which reflect the nature of the available information.

Finally the next few years should see more focus on the problem of how interpretations are constructed incrementally during on-line comprehension. Investigations are likely to be informed by developments in lexical and formal semantics, as well as in pragmatics, including an increase in our understanding of the syntactic/pragmatic interface.

As we pointed out earlier, current work in sentence processing began in the "language-as-product" tradition, with transformational grammar defining the representations that a comprehender develops in encoding the grammatical structure of a sentence. As the field has developed, attention has shifted away from the sentence as a linguistic entity. As this trend continues, we expect to see constraints from competence grammars embedded within models of language processing, but not as an encapsulated component of the system. Thus, linguistic representations will play a central role in sentence processing, but as part of a more integrated system that coordinates linguistic and nonlinguistic information as the input unfolds over time. This will pave the way for models of language processing that integrate the language-as-product tradition with the "language-as-action" tradition (see Clark, 1993, and Clark and Bly, Chapter 11, this volume).

Acknowledgments

The first author's research during preparation of this chapter was supported by Grant HD-27206 from the NICHD. We would like to express our appreciation to Joanne Miller for editorial advice that improved the readability and the organization of the chapter, and to Kathy Eberhard, Julie Sedivy, and Joy Hanna for helpful comments. Special thanks to Sheryl Knowlton-Spivey for assistance with references.

References

Ades, A., & Steedman, M. (1982). On the order of words. *Linguistics and Philosophy, 4,* 517–558.

Allen, J. F. (1994). *Natural language understanding.* Redwood City, CA: Benjamin/Cummings.

Altmann, G. (1989). Parsing and interpretation: A introduction. *Language and Cognitive Processes, 4,* 1–19.

Altmann, G., Garnham, A., & Dennis, Y. (1992). Avoiding the garden-path: Eye movements in context. *Journal of Memory and Language, 31*, 685–712.

Altmann, G., & Steedman, M. (1988). Interaction with context during human sentence processing. *Cognition, 30*, 191–238.

Bates, E., & MacWhinney, B. (1989). Functionalism and the competition model. In B. MacWhinney & E. Bates (Eds.), *The crosslinguistic study of sentence processing*. Cambridge, UK: Cambridge University Press.

Beach, C. (1991). The interpretation of prosodic patterns at points of syntactic structure ambiguity: Evidence for cue trading relations. *Journal of Memory and Language, 30*, 644–663.

Berwick, R. C., & Weinberg, A. (1984). *The grammatical basis of linguistic performance: Language use and acquisition*. Cambridge, MA: MIT Press.

Bever, T. G. (1970). The cognitive basis for linguistic structures. In J. R. Hayes (Ed.), *Cognition and the development of language*. New York: Wiley.

Bever, T. G. (1988). The psychological reality of grammar: A student's eye view of cognitive science. In G. Hirst (Ed.), *The making of cognitive science: A festschrift for George A. Miller*. Cambridge, UK: Cambridge University Press.

Bever, T. G., Garrett, M. F., & Hurtig, R. R. (1973). Ambiguity increases complexity of perceptually incomplete clauses. *Memory & Cognition, 1*, 279–286.

Bever, T. G., & Hurtig, R. R. (1975). Detection of a non-linguistic stimulus is poorest at the end of a clause. *Journal of Psycholinguistic Research, 4*, 1–7.

Bever, T. G., & McElree, B. (1988). Empty categories access their antecedents during comprehension. *Linguistic Inquiry, 19*, 35–43.

Blumenthal, A. L. (1967). Prompted recall of sentences. *Journal of Verbal Learning and Verbal Behavior, 6*, 203–206.

Bock, J. K. (1986). Syntactic persistence in language production. *Cognitive Psychology, 18*, 355–387.

Boland, J. E. (1993). The role of verb argument structure in sentence processing: Distinguishing between syntactic and semantic effects. *Journal of Psycholinguistic Research, 22*, 135–152.

Boland, J. E., Tanenhaus, M. K., & Garnsey, S. M. (1990). Evidence for the immediate use of verb control information in sentence processing. *Journal of Memory and Language, 29*, 413–432.

Bransford, J. D., Barclay, J., & Franks, J. J. (1972). Sentence memory: A constructive versus interpretive approach. *Cognitive Psychology, 3*, 193–209.

Bransford, J. D., & Franks, J. J. (1971). The abstraction of linguistic ideas. *Cognitive Psychology, 2*, 331–350.

Brennan, S. E. (in press). Centering attention in discourse. *Language and Cognitive Processes*.

Bresnan, J. W. (1978). A realistic transformational grammar. In M. Halle, J. W. Bresnan, & G. A. Miller (Eds.), *Linguistic theory and psychological reality*. Cambridge, MA: MIT Press.

Bresnan, J. W., & Kaplan, R. M. (1982). Introduction: Grammars as mental representations of language. *The mental representation of grammatical relations*. Cambridge, MA: MIT Press.

Britt, M. A. (1994). The interaction of referential ambiguity and argument structure. *Journal of Memory and Language, 33*, 251–283.

Britt, M. A., Perfetti, C. A., Garrod, S., & Rayner, K. (1992). Parsing and discourse: Context effects and their limits. *Journal of Memory and Language, 31*, 293–314.

Burgess, C. (1991). *The interaction of syntactic semantic and visual factors in syntactic ambiguity resolution*. Unpublished doctoral dissertation, University of Rochester, Rochester, NY.

Cacciari, C., & Tabossi, P. (Eds.). (1993). *Idioms: Processing, structure and interpretation*. Hillsdale, NJ: Erlbaum.

Carey, P. W., Mehler, J., & Bever, T. G. (1970). Judging the veracity of ambiguous sentences. *Journal of Verbal Learning and Verbal Behavior, 9,* 243–254.

Carlson, G. N., & Tanenhaus, M. K. (1988). Thematic roles and language comprehension. In W. Wilkins (Ed.), *Syntax and semantics: Vol. 21. Thematic relations.* London: Academic Press.

Carreiras, M., & Clifton, C. (in press). Relative clause interpretation preferences in Spanish and English. *Language and Speech.*

Carreiras, M., & Gernsbacher, M. A. (1992). Comprehending conceptual anaphors in Spanish. *Language and Cognitive Processes, 7,* 281–300.

Carroll, J. M., & Bever, T. G. (1978). Sentence comprehension: A case study in the relation of knowledge and perception. In E. C. Carterette & M. P. Friedman (Eds.), *Handbook of perception* (Vol. 7, pp. 299–317). New York: Academic Press.

Carroll, J. M., Tanenhaus, M. K., & Bever, T. G. (1978). The perception of relations: The interaction of structural, functional and contextual factors in the segmentation of speech. In W. J. M. Levelt & G. B. Flores d'Arcais (Eds.), *Studies in the perception of language* (pp. 187–218) New York: Wiley.

Chomsky, N. (1957) *Syntactic structures.* The Hague: Mouton.

Chomsky, N. (1965). *Aspects of the theory of syntax.* Cambridge, MA: MIT Press.

Chomsky, N. (1970). Remarks on nominalization. In R. Jacobs & P. Rosenbaum (Eds.), *Reading in English transformational grammar.* Waltham, MA: Ginn.

Chomsky, N. (1981). *Lectures on government and binding.* Dordrecht: Foris.

Clark, H. H. (1993). *Arenas of language use.* Chicago: University of Chicago Press.

Clifton, C. (1993). Thematic roles in sentence parsing. *Canadian Journal of Experimental Psychology, 47,* 222–246.

Clifton, C., & DeVincenzi, M. (1990). Comprehending sentences with empty elements. In D. A. Balota, G. B. Flores d'Arcais, & K. Rayner (Eds.), *Comprehension processes in reading* (pp. 265–283). Hillsdale, NJ: Erlbaum.

Clifton, C. & Ferreira, F. (1989). Ambiguity in context. *Language and Cognitive Processes, 4,* (SI), 77–104.

Clifton, C., & Frazier L. (1989). Comprehending sentences with long-distance dependencies. In G. N. Carlson & M. K. Tanenhaus (Eds.), *Linguistic structure in language processing.* Dordrecht: Kluwer.

Clifton, C., Frazier, L., & Connine, C. (1984). Lexical and syntactic expectations in sentence comprehension. *Journal of Verbal Learning and Verbal Behavior, 23,* 696–708.

Clifton, C., Kurcz, I., & Jenkins, J. (1965). Grammatical relations as determinants of sentence similarity. *Journal of Verbal Learning and Verbal Behavior, 4,* 112–117.

Clifton, C., Speer, S. R., & Abney, S. (1991). Parsing arguments: Phrase structure and argument structure as determinants of initial parsing decisions. *Journal of Memory and Language, 30,* 251–271.

Cloitre, M., & Bever, T. G. (1988). Linguistic anaphors, levels of representation, and discourse. *Language and Cognitive Processes, 3,* 293–322.

Cooper, W. E., & Paccia-Cooper, J. (1980). *Syntax and speech.* Cambridge, MA: Harvard University Press.

Cowart, W., & Cairns, H. S. (1987). Evidence for an anaphoric mechanism within syntactic processing: Some reference relations defy semantic and pragmatic constraints. *Memory & Cognition, 15,* 318–331.

Crain, S., & Fodor, J. D. (1985). How can grammars help parsers? In D. R. Dowty, L. Karttunen, & A. Zwicky (Eds.), *Natural language parsing: Psychological, computational, and theoretical perspectives.* Cambridge, UK: Cambridge University Press.

Crain, S., & Steedman, M. (1985). On not being led up the garden path: The use of context by the psychological parser. In D. R. Dowty, L. Kartunnen, & A. Zwicky (Eds.), *Natural language parsing: Psychological, computational and theoretical perspectives*. Cambridge, UK: Cambridge University Press.

Cuetos, F., & Mitchell, D. C. (1988). Cross-linguistic differences in parsing: Restrictions on the use of the late closure strategy in Spanish. *Cognition, 30,* 73–105.

Cutler, A., & Norris D. (1979). Monitoring sentence comprehension. In W. E. Cooper & E. C. T. Walker (Eds.), *Sentence processing: Psycholinguistic studies presented to Merrill Garrett* (pp. 113–134). Hillsdale, NJ: Erlbaum.

Dell, G. S., McKoon, G., & Ratcliff, R. (1983). The activation of antecedent information during the processing of anaphoric reference in reading. *Journal of Verbal Learning and Verbal Behavior, 22,* 121–132.

Duffy, S. A., Morris, R. K., & Rayner, K. (1988). Lexical ambiguity and fixation times in reading. *Journal of Memory and Language, 27,* 429–446.

Farrar, W., & Kawamoto, A. (1993). The return of "visiting relatives": Pragmatic effects in sentence processing. *Quarterly Journal of Experimental Psychology, 46A,* 463–487.

Ferreira, F., & Clifton, C. (1986). The independence of syntactic processing. *Journal of Memory and Language, 25,* 348–368.

Ferreira, F., & Henderson, J. (1990). The use of verb information in syntactic parsing: A comparison of evidence from eye movements and segment-by-segment self-paced reading. *Journal of Experimental Psychology; Learning, Memory and Cognition, 16,* 555–568.

Ferreira, F., & Henderson, J. (1991). Recovery from misanalyses of garden-path sentences. *Journal of Memory and Language, 30,* 461–476.

Fodor, J. A. (1983). *Modularity of mind*. Cambridge, MA: MIT Press.

Fodor, J. A., Bever, T. G., & Garrett, M. F. (1974). *The psychology of language*. New York: McGraw-Hill.

Fodor, J. A., & Garrett, M. F. (1966). Some reflections on competence and performance. In J. Lyons & R. J. Wales (Eds.), *Psycholinguistic papers: Proceedings of the 1966 Edinburgh Conference*. Edinburgh: Edinburgh University Press.

Fodor, J. D. (1978). Parsing strategies and constraints on transformations. *Linguistic Inquiry, 9,* 427–473.

Fodor, J. D. (1989). Empty categories in sentence processing. *Language and Cognitive Processes, 4,* 155–209.

Ford, M., Bresnan, J. W., & Kaplan, R. M. (1982). A competence-based theory of syntactic closure. In J. W. Bresnan (Ed.), *The mental representation of grammatical relations*. Cambridge, MA: MIT Press.

Forster, K. I. (1979). Levels of processing and the structure of the language processor. In W. E. Cooper & E. C. T. Walker (Eds.), *Sentence processing: Psycholinguistic studies presented to Merrill Garrett*. Hillsdale, NJ: Erlbaum.

Forster, K. I., & Olbrei, I. (1973). Semantic heuristics and syntactic analysis. *Cognition, 2,* 319–348.

Frazier, L. (1987). Sentence processing: A tutorial review. In M. Coltheart (Ed.), *Attention and performance XII: The psychology of reading*. London: Erlbaum.

Frazier, L. (1989). Against lexical generation of syntax. In W. Marslen-Wilson (Ed.), *Lexical representation and process*. Cambridge, MA: MIT Press.

Frazier, L., & Clifton, C. (1994). *Construal*. Manuscript, University of Massachusetts, Amherst.

Frazier, L., & Fodor, J. D. (1978). The sausage machine: A new two-stage parsing model. *Cognition, 6,* 291–325.

Frazier, L., & Rayner, K. (1982). Making and correcting errors during sentence comprehension: Eye movements in the analysis of structurally ambiguous sentences. *Cognitive Psychology, 14,* 178–210.

Frazier, L., & Rayner, K. (1987). Resolution of syntactic category ambiguities: Eye movements in parsing lexically ambiguous sentences. *Journal of Memory and Language, 26,* 505–526.

Garfield, J. (Ed.). (1987). *Modularity in knowledge representation and natural language understanding.* Cambridge, MA: MIT Press.

Garnham, A. (1981). Mental models as representations of text. *Memory & Cognition, 9,* 560–565.

Garnham, A., & Oakhill, J. (1987). Interpreting elliptical verb phrases. *Quarterly Journal of Experimental Psychology, 39A,* 611–627.

Garnham, A., & Oakhill, J. (1992). Discourse processing and text representation from a "mental models" perspective. *Language and Cognitive Processes, 7,* 193–204.

Garnsey, S. M. (1993). Event-related brain potentials in the study of language: An introduction. *Language and Cognitive Processes: Special Issue, 8,* 337–356.

Garnsey, S. M., Lotocky, M., & McConkie, G. (1992). *Verb-usage knowledge in sentence comprehension.* Poster presented at the 33rd annual meeting of the Psychonomics Society.

Garnsey, S. M., Tanenhaus, M. K., & Chapman, R. M. (1989). Evoked potentials and the study of sentence comprehension. *Journal of Psycholinguistic Research, 18,* 51–60.

Gazdar, G., Klein, E., Pullum, G. K., & Sag, I. A. (1985). *Generalized phrase structure grammar.* Cambridge, MA: Harvard University Press.

Gernsbacher, M. A. (1985). Surface information loss in comprehension. *Cognitive Psychology, 17,* 324–363.

Gernsbacher, M. A. (1989). Mechanisms that improve referential access. *Cognition, 32,* 99–156.

Gernsbacher, M. A. (1991). Comprehending conceptual anaphors. *Language and Cognitive Processes, 6,* 81–105.

Gibbs, R. W. (1984). Literal meaning and psychological theory. *Cognitive Science, 8,* 275–304.

Gibson, E. (1991). *A computational theory of linguistic processing: Memory limitations and processing breakdown.* Unpublished doctoral dissertation, Carnegie Mellon University, Pittsburgh, PA.

Gibson, E., & Hickok, G. (1993). Sentence processing with empty categories. *Language and Cognitive Processes, 8,* 147–161.

Gibson, E., Pearlmutter, N., Canseco-Gonzalez, E., & Hickok, G. (in press). Cross-linguistic attachment preferences: Evidence from English and Spanish. *Cognition.*

Gordon, P. C., Grosz, B. J., & Gilliom, L. A. (1993). Pronouns, nouns, and the centering of attention in discourse. *Cognitive Science, 17,* 311–349.

Gorrell, P. (1989). Establishing the loci of serial and parallel effects in syntactic processing. *Journal of Psycholinguistic Research, 18,* 61–73.

Greene, J. M. (1970). The semantic function of negatives and positives. *British Journal of Psychology, 61,* 17–22.

Greene, S. B., McKoon, G., & Ratcliff, R. (1992). Pronoun resolution and discourse models. *Journal of Experimental Psychology: Learning, Memory, and Cognition, 18,* 266–283.

Grosz, B. J., Joshi, A. K., & Weinstein, S. (1983). Providing a unified account of definite noun phrases in discourse. In *Proceedings of the 21st annual meeting of the Association for Computational Linguistics.* Cambridge, MA: MIT Press.

Hagoort, P., Brown, C., & Groothusen, J. (1993). The syntactic positive shift (SPS) as an ERP measure of syntactic processing. *Language and Cognitive Processes, 8,* 439–484.

Halpern, A., Mauner, G., & Tanenhaus, M. K. (1993). Priming of structural and conceptual verb-phrase anaphors. In *Proceedings of the 23rd annual meeting of the Northeastern Linguistics Society.* Amherst, MA: Graduate Student Linguistic Association.

Hankamer, J., & Sag, I. A. (1976). Deep and surface anaphor. *Linguistic Inquiry, 7,* 391–428.

Haviland, S. E., & Clark, H. H. (1974). What's new? Acquiring new information as a process in communication. *Journal of Verbal Learning and Verbal Behavior, 13,* 512–521.

Holmes, V., Stowe, L., & Cupples, L. (1989). Lexical expectations in parsing complement-verb sentences. *Journal of Memory and Language, 28,* 668–689.

Hudson-D'Zmura, S., & Tanenhaus, M. K. (in press). Assigning antecedents to ambiguous pronouns: The role of the center of attention as the default assignment. In E. Prince, A. Joshi, & M. Walker (Eds.), *Centering in discourse.* Oxford: Oxford University Press.

Jarvella, R. J. (1971). Syntactic processing of connected speech. *Journal of Verbal Learning and Verbal Behavior, 10,* 409–416.

Johnson-Laird, P. (1983). *Mental models.* Cambridge, UK: Cambridge University Press.

Johnson-Laird, P. (1984). Linguistics and psychology. In M. H. Bornstein (Ed.), *Cross currents in contemporary psychology.*

Johnson-Laird, P., & Stevenson, R. (1970). Memory for syntax. *Nature (London) 227,* 412.

Juliano, C., & Tanenhaus, M. K. (1993). Contingent frequency effects in syntactic ambiguity resolution. In *Proceedings of the 15th annual conference of the Cognitive Science Society* (pp. 593–598). Hillsdale, NJ: Erlbaum.

Juliano, C., & Tanenhaus, M. K. (1994). A constraint-based lexicalist account of the subject/object attachment preference. *Journal of Psycholinguistic Research.*

Just, M. A., & Carpenter, P. A. (1980). A theory of reading: From eye fixations to comprehension. *Psychological Review, 87,* 329–354.

Just, M. A., & Carpenter, P. A. (1992). A capacity theory of comprehension: Individual differences in working memory. *Psychological Review, 99,* 122–149.

Just, M. A., Carpenter, P. A., & Woolley, J. (1982). Paradigms and processes in reading comprehension. *Journal of Experimental Psychology: General, 111,* 228–238.

Kawamoto, A. (1993). Nonlinear dynamics in the resolution of lexical ambiguity: A parallel distributed processing account. *Journal of Memory and Language, 32,* 474–516.

Kimball, J. (1973). Seven principles of surface structure parsing in natural language. *Cognition, 2,* 15–47.

King, J., & Just, M. A. (1991). Individual differences in syntactic processing: The role of working memory. *Journal of Memory and Language, 30,* 580–602.

Kleunder, R., & Kutas, M. (1993). Bridging the gap: Evidence from ERPs on the processing of unbounded dependencies. *Journal of Cognitive Neuroscience, 5,* 196–214.

Kurtzman, H. (1985). *Studies in syntactic ambiguity resolution.* Doctoral dissertation, MIT, Cambridge, MA. (Distributed by Indiana University Linguistics Club)

Levelt, W. J. M. (1978). A survey of studies is sentence perception: 1970–1976. In W. J. M. Levelt & G. B. Flores d'Arcais (Eds.), *Studies in the perception of language.* Chichester: Wiley.

Lucas, M., Tanenhaus, M. K., & Carlson, G. N. (1990). Levels of representation in the interpretation of anaphoric reference and instrument inference. *Memory & Cognition, 18,* 611–631.

MacDonald, M. C. (1989). Priming effects from gaps to antecedents. *Language and Cognitive Processes, 4,* 35–56.

MacDonald, M. C. (1993). The interaction of lexical and syntactic ambiguity. *Journal of Memory and Language, 32,* 692–715.

MacDonald, M. C. (1994). Probabilistic constraints and syntactic ambiguity resolution. *Language and Cognitive Processes, 9,* 157–201.

MacDonald, M. C., Just, M. A., & Carpenter, P. A. (1992). Working memory constraints on the processing of syntactic ambiguity. *Cognitive Psychology, 24,* 56–98.

MacDonald, M. C., & MacWhinney, B. (1991). Measuring inhibition and facilitation from pronouns. *Journal of Memory and Language, 29,* 469–492.

MacDonald, M. C., Pearlmutter, N., & Seidenberg, M. S. (1994). Syntactic ambiguity resolution as lexical ambiguity resolution. In C. Clifton, L. Frazier, & K. Rayner (Eds.), *Perspectives on sentence processing.* Hillsdale, NJ: Erlbaum.

MacDonald, M. C., Pearlmutter, N., & Seidenberg, M. S. (1994). The lexical nature of syntactic ambiguity resolution. *Psychological Review. 101,* 676–703.

Marcus, M. P. (1980). *A theory of syntactic recognition for natural language.* Cambridge, MA: MIT Press.

Marcus, M. P., Hindle, D., & Fleck, M. (1983). D-theory: Talking about talking about trees. In *Proceedings of the 21st annual meeting of the Association for Computational Linguistics* (pp. 129–136). Hillsdale, NJ: Erlbaum.

Marcus, M. P., Santorini, B., & Marcinkiewicz, M. A. (1993). Building a large annotated corpus of English: The Penn Treebank. *Computational Linguistics, 19,* 313–330.

Marslen-Wilson, W. (1973). Linguistic structure and speech shadowing at very short latencies. *Nature (London), 244,* 522–523.

Marslen-Wilson, W. (1975). Sentence perception as an interactive parallel process. *Science, 189,* 226–228.

Marslen-Wilson, W. (1987). Functional parallelism in spoken word recognition. *Cognition, 25,* 71–102.

Marslen-Wilson, W. (1989). Access and integration: Projecting sound onto meaning. In W. Marslen-Wilson (Ed.), *Lexical representation and process.* Cambridge, MA: MIT Press.

Marslen-Wilson, W., Brown, C., & Tyler, L. K. (1988). Lexical representations in language comprehension. *Language and Cognitive Processes, 3,* 1–16.

Marslen-Wilson, W., & Tyler, L. K. (1987). Against modularity. In J. L. Garfield (Ed.), *Modularity in knowledge representation and natural language understanding.* Cambridge, MA: MIT Press.

Marslen-Wilson, W., Tyler, L. K., & Seidenberg, M. S. (1978). Sentence processing and the clause boundary. In W. J. M. Levelt & G. B. Flores d'Arcais (Eds.), *Studies in the perception of language.* New York: Wiley.

Marslen-Wilson, W., Tyler, L. K., Warren, P., Grenier, P., & Lee, C. S. (1992). Prosodic effects in minimal attachment. *Quarterly Journal of Experimental Psychology, 45A,* 73–87.

Marslen-Wilson, W., & Welsh, A. (1978). Processing interactions and lexical access during word recognition in continuous speech. *Cognitive Psychology, 10,* 29–63.

Mauner, G., Tanenhaus, M. K., & Carlson, G. (in press-a). Implicit arguments in sentence processing. *Journal of Memory and Language.*

Mauner, G., Tanenhaus, M. K., & Carlson, G. N. (in press-b). A note on parallelism effects in processing deep and surface verb-phrase anaphors. *Language and Cognitive Processes.*

McClelland, J. L., & Rumelhart, D. E. (1981). An interactive activation model of context effects in letter perception: Part 1. An account of basic findings. *Psychological Review, 88,* 375–407.

McElree, B. (1993). The locus of lexical preference effects in sentence comprehension: A time-course analysis. *Journal of Memory and Language, 32,* 536–571.

McElree, B., & Bever, T. G. (1989). The psychological reality of linguistically defined gaps. *Journal of Psycholinguistic Research, 18,* 21–35.

McElree, B., & Griffith, T. (in press). Syntactic and thematic processing in sentence comprehension: Evidence for a temporal dissociation. *Journal of Experimental Psychology: Learning, Memory, and Cognition.*

McKoon, G., & Ratcliff, R. (1979). Priming in episodic memory. *Journal of Verbal Learning and Verbal Behavior, 18,* 463–480.

McKoon, G., & Ratcliff, R. (1992). Inference during reading. *Psychological Review, 99,* 440–466.

McKoon, G., & Ratcliff, R. (1994). Sentential context and on-line lexical decision. *Journal of Experimental Psychology: Learning, Memory, and Cognition, 20,* 1239–1243.

McKoon, G., Ratcliff, R., & Ward, G. (1994). Testing theories of language processing: An empirical investigation of the on-line lexical decision task. *Journal of Experimental Psychology: Learning, Memory, and Cognition, 20,* 1219–1228.

McKoon, G., Ratcliff, R., Wad, G., & Sproat, R. (1993). Morphosyntactic and pragmatic factors affecting the accessibility of discourse entities. *Journal of Language and Memory, 32,* 56–75.

Mehler, J. (1963). Some effects of grammatical transformations on the recall of English sentences. *Journal of Verbal Learning and Verbal Behavior, 2,* 346–351.

Miller, G. A. (1956). The magical number seven, plus or minus two: Some limits on our capacity for processing information. *Psychological Review, 63,* 81–97.

Miller, G. A. (1962). Some psychological studies of grammar. *American Psychologist, 17,* 748–762.

Miller, G. A., & Chomsky, N. (1963). Finitary models of language users. In R. D. Luce, R. R. Bush, & E. Galanter (Eds.), *Handbook of mathematical psychology.* New York: Wiley.

Miller, G. A., & Isard, S. D. (1963). Some perceptual consequences of linguistic rules. *Journal of Verbal Learning and Verbal Behavior, 2,* 217–228.

Mitchell, D. C. (1987). Lexical guidance in human parsing: Laws and processing characteristics. In M. Coltheart (Ed.), *Attention and performance XII: The psychology of reading.* London: Erlbaum.

Mitchell, D. C. (1989). Verb guidance and other lexical effects in parsing. Special issue: Parsing and interpretation. *Language and Cognitive Processes, 4,* (SI), 123–154.

Mitchell, D. C., Corley, M. M. B., & Garnham, A. (1992). Effects of context in human sentence parsing: Evidence against a discourse-based proposal mechanism. *Journal of Experimental Psychology: Learning, Memory, and Cognition, 18,* 69–88.

Mitchell, D. C., & Cuetos, F. (1991). The origins of parsing strategies. *Conference proceedings: Current issues in natural language processing.* Austin: University of Texas.

Mitchell, D. C., & Holmes, V. (1985). The role of specific information about the verb in parsing sentences with local structure ambiguity. *Journal of Memory and Language, 24,* 542–559.

Morrow, D. G.,& Bower, G. H. (1989). Updating situation models during narrative comprehension. *Journal of Memory and Language, 28,* 292–312.

Murphy, G. L. (1985). Processes of understanding anaphora. *Journal of Memory and Language, 24,* 290–303.

Murphy, G. L. (1990). Interpretation of verb-phrase anaphora: Influences of task and syntactic context. *Quarterly Journal of Experimental Psychology, 42A,* 675–692.

Murphy, G. L., & Shapiro, A. (1994). Forgetting verbatim information in discourse. *Memory & Cognition, 22,* 85–94.

Murray, W., & Liversedge, S. (1994). Referential context and syntactic processing. In C. Clifton, L. Frazier, & K. Rayner (Eds.), *Perspectives on sentence processing.* Hillsdale, NJ: Erlbaum.

Ni, W., & Crain, S. (1990). How to resolve structural ambiguities. In *Proceedings of the North East Linguistic Society,* (Vol. 20). Amherst, MA: Graduate Student Linguistics Association.

Nicol, J. (1993). Reconsidering reactivation. In G. Altmann & R. Shillcock (Eds.), *Cognitive models of speech processing: The second Sperlonga meeting.* Hillsdale, NJ: Erlbaum.

Nicol, J., Fodor, J. D., & Swinney, D. A. (in press). Using cross-modal lexical decision tasks to investigate sentence processing. *Journal of Experimental Psychology: Learning, Memory, and Cognition, 20,* 1229–1238.

Nicol, J., & Swinney, D. A. (1989). The role of structure in coreference assignment during sentence comprehension. *Journal of Psycholinguistic Research, 18,* 5–19.

Oakhill, J., Garnham, A., Gernsbacher, M. A., & Cain, K. (1992). How natural are conceptual anaphors? *Language and Cognitive Processes, 7,* 257–280.

Oden, G. C. (1978). Semantic constraints and judged preference for interpretations of ambiguous sentences. *Memory & Cognition, 6,* 26–37.

Osterhout, L., & Holcomb, P. (1992). Event-related brain potentials elicited by syntactic anomaly. *Journal of Memory and Language, 31,* 785–806.

Pickering, M., & Barry, G. (1991). Sentence processing without empty categories. *Language and Cognitive Processes, 6,* 229–259.

Pierrehumbert, J., & Hirschberg, J. (1990). The meaning of intonational contours in discourse. In P. R. Cohen, J. Morgan and M. Pollack (Eds.), *Intentions in communication.* Cambridge, MA: MIT Press.

Pollard, C. J., & Sag, I. A. (1993). *Head-driven phrase structure grammar.* Chicago: University of Chicago Press.

Potter, M., & Lombardi, L. (1990). Regeneration in the short term recall of sentences. *Journal of Memory and Language, 29,* 633–654.

Price, P. J., Ostendorf, M., Shattuck-Hufnagel, S., & Fong, C. (1991). The use of prosody in syntactic disambiguation. *Journal of the Acoustical Society of America, 90,* 2956–2970.

Pritchett, B. L. (1992). *Grammatical competence and parsing performance.* Chicago: University of Chicago Press.

Rayner, K., Carlson, M., & Frazier, L. (1983). The interaction of syntax and semantics during sentence processing: Eye movements in the analysis of semantically biased sentences. *Journal of Verbal Learning and Verbal Behavior, 22,* 358–374.

Rayner, K., & Frazier, L. (1987). Parsing temporarily ambiguous complements. *Quarterly Journal of Experimental Psychology, 39A,* 657–673.

Rayner, K., Garrod, S. C., & Perfetti, C. A. (1992). Discourse influences during parsing are delayed. *Cognition, 45,* 109–139.

Rayner, K., McConkie, G., & Zola, D. (1980). Integrating information across eye movements. *Cognitive Psychology, 12,* 206–226.

Rayner, K., & Morris, R. (1991). Comprehension processes in reading ambiguous sentences: Reflections from eye movements. In G. B. Simpson (Ed.), *Advances in psychology: Understanding word and sentence* (pp. 175–198). Amsterdam: Elsevier/North-Holland.

Rayner, K., & Pollatsek, A. (1987). Eye movements in reading: A tutorial review. In M. Coltheart (Ed.), *Attention and performance XII: The psychology of reading.* London: Erlbaum.

Rayner, K., Sereno, S. C., Morris, R. K., Schmauder, A. R., & Clifton, C. (1989). Eye movements and on-line language comprehension. *Language and Cognitive Processes, Special Issue: Parsing and Interpretation, 4,* (SI), 21–49.

Sachs, J. S. (1967). Recognition memory for syntactic and semantic aspects of connected discourse. *Perception & Psychophysics, 2,* 437–442.

Sag, I. A., & Hankamer, J. (1984). Toward a theory of anaphoric processing. *Linguistics and Philosophy, 7,* 325–345.

Sanford, A. J., & Garrod, S. C. (1989). What, when and how? Questions of immediacy in anaphoric reference resolution. *Language and Cognitive Processes, Special Issue: Parsing and Interpretation, 4,* (SI), 235–262.

Schmauder, R., Kennison, S. M., & Clifton, C. (1991). On the conditions necessary for obtaining argument structure complexity effects. *Journal of Experimental Psychology: Learning, Memory, and Cognition, 17,* 1188–1192.

Schwanenflugel, P. J. (Ed.). (1991). *The psychology of word meanings.* Hillsdale, NJ: Erlbaum.

Sedivy, J. C., Carlson, G. N., Tanenhaus, M. K., Spivey-Knowlton, M. J., & Eberhard, K. (in press). The cognitive function of contrast sets in processing focus constructions. In *Proceedings of the IBM Conference on Focus and Natural Language Processing.*

Seidenberg, M. S., & McClelland, J. L. (1989). A distributed, developmental model of word recognition and naming. *Psychological Review, 96,* 447–452.

Seidenberg, M. S., Tanenhaus, M. K., Leiman, J. M., & Bienkowski, M. A. (1982). Automatic access of the meanings of ambiguous words in context: Some limitations of knowledge-based processing. *Cognitive Psychology, 14,* 489–537.

Shapiro, L. P., Nagel, N. H., & Levine, B. A. (1993). Preferences for a verb's complements and their use in sentence processing. *Journal of Memory and Language, 32,* 96–114.

Shapiro, L. P., Zurif, E., & Grimshaw, J. (1989). Verb processing during sentence comprehension: Contextual impenetrability. *Journal of Psycholinguistic Research, 18,* 223–243.

Shillcock, R., & Bard, E. (1993). Modularity and the processing of closed-class words. In G. Altmann & R. Shillcock (Eds.), *Cognitive models of speech processing: The second Sperlonga meeting.* Hillsdale, NJ: Erlbaum.

Simpson, G. B. (1984). Lexical ambiguity and its role in models of word recognition. *Psychological Bulletin, 96,* 316–340.

Slobin, D. I. (1966). Grammatical transformations and sentence comprehension in childhood and adulthood. *Journal of Verbal Learning and Verbal Behavior, 5,* 219–227.

Speer, S. R., Crowder, R. G., & Thomas, L. M. (1993). Prosodic structure and sentence recognition. *Journal of Memory and Language, 32,* 336–358.

Speer, S. R., & Kjelgaard-Bernstein, M. (1992). *The influence of prosodic structure on processing temporary syntactic ambiguity.* Poster presented at the 33rd annual meeting of the Psychonomics Society, St. Louis, MO.

Spivey-Knowlton, M. J., & Sedivy, J. C. (in press). Resolving attachment ambiguities with multiple constraints. *Cognition.*

Spivey-Knowlton, M. J. & Tanenhaus, M. K. (1994). Referential context and syntactic ambiguity resolution. In C. Clifton, L. Frazier, & K. Rayner (Eds.), *Perspectives on sentence processing.* Hillsdale, NJ: Erlbaum.

Spivey-Knowlton, M. J., Trueswell, J. C., & Tanenhaus, M. K. (1993). Context effects in syntactic ambiguity resolution: Discourse and semantic influences in parsing reduced relative clauses. *Canadian Journal of Experimental Psychology, 47,* 276–309.

Stowe, L. (1986). Evidence for on-line gap location. *Language and Cognitive Processes, 1,* 227–245.

Stowe, L. (1989). Thematic structures in sentence comprehension. In G. N. Carlson & M. K. Tanenhaus (Eds.), *Linguistic structure in language processing.* Dordrecht: Kluwer.

Stowe, L., Tanenhaus, M. K., & Carlson, G. N. (1991). Filling gaps on-line: Use of lexical and semantic information in sentence processing. *Language and Speech, 34,* 319–340.

Swinney, D. A. (1979). Lexical access during sentence comprehension: (Re)consideration of context effects. *Journal of Verbal Learning and Verbal Behavior, 18,* 645–660.

Swinney, D. A. (1991). The resolution of indeterminacy during language comprehension: Perspectives on modularity in lexical, structural, and pragmatic processing. In G. B. Simpson (Ed.), *Advances in psychology: Understanding word and sentence.* Amsterdam: Elsevier/North-Holland.

Swinney, D. A., Ford, M., Frauenfelder, U. H., & Bresnan, J. W. (1989). On the temporal course of gap-filling and antecedent assignment during sentence comprehension. In B. Grosz, R. M. Kaplan, M. Macken, & I. A. Sag (Eds.), *Language structure and processing.* Stanford, CA: Center for the Study of Language and Information.

Swinney, D. A., Onifer, W., Prather, P., & Hirschkowitz, M. (1978). Semantic facilitation across sensory modalities in the processing of individual words and sentences. *Memory & Cognition, 7,* 165–195.

Tabossi, P., Spivey-Knowlton, M. J., McRae, K., & Tanenhaus, M. K. (1994). Semantic effects on syntactic ambiguity resolution: Evidence for a constraint-based resolution process. In C. Umilta & M. Moscovitch (Eds.), *Attention and performance XV.* Hillsdale, NJ: Erlbaum.

Tanenhaus, M. K., Boland, J. E., Mauner, G., & Carlson, G. N. (1993). More on combinatory lexical information: Thematic structure in parsing and interpretation. In G. Altmann & R. Shillcock (Eds.), *Cognitive models of speech processing:* The second Sperlonga Meeting. Hillsdale, NJ: Erlbaum.

Tanenhaus, M. K., & Carlson, G. N. (1989). Lexical structure and language comprehension.

In W. Marslen-Wilson (Ed.), *Lexical representation and process* (pp. 529–561). Cambridge, MA: MIT Press.

Tanenhaus, M. K., & Carlson, G. N. (1990). Comprehension of deep and surface verb phrase anaphors. *Language and Cognitive Processes, 5,* 257–280.

Tanenhaus, M. K., Dell, G. S., & Carlson, G. N. (1987). Context effects and lexical process-ing: A connectionist approach to modularity. In J. L. Garfield (Ed.), *Modularity in knowl-edge representation and natural language understanding* (pp. 83–108). Cambridge: MA: MIT Press.

Tanenhaus, M. K., & Donnenwerth-Nolan, S. (1984). Syntactic context and lexical access. *Quarterly Journal of Experimental Psychology, 36A,* 649–661.

Tanenhaus, M. K., Garnsey, S. M., & Boland, J. E. (1991). Combinatory lexical information and language comprehension. In G. T. M. Altmann (Ed.), *Cognitive models of speech processing: Psycholinguistic and computational perspectives.* Cambridge, MA: MIT Press.

Tanenhaus, M. K., Leiman, J. M., & Seidenberg, M. S. (1979). Evidence for multiple stages in the processing of ambiguous words in syntactic contexts. *Journal of Verbal Learning and Verbal Behavior, 18,* 645–659.

Tanenhaus, M. K., & Seidenberg, M. S. (1981). Discourse context and sentence perception. *Discourse Processes, 26,* 197–220.

Tanenhaus, M. K., Spivey-Knowlton, M. J., Eberhard, K., & Sedivy, J. C. (in press). Using eye-movements to study spoken language comprehension: Evidence for visually-mediated incremental interpretation. In T. Inoue & J. L. McClelland (Eds.), *Attention and performance XVI: Integration in perception and communication.* Cambridge, MA: MIT Press.

Taraban, R., & McClelland, J. (1988). Constituent attachment and thematic role expectations. *Journal of Memory and Language, 27,* 597–632.

Townsend, D. J., & Bever, T. G. (1978). Interclause relationships and clausal processing. *Journal of Verbal Learning and Verbal Behavior, 17,* 509–521.

Townsend, D. J., & Bever, T. G. (1982). Natural units interact during language comprehen-sion. *Journal of Verbal Learning and Verbal Behavior, 28,* 681–703.

Trueswell, J. C., & Tanenhaus, M. K. (1991). Tense, temporal context and syntactic ambiguity resolution. *Language and Cognitive Processes, 6,* 339–350.

Trueswell, J. C., & Tanenhaus, M. K. (1992). Consulting temporal context in sentence com-prehension: Evidence from the monitoring of eye movements in reading. In *Proceedings of the 14th annual meeting of the Cognitive Science Society* (pp. 492–497). Hillsdale, NJ: Erlbaum.

Trueswell, J. C., & Tanenhaus, M. K. (1994). Toward a constraint-based lexicalist approach to syntactic ambiguity resolution. In C. Clifton, L. Frazier, & K. Rayner (Eds.), *Perspectives on sentence processing.* Hillsdale, NJ: Erlbaum.

Trueswell, J. C., Tanenhaus, M. K., & Garnsey, S. M. (1994). Semantic influences on parsing: Use of thematic role information in syntactic disambiguation. *Journal of Memory and Language, 33,* 285–318.

Trueswell, J. C., Tanenhaus, M. K., & Kello, C. (1993). Verb-specific constraints in sentence processing: Separating effects of lexical preference from garden-paths. *Journal of Experi-mental Psychology: Learning, Memory, and Cognition, 19,* 528–553.

Tyler, L. K., & Marslen-Wilson, W. D. (1977). The on-line effects of semantic context on syntactic processing. *Journal of Verbal Learning and Verbal Behavior, 16,* 683–692.

Tyler, L. K., & Marslen-Wilson, W. D. (1982). The resolution of discourse anaphors: Some on-line studies. *Text, 2,* 263–291.

Wanner, E. (1974). *On remembering, forgetting and understanding sentences.* The Hague: Mouton.

Wanner, E. (1977). Review of Fodor, et al. (1974). *Psycholinguistic Research, 6,* 261–270.

Wanner, E. (1980). The ATN and the sausage machine: Which one is baloney? *Cognition, 8,* 209–225.

Wanner, E., & Maratsos, M. (1978). An ATN approach to comprehension. In M. Halle, J. W.

Bresnan, & G. A. Miller (Eds.), *Linguistic theory and psychological reality*. Cambridge, MA: MIT Press.

Webber, B. L. (1979). *A formal approach to discourse anaphora*. New York: Garland.

Webber, B. L. (1988). Tense as a discourse anaphor. *Computational Linguistics, 14*, 61–73.

Weinberg, A. (in press). Minimal commitment: A parsing theory for the 90s. *Language and Cognitive Processes*.

West, R. F., & Stanovich, K. E. (1986). Robust effects of syntactic context on naming. *Memory & Cognition, 14*, 104–112.

Wright, B., & Garrett, M. F. (1984). Lexical decision in sentences: Effects of syntactic structure. *Memory & Cognition, 12*, 31–45.

CHAPTER 8

Language Acquisition: Speech Sounds and the Beginning of Phonology

Peter W. Jusczyk

I. INTRODUCTION

For close to fifty years, scientists and engineers have been trying to develop machines that could take a speech input and produce an acceptable written transcript of it. Despite the efforts of many bright minds, success in this endeavor has been a long time coming and still seems years away. Yet human infants typically manage to crack the speech code in a way that allows them to achieve reasonable fluency in a native language by 3 years of age (see Clark, Chapter 9, this volume). Why is speech so hard for machines, but easy for infants? What hurdles lie in the path of successful speech recognition that infants manage to surmount (see Nygaard and Pisoni, Chapter 3, this volume)?

One basic problem that any speech recognition system has to solve is to recover the appropriate units from the speech signal. This has been termed the segmentation problem. Although fluent perceivers of a language tend to hear speech as a sequence of discrete words, there is often considerable acoustic overlap between successive items in the speech stream. Consequently, even boundaries between words (let alone between units such as syllables or phones) typically are not clearly marked in the input. It is likely that knowledge of native language sound patterns, along with other information about its grammatical organization, play some role in solving the

Speech, Language, and Communication

segmentation problem for fluent perceivers. When listeners do not have access to this information, such as when they listen to an unfamiliar foreign language, they often have difficulty determining where one word leaves off and another begins.

Another major obstacle to successful speech recognition is what has been termed the invariance problem. This has to do with the fact that there is considerable variability in the speech signal, and it seems to occur at every possible level of analysis. The acoustic properties associated with a particular phone depend on the nature of the surrounding phonetic segments. Speech researchers have met with only limited success in their efforts to identify invariant acoustic features that could signal the presence of a particular phoneme in all its possible contexts (Blumstein & Stevens, 1978, 1980; Delattre, Liberman, & Cooper, 1955; Klatt, 1989; Liberman, Cooper, Shankweiler, & Studdert-Kennedy, 1967; Searle, Jacobson, & Rayment, 1979; Stevens & Blumstein, 1981). Not only must speech recognition systems cope with variability in how a particular phonetic segment is realized in different contexts, but they must also deal with talker variability. Owing to differences in vocal tract shape and size, and the speed and accuracy with which talkers can execute articulatory movements, there may be marked acoustic differences in the same utterance produced by different talkers. Listeners must be able to compensate for these kinds of talker differences in order to correctly identify words and phonetic segments (Bladon, Henton, & Pickering, 1984; Rand, 1971; Verbrugge, Strange, Shankweiler, & Edman, 1976). Finally, even within the same talker, changes in speaking rate can have an important impact on the mapping between acoustic cues and phonetic segments (Miller & Liberman, 1979).

There is also a third task facing language learners even if they make headway in dealing with the segmentation and invariance problems. This has to do with discovering the particular kinds of units that are being manipulated in the speech signal and any ordering constraints on these units. Each language draws on only a subset of the possible sounds that are used in forming words in natural languages. To become a fluent perceiver of a particular language, the learner has to determine which elements are used in the language and just how these can be combined. Moreover, because languages differ not only in their segmental structures, but also in their prosodic structures, the learner needs to discover the organization of both these levels within the native language.

What we do know about when infants begin to deal effectively with these kinds of obstacles to successful speech recognition? In what follows, I outline some of the basic capacities that infants have for perceiving speech and when some of the major milestones appear to be achieved. I also discuss how these capacities evolve as the infant becomes engaged in acquiring a native language and relate some of these developments to concurrent changes in speech production. (For detailed models regarding the development of speech perception capacities, see Best, 1993; Jusczyk, 1992, 1993b, in press; Suomi, 1993.)

II. BASIC CAPACITIES FOR PERCEIVING PHONETIC CONTRASTS

Although speech research with infants began in earnest only about twenty-five years ago, there is much information about the ability of infants to discriminate contrasts between different speech sounds. Investigators have tested a wide range of contrasts, from language spoken within and outside the infants' native environment. In addition, much research has been directed at the nature of the mechanisms underlying infants' speech perception abilities.

A. Native Language Contrasts

When Eimas, Siqueland, Jusczyk, and Vigorito (1971) undertook their study, there was some doubt as to whether infants could perceive speech contrasts before they began producing them in their own babbling. Moreover, these investigators also wished to explore how closely infants' speech perception capacities parallel those of adults. For this reason, they examined not only whether infants could detect a voicing distinction between the syllables [ba] and [pa], but also whether their perception of this distinction was categorical, as is the case for adult listeners (Abramson & Lisker, 1970; Liberman, Harris, Hoffman, & Griffith, 1957). Categorical perception of speech refers to a situation in which the ability to discriminate two different sounds is only about as good as the ability to assign them to different phoneme categories, such as [b] and [p] (Studdert-Kennedy, Liberman, Harris, & Cooper, 1970).

Eimas et al. tested both 1- and 4-month-old infants using the high-amplitude sucking procedure (Jusczyk, 1985; Siqueland and DeLucia, 1969). After obtaining a base-line measure of the infant's sucking, they made the presentation of a speech syllable (e.g., [ba]) contingent on the infant's sucking rate. During this preshift phase, the more often the infant sucked, the more often the syllable was played. When the infant's sucking rate to this first stimulus declined to a predetermined habituation criterion, the postshift phase began. There were three different types of treatment conditions during this postshift phase. Infants in the control condition continued to hear exactly the same syllable as they heard in the preshift phase. Infants in the "between-categories" condition heard a new syllable from the other phonemic category (e.g., [pa]), which differed in its voicing from the syllable in the preshift period (e.g., [ba]). Infants in the "within-categories" condition also heard a new syllable, which differed by the same amount from the preshift syllable in its acoustic characteristics, but the new syllable was a different member of the same phonemic category (e.g., two different [ba] stimuli). The results indicated that only the infants in the between-categories condition showed significant increases in sucking during the postshift period. Eimas et al. interpreted these results as an indication that infants as young as 1 month old are able to perceive the difference between [ba] and [pa]. Moreover, like adults, their discrimination of this voicing distinction is categorical in that they respond to between-category differences, but not to within-category differences.

Reports from other laboratories indicated that young infants' capacities for discriminating speech contrasts were not limited solely to ones involving voicing distinctions. Moffitt (1971) used a heart-rate dishabituation procedure and found that 5-month-olds were able to discriminate a place of articulation contrast between the syllables [ba] and [ga]. Morse (1972) used the HAS procedure to investigate the same contrast with 2-month-olds and found similar results. A subsequent investigation by Eimas (1974) demonstrated that place of articulation distinctions like the one between [bæ] and dæ] are discriminated in a categorical manner. Moreover, an investigation with newborns by Bertoncini, Bijeljac-Babic, Blumstein, and Mehler (1987) demonstrated that the ability to discriminate place of articulation differences among stop consonants is present right from birth.

Other types of consonantal contrasts were also investigated. Eimas (1975a) tested 2- to 3-month-old infants on the distinction between [ra] and [la]. This contrast is one that children often master late in speech production (Strange & Broen, 1981; Templin, 1957), and also one that certain non-native speakers of English have difficulty with (Miyawaki et al., 1975). Nevertheless, Eimas found that infants reliably discriminated this contrast and, like native English speakers, gave evidence of categorical discrimination along this speech continuum. Other types of manner of articulation contrasts were also investigated. Several studies focused on infants' discrimination of stop/glide distinctions (e.g., [ba] vs. [wa]). Hillenbrand, Minifie, and Edwards (1979) found that 6- to 8-month-old infants are able to discriminate these syllables, and subsequent research by Eimas and Miller (1980a; Miller & Eimas, 1983) demonstrated categorical discrimination of the same contrast by 2-month-olds. The oral/nasal distinction between syllables like [ba] and [ma] was tested by Eimas and Miller (1980b). Once again, 2- to 4-months-old infants discriminated this contrast. However, unlike the earlier consonantal contrasts examined, the infants also were able to discriminate within-category distinctions for these stimuli. Hence, perception of this distinction is apparently not categorical for infants.

The studies reviewed thus far have all included contrasts involving at least one stop consonant. Data also exist regarding the abilities of infants to discriminate contrasts involving other types of speech segments. Fricative contrasts have been studied by a number of investigators. Eilers (1977) reported that 3-month-olds were able to discriminate a voicing contrast between [s] and [z] in syllable-final position (i.e., [as] vs. [az]), but not in syllable-initial position ([sa] vs. [za]). However, the latter result has been criticized on methodological grounds (Aslin, Pisoni, & Jusczyk, 1983). Place of articulation differences between fricatives have also been investigated. Holmberg, Morgan, and Kuhl (1977) reported that 6-month-olds were able to detect a contrast between [fa] and [θa]. A. Levitt, Jusczyk, Murray, and Carden (1988) investigated the same contrast with 2-month-olds and found evidence for categorical discrimination of place of articulation differences with fricatives. Findings have also been reported demonstrating that 2-month-olds can distinguish place of articulation contrasts between nasal consonants, such as [ma] and [na] (Eimas & Miller, 1980b), and between glides, such as [wa] and [ja] (Jusczyk, Copan, & Thompson, 1978).

Along with their abilities to detect subtle contrasts among consonants, infants can distinguish native language vowel contrasts. Trehub (1973) found evidence for the discrimination of [a] from [i] and [i] from [u] in infants 1 to 4 months of age (Kuhl & Miller, 1982). Evidence that infants are capable of detecting even more subtle contrasts between vowels was reported by Swoboda, Morse, and Leavitt (1976). These investigators presented 2-month-olds with contrasts from a vowel continuum extending from [i] to [I]. Not only were infants able to discriminate between-category distinctions from this continuum, but, like adults, they were also able to detect within-category vowel contrasts. Evidence for the discrimination of another subtle vowel distinction (between [a] and [ɔ]) has been reported by Kuhl (1983). However, in a recent study with Swedish infants, Lacerda (1992) found that a contrast between the Swedish vowel pair [a] and [ɑ] was not discriminated, even though another Swedish contrast, between [a] and [ʌ], was discriminated.

In summary, from a very early age, infants discriminate many, if not all, of the contrasts that are likely to occur among words in the native language. Moreover, at least on a general level, there are some striking similarities between the way that infants and adults respond to the same kinds of speech contrasts. Like adults, infants tend to discriminate contrasts between consonants categorically, whereas they show a greater ability to discriminate within-category vowel differences.

B. Foreign Language Contrasts

Soon after the first reports about infants' speech perception capacities, there was much interest as to whether the emergence of these capacities actually demands some period of familiarization or experience with a particular language. Consequently, attempts were made to gather information about how infants perceive speech contrasts that do not appear in their native language environments. Streeter (1976) used the HAS procedure to investigate Kikuyu infants' perception of English voicing contrasts. The contrast between [ba] and [pa] is not one found in Kikuyu (although the language does include contrasts between prevoiced and voiced consonants). Despite their lack of familiarity with the contrast, 1- to 4-month-old Kikuyu infants were able to discriminate the voiced/voiceless pair. A similar finding was reported by Lasky, Syrdal-Lasky, and Klein (1975) who used a heart rate measure and found that 4½- to 6-month-old Guatemalan infants discriminated the English voicing contrast between [ba] and [pa]. Although Spanish does have a voicing distinction, it is not the same one that occurs in English (Lisker & Abramson, 1970; Williams, 1977b). Despite the fact that Spanish was the language spoken in the home of these infants, they discriminated the English voicing contrast, but not the Spanish one. The behavior of the Guatemalan infants did contrast in an interesting way with that of the Kikuyu infants in Streeter's study. The latter group gave evidence of discriminating the prevoiced/voiced contrast that does occur in their native language, whereas the former group did not discriminate the voicing contrast that occurs in Spanish. One possible explanation for this is that the Kikuyu and English contrasts occur closer to the infants' innate perceptual boundaries than does the Spanish contrast. Discriminating the Spanish voicing contrast may require some realignment of the infant's perceptual categories (Aslin & Pisoni, 1980). In any event, the findings from these studies suggest that both innate and experiential factors contribute to where the perceptual boundaries are set for fluent speakers of a language.

A number of studies have also investigated how infants from English-speaking homes perceive foreign language contrasts. One of the first attempts was reported by Eimas (1975b) who investigated whether American infants could discriminate the prevoiced/voiceless distinction that occurs between stop consonants in languages like Thai (Lisker & Abramson, 1964). Eimas found that only when the voicing difference was large (on the order of 80 ms) did the American infants discriminate it. More convincing evidence that American infants can discriminate the prevoiced/voiced contrast comes from a study by Aslin, Pisoni, Hennessy, and Perey (1981) who used the operant headturn procedure to test 6-month-olds. They found that although the smallest difference to discriminate the prevoiced/voiced contrast was larger than that for the voiced/voiceless contrast, all of their subjects discriminated both contrasts.

Although many early studies investigated voicing contrasts, information is also available about how infants respond to other types of foreign language contrasts. Trehub (1976) examined 1- to 4-month-old English Canadian infants' responsiveness to an oral/nasal vowel contrast ([pa] vs. [pā]), found in languages like Polish and French, and a contrast between [řa] and [za], which occurs in Czech. Despite their lack of experience with these contrasts, infants discriminated each one. There are also indications that 6-month-old English Canadian infants can discriminate a retroflex/dental place of articulation contrast from Hindi and a glottalized velar/uvular contrast from Nthlakapmx (Werker & Tees, 1984). Best, McRoberts, and Sithole (1988) also found that English-learning 6-month-olds could discriminate a lateral versus a medial click contrast from Zulu. Subsequently, Best (1991) reported similar findings with respect to a place of articulation distinction between ejectives in Ethiopian. Moreover, at $4\frac{1}{2}$ months of age, English-learning infants are sensitive to the German vowel contrasts [U] versus [Y] and [u:] versus [y:] (Werker, Lloyd, & Pegg, 1993).

Taken together, these studies of the perception of foreign language contrasts suggest that young infants' capacities for discriminating speech contrasts extend beyond those sounds that they are likely to have encountered in their native environment. Thus, for at least some speech contrasts, infants do not require prior experience in order to discriminate them. Findings of this sort have led to the view that infants are born with the capacity to discriminate contrasts that could potentially appear in any of the world's languages (Eimas, Miller, & Jusczyk, 1987; Werker & Pegg, 1992). Experience with language appears to have its impact by getting the infant to focus on those contrasts that play a critical role in distinguishing words in the native language.

C. Coping with Variability in the Speech Signal

1. Talker Variability

An important aspect of fluent speech perception is being able to compensate for the acoustic differences that arise when different talkers pronounce the same items. Without some ability to recognize the same word produced by different talkers, it is hard to see how the infant could ever learn the meanings of words. Without normalization for different talkers, every acoustic difference could potentially signal a difference in meaning and the task of acquiring a language would be insurmountable.

The first attempt to explore how infants deal with variability in speech occurred in a study conducted by Kuhl using the HAS procedure (Kuhl, 1976; Kuhl & Miller, 1982). Infants, 1 to 4 months old, were exposed in the preshift phase to two different tokens of the vowel [a]. One of these was produced with a monotone; the other with a rise–fall pitch contour. During the postshift phase, infants in the experimental group heard two comparable tokens of the vowel [i]. At issue was whether infants could successfully discriminate the vowel contrast despite the irrelevant variation in the pitch contour of the syllables. A different set of infants had to detect a pitch change when vowel identity was varying. This group heard the monotonic versions of the two vowels during the preshift phase and the rise–fall versions during the postshift phase. The results indicated that infants detected a vowel change in the face of irrelevant pitch variation, but they did not detect the pitch change when vowel variation was present. However, because the size of the pitch changes were not necessarily equivalent to the size of the vowel changes, it is difficult to say whether infants are simply more attuned to vowel changes than to pitch changes (Carrell, Smith, & Pisoni, 1981). Nevertheless, the important point is that infants this age display some ability to cope with variability in speech.

Kuhl (1979) conducted a more extensive investigation of infants' ability to handle variability in a study with 6-month-olds. She explored the consequences of both talker and pitch variability. Infants were trained using the operant headturning procedure to discriminate a contrast between [a] and [i] when both talker's voice and pitch contour were held constant. Once the infants demonstrated discrimination of this contrast, they were tested for their ability to maintain the discrimination in the face of variability in pitch and talker's voice. Variability was increased gradually over a series of training stages. In the final stage, there were tokens of each vowel produced by three different talkers using two different pitch contours. Even with this degree of variability, the infants continued to successfully detect the vowel contrast. In another study (Kuhl, 1983), 6-month-olds were tested on a more difficult vowel contrast, [a] versus [ɔ]. What makes this contrast particularly difficult in this situation is the fact that productions of these vowels by different talkers often result in considerable acoustic overlap. What counts as a [ɔ] for one talker may be an [a] for another talker. Although there were indications that infants had more difficulty with variability for this vowel contrast than the previous one, they still were able to reliably detect the [a]/[ɔ] contrast even with the maximum degree of variability present. Thus, by 6 months of age, infants clearly do possess some ability to deal with the kind of variability attributable to different talkers.

More recently, Jusczyk, Pisoni, and Mullennix (1992) found that infants as young as 2 months old display some capacity for handling talker variability. Using the HAS procedure, Jusczyk et al. presented infants with tokens of the words *bug* and *dug* produced by 6 male and 6 female talkers. During the preshift phase one group heard all 12 tokens of one of the two words, and in the postshift phase they heard the tokens of the other word. Infants in this group significantly increased their postshift sucking, indicating that they detected the change from one word to the other despite the talker variation. In fact, the postshift performance of this group did not differ significantly from that of a group exposed to only a single token of each word produced by the same talker. These results, showing that 2-month-olds can detect a stop consonant difference in the face of talker variability, parallel Kuhl's findings for 6-month-olds' capacities with respect to vowel differences. Thus, at the very least, the rudiments of perceptual normalization seem to be present at a very early point in infancy.

To learn whether handling talker variability has any costs associated with it for infants' speech processing capacities, Jusczyk et al. conducted several additional experiments. Studies have indicated that talker variability can affect adult listeners' retention of speech (Martin, Mullennix, Pisoni, & Summers, 1989). Jusczyk et al. explored whether infants' memories for speech information might also be affected by talker variability. They introduced a 2-min delay period between the preshift and postshift phase of the HAS procedure. Infants who heard only a single token of each word produced by the same talker continued to discriminate the contrast between *bug* and *dug* despite the delay. However, infants who heard all 12 tokens of the words produced by different talkers did not show evidence of discrimination following the delay. Evidently, talker variability affected the infants' retention of the speech sounds. Moreover, the results of another follow-up study suggest that even variability among tokens produced by a single talker can affect infants' retention of speech. Although infants detected a contrast between *bug* and *dug* without a delay period when 12 tokens from the same talker were used, they did not detect the same contrast when a 2-min delay period was imposed. Note that the delay period does not significantly affect infants' performance when there is no variability among stimulus tokens. Only when there is variability among tokens does infants' retention of information suffer. Overall, the results show that although 2-month-olds can cope with variability in speech, their processing resources available for the encoding and retrieval of speech information are likely to be affected.

2. Variability in Speaking Rate

Talker differences are not the only source of variability that infants must cope with in processing speech. Changes in speaking rate can also affect the acoustic characteristics of speech sounds. Eimas and Miller (1980a; Miller & Eimas, 1983) investigated whether infants' perception of phonetic contrasts is affected by changes in speaking rate. To test this, they used syllables having either short (80 ms) or long (296 ms) durations. The former typically occur in fast rates of speech and the latter in slower speech. The speech contrast chosen ([ba] vs. [wa]) is one known to depend on the rate of change of the initial formant transitions. Short, rapidly changing formant transitions are associated with the production of stop consonants like [ba], whereas longer, gradually changing formant transitions are present in glides like

[wa]. However, the point at which adult listeners decide that a given syllable is either [ba] or [wa] has been shown to be dependent on speaking rate (Miller & Liberman, 1979). Eimas and Miller designed their stimuli so that a pair that constituted a between-category distinction at one rate was a within-category pair at the other rate. Infants tested on these behaved analogously to adults. They discriminated between-category, but not within-category pairs from each series. Regardless of whether the mechanism responsible is specific to speech, as Eimas and Miller concluded, or more general (Jusczyk, Pisoni, Fernald, Reed, & Myers, 1983), infants' perception of speech is apparently sensitive to changes in speaking rate.

3. Contextual Variability of Phonetic Segments

As mentioned at the outset, the specific acoustic properties associated with a particular phoneme can vary greatly depending on their context (Liberman et al., 1967). Thus, different sources of information could signal the presence of the same phonetic contrast in different contexts (Lisker, 1986). The availability of different acoustic correlates of phonetic contrasts suggests that listeners "trade off" these cues in different contexts. Indeed, evidence for trading relations has been observed for adults (Best, Morrongiello, & Robson, 1981; Repp, 1982).

These facts about the contextual variability of phonetic segments raise some interesting questions with respect to infants' behavior. First, are infants sensitive to the kind of cue-trading relations observed in adult speech perception? Second, do infants recognize the phonetic identity of a particular segment across the various contexts it appears in? Third, what capacities do infants have for integrating acoustic information pertaining to a particular phonetic segment?

With respect to the first of these questions, there is some indication that infants are sensitive to certain trading relations in speech (Eimas, 1985; Miller & Eimas, 1983). In particular, Eimas (1985) tested 2- to 4-month-old infants on stimulus series ranging from *say* to *stay*. For this series, spectral cues relating to formant transitions were traded with temporal cues relating to the duration of a silent gap. By comparing how infants responded to the stimuli when the spectral and temporal cues either conflicted or cooperated, he found evidence to support the view that infants treat these cues as perceptually equivalent. Specifically, only when the cues cooperated did infants discriminate the speech stimuli. Hence, infants appear to be sensitive to how these spectral and temporal cues enter into cue-trading relations in speech.

Another indication that infants are sensitive to the contexts in which acoustic cues are embedded comes from a study by A. Levitt et al. (1988). Previous work with adults had shown that listeners apparently interpret formant transition information relating to place of articulation distinctions as a contextually dependent manner (Carden, Levitt, Jusczyk, & Walley, 1981). Formant transition differences that signaled a change of place of articulation difference for stop consonants did not indicate a place distinction when it occurred in the context of fricatives. Levitt et al. tested 2-month-olds on the same series of sounds. Their results suggested that infants' perception of the formant transition differences in the speech sounds depended on the presence or absence of accompanying frication noises. Contrasts that were not discriminated without accompanying frication were discriminated when frication was present, and vice versa. These results paralleled the kinds of context effects that Carden et al. observed for adults' perception of the same contrasts. Levitt et al. concluded that the source of these effects does not depend on long experience in producing and perceiving speech, but rather is a consequence of the inherent organization of the underlying perceptual mechanisms.

Given that even 2-month-olds' displays are influenced by the context in which a particular phone occurs, do they perceive a similarity among the different instances of the same phonetic segment in these different contexts? Jusczyk and Derrah (1987) used a modification of the HAS procedure to investigate this possibility. They familiarized 2-month-olds during the preshift phase with a series of syllables sharing a common phonetic segment (e.g., [bi], [ba], [bo], [bɚ]). During the postshift phase, a new syllable was added to the set, which either shared (e.g., [bu]) or did not share (e.g., [du]) a phoneme in common with the other syllables. Jusczyk and Derrah hypothesized that if infants recognized the occurrence of a common [b] segment across all of the syllables, they might respond differently in the postshift period depending on whether the novel syllable shared the same phonetic segment or not. For example, they might display higher sucking rates to a more novel stimulus like [du], which did not share a common segment. In fact, infants did not respond in this fashion. Both types of changes were detected and there was no indication of increased responding to the syllable from the novel phonetic category. These results were replicated with 2-month-olds and extended to newborns in a study by Bertoncini, Bijeljac-Babic, Jusczyk, Kennedy, and Mehler (1988). They not only replicated the result for syllables with common consonant segments, but found a comparable result for syllables with common vowel segments (e.g., [bi], [si], [li], [mi]). In the latter case, the novel item added in the postshift phase either shared ([di]) or did not share ([da]) the same vowel as the other stimuli. Results of several other investigations along these lines (Jusczyk, Bertoncini, Bijeljac-Babic, Kennedy, & Mehler, 1990; Jusczyk, Kennedy, & Jusczyk, in press; Jusczyk, Kennedy, Jusczyk, Schomberg, & Koenig, in press), which will be discussed further in another context, also yielded little indication that infants this age recognize the identity of the same phonetic segment in different contexts.

We now turn our attention to the third question. What capacities do infants have for integrating acoustic information relating to the perception of a phonetic segment? There are several indications that infants do possess some capacities for integrating information in the speech signal. First, Miller and Eimas (1979) found that 3- to 4-month-old infants detect syllable contrasts that involve rearrangements of the same phonetic features. This result implies that infants are sensitive not only to the particular features present, but also the order and combination in which the features occur. A different facet of the infant's capacity to integrate different portions of the acoustic signal into a coherent speech percept comes from a more recent study by Eimas and Miller (1992). They presented 3- to 4-month-old infants with speech information dichotically, so that information about the third formant transition alone went to one ear, while information about the remainder of the syllable went to the other ear. The third formant contained the critical information for distinguishing the syllable [da] from [ga]. The infants not only discriminated these dichotic patterns, but did so even when the third formant transitions were greatly attenuated. In the latter case, the infants' performance with the dichotic stimuli was significantly better than their capacity to discriminate the attenuated third formant transitions when they were presented in isolation. Eimas and Miller concluded that these young infants already possess the means to integrate disparate sources of information into coherent speech percepts. Indeed, the operation of mechanisms of this sort could underlie infants' abilities to cope with some of the variability present in the speech signal. In any case, it appears that at an early age, infants do possess some important capacities that help them to deal with the different sources of acoustic variability associated with speech sounds.

D. The Role of Memory and Attention in Infant Speech Perception

For most typical speech perception experiments with infants, researchers work hard to eliminate possible sources of distraction. Testing usually takes place under quiet conditions, in sound-insulated and dimly lit rooms. Such precautions are especially important if the objective is to determine the limits of infants' capacities for perceiving speech contrasts. The information gained from such studies informs us about what infants can do under the best of circumstances. Nevertheless, if our goal is to understand how these capacities are used in acquiring a native language, then we have to understand how these capacities function in the midst of the distractions that occur in everyday life. Investigations of how the infant handles variability do give some indication about how robust speech perception capacities are when distracting information is present. Similarly, studies of the perception of speech in noise further help to specify the limits of infants' speech processing capacities. Infants can discriminate speech sounds under such conditions, although they require signal-to-noise ratios 6–12 dB higher than do adults (Nozza, Rossman, Bond, & Miller, 1990).

One way of better understanding how attentional processes affect infants' speech perception capacities is to look for situations in which attention is likely to affect the discriminability of certain contrasts. One such example is to compare how infants process the same kinds of contrasts in both stressed and unstressed syllables. Several early studies explored this issue by using two-syllable stimuli and embedding a critical phonetic contrast in either a stressed (e.g., [da ba'] vs. [da ga']) or unstressed ([da' ba] vs. [da' ga]) syllable. Two-month-olds were equally adept at discriminating the contrast regardless of whether it occurred in the stressed or unstressed syllable (Jusczyk et al., 1978; Jusczyk & Thompson, 1978). However, Karzon (1985) reported that when the number of syllables was increased to three ([malana] vs. [marana]), the infants only discriminated a contrast provided that it occurred in syllables that received stress characteristic of child-directed speech. Perhaps when processing load becomes sufficiently great for the infant, exaggerating the syllable stress may help in directing attention to the contrast. The notion that children may attend to and imitate information in stressed syllables is one that has been popular with child language researchers (Brown & Fraser, 1964; Gerken, Landau, & Remez, 1989; Gleitman & Wanner, 1982).

Another factor that could possibly affect infants' ability to attend to phonetic contrasts has to do with the position of the contrast within the utterance. All other things being equal, contrasts located medially in utterances might be expected to be more difficult for the infant than those located syllable-initially or finally. However, studies examining this issue have reported that discriminability of phonetic contrasts does not appear to vary with their location within utterances (Goddsitt, Morse, Ver Hoove, & Cowan, 1984; Jusczyk et al., 1978; Jusczyk & Thompson, 1978; Williams, 1977a).

A different means of manipulating infants' attentional focus was adopted by Jusczyk et al. (1990). They tested 2-month-olds using a modified version of the HAS procedure. The attentional focus of the infants was manipulated by varying the perceptual similarity of items in the stimulus set. Some infants were exposed to a set of syllables with perceptually similar consonants ([pa], [ka], [ma]) during the preshift phase. Other infants were exposed to a set of syllables that included three perceptually dissimilar vowels ([bi], [ba], [bu]). Jusczyk et al. (1990) hypothesized that when the items were highly similar, as in the first set, infants would be more apt to focus on finer-grained details of the syllables. However, when the items were very dissimilar, as in the second set, the infants would tend to focus on coarser distinctions among the syllables. They predicted that when focusing on fine distinctions (i.e., for items closely clustered in perceptual space), infants would be more apt to notice the addition of a new syllable to the set than when focused on coarser distinctions (i.e., for items greatly separated in perceptual space). These predictions were borne out in the behavior of 4-day-olds. When these infants were exposed to the coarse distinction set (i.e., [bi], [ba], [bu]), they did not detect the addition of a new syllable [bʌ] which was perceptually very similar to one of the original set members (i.e., [ba]). By comparison, for the familiarization sets containing some fine-grained distinctions (e.g., [pa], [ka], [ma]), the 4-day-olds were able to detect the addition of even a highly similar syllable ([ta]) to the set. By 2 months of age, infants are apparently more resistant to this type of attentional manipulation. They detected the new syllable regardless of being focused on fine- or coarse-grained distinctions during the preshift period. One possible explanation for this change in susceptibility to the attentional manipulation is that the older groups are better able to cope with the processing demands of the task. Alternatively, the greater experience of 2-month-olds with native language input (including many fine-grained phonetic contrasts) may render them more resistant to the attentional focus manipulation.

Much remains to be learned about the role of attentional processes in developing speech perception capacities. Understanding the relationship between attention and speech perception in infants is also critical to determining the use to which such capacities are put in acquiring language. It is one thing to know what the limits of infants speech perception capacities are under ideal circumstances; it is another to know how these capacities function in a language learning situation. Certainly, the way in which infants attend to speech could influence the development of a mental lexicon for native language words (Jusczyk, 1993a). Moreover, it is possible that information present in the speech signal could provide cues to syntactic organization (Gleitman & Wanner, 1982; Morgan, 1986; Peters, 1983).

A key to understanding the role of speech perception in language acquisition is to learn more about what information infants retain about speech sounds. Such information is valuable not only in understanding the development of the lexicon, but also in delineating the growth of word recognition processes during language acquisition. Consider that developing a lexicon requires long-term storage of the sound pattern associated with each lexical item. Consequently, any immediate perceptual representation of an utterance must eventually be encoded in long-term memory in order to be retrieved in recognizing words in fluent speech.

There are some indications that infants can retain at least gross features of speech that they have been exposed to repeatedly. Even human newborns apparently retain some memory for speech they were exposed to prenatally. DeCasper and Spence (1986) found that infants preferred listening to stories that their mothers had recited to them prenatally as opposed to unfamiliar stories. Mehler et al. (1988) also noted that 4-day-olds show a preference for speech in their mothers' native language. Nevertheless, because long passages of fluent speech were used in both studies, it cannot be determined whether infants remembered more than gross rhythmic features of the input.

Several recent studies have attempted to gain a more precise estimate of the kind of detail that infants are able to retain about speech sounds. Jusczyk, Kennedy, and Jusczyk (in press) tested 2-month-olds with a modified version of the HAS procedure that included a delay period between the preshift and postshift phases of the experiment. During the delay, a series of slides was shown without any accompanying auditory stimulation. The infants gave evidence of remembering considerable detail about the preshift stimuli. Even minimal changes of a single phonetic feature were detected. More recently, Jusczyk, Kennedy, Jusczyk, Schomberg, and Koenig (in press) examined the ability of infants' to retain information about bisyllabic utterances. During the preshift phase, 2-month-olds were exposed to a set of bisyllabic utterances that either shared (i.e., [ba' mɪt], [ba' zi], [ba' lo], [ba' des]) or did not share (i.e., [nɛ' lo], [pæ' zi], [chu' des], [ko' mɪt]) a common syllable. The presence of a common syllable during the preshift phase did lead to a significant improvement in the infants' ability to detect the addition of a new item to the set during the postshift phase. Only infants who had heard the set with the common syllable detected the addition of a new bisyllable (e.g., [ba' nʌ] or [na' bʌ]) to the postshift set. Jusczyk et al. took this as an indication that the presence of a common syllable enhanced the encoding of these items during the delay period, allowing them to be better remembered. The information that infants remember about speech is not limited solely to phonetic or prosodic features. In their examination of how variability affects infants' memory for speech sounds, Jusczyk, Pisoni, and Mullennix (1992) found evidence that infants encode information that permits them to detect, after a 2-min delay, gender changes in voice quality.

As with the role of attention, research on memory processes connected with infant speech perception has only recently begun. What information is available suggests that in the first few months of life infants are apparently able to encode detailed information about speech syllables and to retain it for at least brief periods of time. Just how these capacities for remembering speech change as the infant acquires more information about the native language and begins to deal with other levels of linguistic organization is not clear at present.

III. LEARNING NATIVE LANGUAGE SOUND PATTERNS

Becoming a fluent perceiver of a language requires more than discriminating and categorizing speech sounds. The listener also needs to segment the stream of speech into words, phrases, and clauses to recover the talker's intended message. The way in which these units of linguistic organization are represented in the speech stream can vary considerably from language to language. Consequently, language learners must discover the organization that governs the formation and transmission of messages in their native language. Innate capacities for perceiving speech may provide a rough categorization of the input that allows the infant to pick up regularities of native language sound patterns. When do infants begin to detect regularities relating to both the phonetic and prosodic organization of the input?

A. Distinguishing between Native and Foreign Language Patterns

1. Tuning Out Foreign Language Categories

The first evidence of important developmental changes in speech perception capacities during the first year of life was reported by Werker and Tees (1984). Although a previous study (Werker, Gilbert, Humphrey, & Tees, 1981) had demonstrated that 6-month-olds from Canadian-English-speaking homes discriminated two Hindi contrasts not found in English, Werker and Tees found that sensitivity to some foreign language contrasts undergoes a decline between 6 and 12 months of age. Infants were tested with an operant headturning procedure on English ([ba]–[da]), Hindi ([ta]–[ta]), and Nthlakapmx ([k'i]–[q'i]) contrasts at three ages: 6–8 months, 8–10 months, and 10–12 months. The youngest age group discriminated all three contrasts. However, by 8–10 months, only some of the infants discriminated the non-native contrasts, and by 10–12 months, the infants discriminated only the English contrast. A longitudinal study involving a new group of Canadian infants verified this developmental trend. To rule out the possibility that the poorer performance of the older infants was not simply an age-related decline in interest, several Hindi- and Nthlakapmx-learning infants were also tested. Even at 11–12 months, these infants were easily able to discriminate the contrast from their native language. Further research with a different, synthetically produced, Hindi contrast ([da]–[Da]), replicated the finding of a developmental decline in sensitivity to non-native contrasts between 6 and 12 months of age (Werker & Lalonde, 1988). In addition, using an entirely different test procedure (visual preference), Best and McRoberts (1989) replicated the finding of a decline in sensitivity by American infants between 6 and 12 months of age to the Nthlakapmx contrast.

When these findings were first reported, the general consensus was that sensitivity declines when contrasts do not appear in the speech input to infants. Moreover, sensitivity to non-native contrasts was thought to drop off somewhere between 8 and 12 months of age. However, the story has proven more complicated than first thought. Best et al. (1988) explored English-learning infants' perception of a Zulu lateral versus medial click contrast. They found that, at all four ages tested (6–8, 8–10, 10–12, and 12–14 months), English-learning infants discriminated the contrast even though it does not appear in English. Hence, the mere absence of experience with the contrast did not lead to a decline in the infants' ability to discriminate. Best (1991) also investigated two additional contrasts, an Ethiopian ejective place of articulation distinction and a Zulu lateral fricative voicing distinction. English-learning infants discriminated the place of articulation distinction for the Ethiopian ejectives. Moreover, performance did not decline between 8 and 12 months of age. This pattern of results matches those of Best et al. for the Zulu click contrasts. However, results for the Zulu lateral fricative voicing distinction were more in line with what Werker and Tees (1984) had observed for Hindi and Nthlakapmx contrasts. Namely, discrimination scores of 10- to 12-month-old infants for the Zulu lateral fricative voicing distinction were significantly lower than those of 6- to 8-month-old infants.

Best (1993) has attempted to account for infants' differing patterns of responsiveness to non-native contrasts in terms of how these contrasts map onto native language contrasts (see Jusczyk, 1992, and Werker, 1991, for alternative views). She suggests that non-native contrasts will remain discriminable when they map onto distinct phonological categories in the native language. Discrimination of non-native contrasts should also remain relatively high if the non-native phonological categories differ significantly in the goodness with which they fit a single phonological category. However, non-native contrasts should be difficult (and therefore be apt to undergo decline) when the non-native phonological categories map equally well onto the same native language phonological category. Results from her most recent investigation with three new Zulu contrasts are largely consistent with this view. In particular, 6- to 8-month-old infants, but not 10- to 12-month-old infants, discriminated a Zulu plosive versus implosive contrast, which maps onto the same English category. Both age groups also discriminated a voiceless versus ejective stop contrast where the Zulu categories differ in the goodness with which they map onto an English category. The one glitch for Best's view came from the Zulu lateral fricative contrast. This should have been a case in which the non-native categories map into two distinct English categories. Consequently, there should have been no developmental decline. However, although the 6- to 8-month-old infants discriminated the contrast, the 10- to 12-month-old infants did not. The decline in performance by the older group deviates from what infants this age did with other contrasts that map onto distinct English categories, for example, the Ethiopian ejective contrast (Best, 1991). It is not clear what the reason is for the discrepancy.

Although most of the research investigating developmental changes in non-native contrasts has focused on consonantal distinctions, there is some limited evidence regarding non-native vowel contrasts. Werker and Polka (1993) reported on an investigation of English-learning infants' perception of two German vowel contrasts ([U] vs. [Y] and [u:] vs. [y:]). Consistent with the reports of a decline in sensitivity to non-native consonant contrasts in 10- to 12-month-old infants, they found no evidence that infants this age discriminated either vowel contrast. However, in sharp contrast to the pattern typically noted for 6- to 8-month-old infants' perception of non-native consonantal contrasts, very few of the English-learning infants discriminated either of the German vowel contrasts. Werker et al. (1993) reported on a follow-up study with infants 4–6 and 6–8 months of age. The 4- to 6-month-old infants, but not the 6- to 8-month-old infants, discriminated the non-native vowel contrasts. Werker et al. interpret this as an indication that native language vowel categories may undergo an earlier reorganization than consonantal categories. Because vowels carry both prosodic and phonetic information, they may be more apt to attract infants' attention to their appearance in the speech stream than are consonants. This might explain an earlier reorganization for vowels than for consonants.

In summary, there is considerable evidence that sensitivity to non-native speech contrasts undergoes some reorganization within the first year of life. The full extent of the reorganization, and the factors responsible for it, are still not fully understood. It seems clear that the nature of the phonological categories that appear in the native language does play some role in the process, but it is not apparent what other factors may help to determine whether sensitivity to non-native language contrasts undergoes a decline or not.

2. Tuning In to Native Language Sound Properties

The process of acquiring the sound structure of a native language could conceivably come about by a process of eliminating any categories that do not appear regularly in the input directed to the infant. However, it is hard to see how this process alone could reveal much about the internal organization of sound categories and patterns within the native language. Rather, it seems more likely that at some point infants draw upon their speech perception capacities to pick up information about patterns and categories that regularly occur in the input. When might such a process begin? Although the decline in sensitivity to non-native contrasts may be tied to a growing knowledge about sound properties and their organization in the native language, it is also possible that the two occur independently of one another. Nevertheless, the available data suggest that infants begin to acquire information about native language sound patterns at the same time that sensitivity to non-native contrasts begin to decline.

In considering how knowledge of native language sound properties develops, it is worth recalling some of the things that the language learner needs to master. At one level, learners need to determine the nature of the elements that make up words in the native language. In addition, they must discover any ordering constraints that hold among these elementary units. Eventually, they must arrive at some notion of when sequences of sounds that appear in the speech steam are grouped together into elementary units of meaning, such as words. We consider the available evidence with respect to each of these domains.

Kuhl and her colleagues (Grieser & Kuhl, 1989; Kuhl, 1991, 1993; Kuhl, Williams, Lacerda, Stevens, & Lindblom, 1992) have suggested that native language vowel categories may get organized around prototypical instances at around 6 months of age. In one study using the operant headturn procedure (Grieser & Kuhl, 1989), American infants were exposed to what adults judged to be either a prototypical instance or a poor instance of the English vowel [i]. The particular instance served as a background stimulus. Novel instances from the category were used as test stimuli. Kuhl measured infants' discrimination of the novel instances from the familiar background stimulus. In effect, the procedure measures infants' ability to generalize from the background stimulus to novel stimuli. When a prototypical instance served as the background stimulus, infants generalized to a significantly larger number of novel instances (i.e., they were less likely to detect a change to one of these). Kuhl (1991) interpreted these findings as an indication that prototypical instances are "perceptual magnets" that shorten perceptual distances between the center and edges of the vowel category (but see Lively, 1993). More recently, Kuhl et al. (1992) extended and replicated the earlier findings by demonstrating that infants' experience with a native language is critical to the formation of vowel prototypes. American and Swedish infants were tested on two vowel prototypes, the English [i] and the Swedish [y]. Infants showed the perceptual magnet effect only for their own native language vowel. Swedish infants demonstrated a magnet effect for [y], but not for [i], whereas American infants showed the reverse pattern.

The finding that infants apparently have begun organizing native language vowel categories by 6 months of age is certainly interesting. However, it would be helpful to know more about the generality of prototypes for vowels. For instance, are all native language vowel categories organized around prototypes? If so, do infants acquire them all at the same time? Are the prototypes talker specific or talker neutral? Finally, how does the apparent failure of Swedish infants, as old as 10 months, to discriminate a native language vowel contrast (Lacerda, 1992) fit with the notion that vowel categories are organized around prototypes by 6 months of age? (For further discussion of these issues, see Jusczyk, 1993b.) Putting aside these questions for the moment, the evidence from Kuhl's studies suggests that by 6 months, infants are beginning to discover the nature of native language vowel categories.

Languages differ not only in the details of their vowel and consonant categories, but also in terms of which sounds regularly appear in words and how these sounds can be ordered (i.e., their phonotactic constraints). Besides discovering meanings and the sound sequences associated with them, learning about native language words involves identifying the sounds that can make up words and the ways in which they may be combined. The infant eventually must learn that the sound [θ], which begins the word *think* does appear regularly in English words, whereas the sound [X] does not (despite the occasional FM announcer's pronunciation of the name *Bach*). Moreover, to be successful in segmenting words from fluent speech, the infant must learn something about the constraints that exist on the sequences of sounds that can appear together in positions within the same syllable. So, although Polish allows clusters such as [kt], [gd], or [db] to begin syllables (as in *kto, gdyby,* and *dba*), English does not.

To investigate when infants first become sensitive to these aspects of native language sound patterns, Jusczyk, Friederici, Wessels, Svenkerud, and Jusczyk (1993) presented infants with lists of unfamiliar words, either from their native language or a foreign language. The aim was to determine whether infants might listen longer to the native language words. If so, it would be an indication that infants had learned something about the phonetic and phonotactic organization of words in their native language. A fluent bilingual Dutch/English talker recorded the materials for the experiment. These two languages were used because they have similar prosodic structures (T. H. Crystal & House, 1988; Ladefoged, 1975; Reitveld, 1988; Reitveld & Koopmans-van Beinum, 1987) but differ in their phonetic properties and phonotactic organization. For instance, Dutch does not allow the vowel that appears in the English word *few,* whereas English does not have the sound that begins the Dutch word *gouda.* Dutch allows sequences like [kn] and [zw] to begin syllables; English does not. English allows voiced stops (i.e., [b], [d], [g]) to appear at the ends of the words, whereas Dutch does not.

Infants were tested using a headturn preference procedure (see Jusczyk, Friederici, et al., 1993, for a detailed description). On a given trial, infants heard a new list of either unfamiliar Dutch or English words and listening times to these were recorded. Each list contained words from one of the languages that violated the phonetic structure or phonotactic constraints in the other language. At 6 months of age, American infants did not listen significantly longer to either the English or Dutch lists. However, American 9-month-olds listened significantly longer to the English lists. To determine if the infants were responding to the items on the basis of their phonetic and phonotactic properties (as opposed to unforeseen prosodic differences), Jusczyk et al. (1993) low-pass filtered their stimuli at 400 Hz. With the low-pass-filtered lists, American 9-month-olds did not listen significantly longer to the English than to the Dutch lists.

To investigate whether the infants were responding because they had learned something about the phonetic and phonotactic properties of native language words, Jusczyk et al. (1993) conducted an additional experiment with both Dutch and American 9-month-olds. One modification was made in the nature of the lists. This time what distinguished the words from the different languages had to do only with their phonotactic properties. Arguably, it is more difficult to pick up the distinction between the native and non-native patterns in this case because each individual phonetic segment can appear in some positions of native language words. Both the Dutch and American 9-month-olds listened longer to the lists in their own native language. Hence, by 9 months of age, infants have picked up some information about the patterns of phonetic sequences that can appear in words in their native language.

Jusczyk, Friederici, et al. (1993) were also curious as to whether infants could use information about prosodic organization to distinguish native language words from non-native ones. They conducted additional experiments comparing American infants' responses to English versus Norwegian word lists. Norwegian differs from English not only in terms of its phonetic and phonotactic properties, but also in its prosodic organization. In contrast to the infants who heard the English and Dutch lists, American 6-month-olds exhibited a significant preference for the English lists. The earlier preference for the native language words appears to be due to sensitivity to prosodic differences. Thus, when the lists were low-pass filtered to remove the phonetic and phonotactic cues, the infants still listened significantly longer to the English lists. Thus, sensitivity to differences involving the prosodic organization of native language words apparently develops sooner than does sensitivity to phonetic and phonotactic organization.

There are indications that the developing sensitivity to sound patterns of native language words goes well beyond what is required to distinguish native from foreign language words. Friederici and Wessels (in press) found that Dutch 9-month-olds show sensitivity to phonotactic legal onset and offset clusters in Dutch words. Not only did the infants listen significantly longer to phonotactically legal Dutch sequences for words occurring in isolation, but they also, under some circumstances, listened longer to word sequences containing phonotactically legal clusters than to ones with phonotactically illegal clusters. The latter finding suggests that they might be able to draw on information about phonotactic sequences to help in segmenting words from the speech stream. Furthermore, another recent investigation suggests that infants are attuned to the frequency with which certain phonotactic sequences occur in native language words (Jusczyk, Charles-Luce, & Luce, in press). Infants were presented with different lists of monosyllables, which contained phonetic sequences that were all phonotactically permissible in English words. However, half of the lists contained monosyllables with sequences that occur with great regularity in English, and the other half were composed of monosyllables with sequences that occur infrequently. Nine-month-olds, but not 6-month-olds, listened significantly longer to the lists with high-frequency phonotactic sequences. These results suggest not only that are infants between 6 and 9 months of age learning about the fine-grained structure of native language word patterns, but that they are remarkably sensitive to how these patterns are distributed in the input. Sensitivity to such properties of the input could well impact on the development and organization of the lexicon and word recognition processes (see Jusczyk, 1992, 1993a, for further discussion).

The infant learning about regularly occurring sound patterns in native language input may also discover information about prosodic patterns that appear with high frequency. Knowledge of regularities related to common word stress patterns in the language could help in segmenting words from fluent speech. Cutler and her colleagues have suggested that fluent English speakers may be able to use such regularities in English word stress patterns to help in word segmentation (Cutler, 1991; Cutler & Butterfield, 1992; Cutler & Carter, 1987; Cutler & Norris, 1988). They note that the overwhelming majority of words in English conversational speech are either monosyllables or multisyllabic words that begin with a strong syllable. Consequently, English listeners could make a plausible first pass at segmenting utterances into words by simply finding the strong syllables and assuming that each one begins a new word.

Might infants learning English benefit from such information about the typical stress patterns of words in the language? A necessary first step for such information to be effective is that they can detect the predominant stress pattern for English words. Jusczyk, Cutler, and Redanz (1993) presented American infants with lists of bisyllabic English words with stress patterns that either followed (i.e., strong/weak) or did not follow (i.e., weak/strong) the predominant ones in the language. Half of the lists were composed of bisyllables with strong/weak patterns (e.g., *final, private*) and the other half consisted of bisyllables with weak/strong patterns (e.g., *affront, inflate*). Although 6-month-olds showed no difference in listening times to either type of list, 9-month-olds listened significantly longer to the lists with strong/weak stress patterns. Moreover, even when the lists were low-pass filtered, 9-month-olds listened significantly longer to the strong/weak patterns, suggesting that they were not simply responding to phonetic or phonotactic properties. Instead, it appears that American infants are also developing sensitivity to the predominant stress patterns of English words at some time between 6 and 9 months of age.

To summarize, infants are developing sensitivity to various aspects of native language sound patterns within the first year of life. Not only are categories for speech sounds beginning to reflect the organization of native language phonetic structure, but infants appear to be influenced by the frequency with which certain phonotactic and prosodic patterns occur in the input. The age at which these developments appear is close to when comprehension of the first words has been noted (Benedict, 1979; Huttenlocher, 1974). Given these developments, one might reasonably expect that infants have at least some minimal capacity for recognizing words in fluent speech. However, most studies of word recognition capacities have used infants well into their second year and have mostly focused only on the degree of detail in infants' representations of words (Pollock & Schwartz, 1990; Werker & Pegg, 1992).

One suggestion as to how infants come to recognize words in fluent speech is that they first learn to recognize isolated words and then match these sound patterns to ones in fluent speech (Suomi, 1993). Although it is doubtful that this procedure could fully explain how words come to be recognized in fluent speech (see Jusczyk, 1993a), this strategy could potentially provide a starting point for the development of word recognition processes. Jusczyk and Aslin (1995) explored whether hearing words in isolation could lead infants to recognize the same words in fluent speech. Four different monosyllabic words were chosen for the study: *feet, cup, dog,* and *bike.* At the start of each experimental session, 7½-month-olds were familiarized with two of the words on alternating trials until they accumulated 30 s of listening time to each word. Half of the infants were familiarized with *cup* and *dog* and the other half with *feet* and *bike.* During the test phase four different passages, each consisting of six sentences, were played for the infants. For a given passage, the same test word appeared in all six sentences (although in different positions within each sentence). Two of the passages contained the words heard in the familiarization period, and the other two contained the other (i.e., not previously heard) test words. Infants listened significantly longer to the passages containing the familiar test words. Moreover, there was no indication that the infants' prior knowledge of the words had any important bearing on the results. Jusczyk and Aslin concluded that the exposure to the target words in isolation made it more likely that infants would attend to the sentences including these words. A second experiment in which infants were first exposed to passages containing two target words, and then tested on repetitions of isolated words, yielded a similar pattern of results. Infants listened longer to isolated words from the passages heard in the familiarization period. Thus, by $7\frac{1}{2}$ months of age, infants have at least some rudimentary ability to detect the appearance of a particular word when it occurs in different fluent speech contexts. Of course, many questions remain about the precise details that infants encode about the sound properties of words in these contexts. Nevertheless, infants' word segmentation abilities are developing as they begin learning about other aspects of the organization of sound patterns in the native language.

B. Learning about Prosodic Organization in the Native Language

Sound patterns of languages differ not only in how they pattern segmental information, but also in suprasegmental aspects of organization relating to the rhythmic and intonational structure. Although the issue of how and when infants learn the way that prosodic information is structured in the native language is important in its own right, interest in this aspect of language acquisition has been heightened by the possibility that prosody provides cues to the syntactic organization of the language. Analyses of fluent speech suggest that boundaries between important grammatical units such as clauses and phrases are often marked by changes in variables related to prosody, such as changes in pitch contour, increases in syllable duration, and pausing (Beckman & Edwards, 1990; Cooper & Paccia-Cooper, 1980; D. Crystal, 1969; Grosjean & Gee, 1987; Klatt, 1975; Lehiste, Olive, & Streeter, 1976; Nakatani & Dukes, 1977; Price, Ostendorf, Shattuck-Hufnagel, & Fong, 1991; Streeter, 1978). Moreover, adult listeners are sensitive to such prosodic markers and may use them to locate syntactic boundaries (Collier & t'Hart, 1975; Lehiste et al., 1976; Luce & Charles-Luce, 1983; Price et al., 1991; Scott, 1982; Scott & Cutler, 1984). These data have led to a number of students of language acquisition to suggest that learners use prosody to determine the location of linguistically relevant units, such as clauses and phrases (Fisher, 1991; Gleitman, Gleitman, Landau, & Wanner, 1988; Gleitman & Wanner, 1982; Hirsh-Pasek et al., 1987; Morgan, 1986; Peters, 1983). This view has come to be known as the Prosodic Bootstrapping Hypothesis. However, for prosodic bootstrapping to be a realistic account of how learners gain access to the syntactic organization of the native language, infants must be sensitive to prosodic markers in the input. Recent studies provide a picture of how sensitivity to native language prosodic structures begins to develop.

At the most basic level, one can ask about when infants have the capacity to distinguish the prosodic patterns of the native language from those of a foreign language. Such a capacity might prove especially important for infants growing up in a multilingual society. Without some ability to separate utterances in one language from utterances in another, discovering the

underlying grammatical organization of a language would be greatly hin-
dered. Mehler et al. (1988) have found that even newborn infants apparently
have some capacity to distinguish utterances in one language from those in
another. Specifically, French newborns distinguished utterances in French
from ones in Russian. One of the remarkable aspects of these results was the
fact that the infants were exposed to a wide variety of different utterances.
Thus, the infants had to extract some general properties that hold across
utterances within a particular language. Moreover, the same pattern of results was obtained even when the speech samples were low-pass filtered at
400 Hz, suggesting that the infants were responding to prosodic differences
(i.e., rhythm, stress, and intonation) between the languages. Additional
experiments by Mehler et al. with American 2-month-olds indicated that
they, too, could distinguish utterances in their own native language (i.e.,
English) from those of a foreign language (i.e., Italian) even when these
were low-pass filtered. In another investigation with American 5-month-
olds, Bahrick and Pickens (1988) found a similar pattern of results for utterances in Spanish versus English.

The results from these investigations demonstrate that, from an early
age, infants are sensitive to the kinds of prosodic differences that serve to
distinguish utterances in one language from those in another. However,
with respect to the prosodic bootstrapping hypothesis, we need to know
when they show signs of detecting potential prosodic markers to grammatical units in the native language. Hirsh-Pasek et al. (1987) investigated
whether infants respond to prosodic marking of clausal units in fluent
speech. They collected speech samples of a mother talking to her 18-month-
old infant, and divided these up into passages that were 15–20 s long. The
passages were modified by inserting 1-s pauses in the passages in one of two
ways. Either the pauses were inserted in the boundary between two successive clauses (Coincident versions) or between two words within each clause
(Noncoincident versions). Hirsh-Pasek et al. reasoned that if infants are
sensitive to prosodic marking of clausal units, they might find the versions
with the pauses at the clause boundaries preferable to those in which the
pauses did not coincide with other prosodic cues for clause boundaries.
Groups of 6- and 9-month-old infants were tested using the headturn preference procedure. Even the 6-month-olds listened significantly longer to
the Coincident than to the Noncoincident versions. Hirsh-Pasek et al. interpreted these findings as an indication that sensitivity to prosodic markers of
clausal units is present in infants as young as 6 months old.

The kinds of prosodic changes observed at clause boundaries in English
are also noted in many other languages (Cruttenden, 1986). Consequently,
American infants' responsiveness to these prosodic changes may not be a
result of something they have learned about English per se, but is rather
attributable to more general processing of the input. Some support for the

latter view comes from other recent investigations. First, $4\frac{1}{2}$-month-old American infants also listened significantly longer to Coincident versions of samples in an unfamiliar language (Polish) than they did to Noncoincident versions (Jusczyk, 1989). Second, studies with musical stimuli (Mozart minuets) also indicate that $4\frac{1}{2}$-month-olds listen significantly longer to samples with pauses inserted at musical phrase boundaries than to samples with pauses in the middle of musical phrases (Jusczyk & Krumhansl, 1993; Krumhansl & Jusczyk, 1990). The cues that appear to signal musical phrase boundaries for infants are a decline in pitch and a lengthening of the final note at the musical phrase boundary. These cues parallel ones associated with clause boundaries (i.e., decline in pitch and clause-final syllable lengthening). Therefore, young infants' sensitivity to prosodic markers of clausal units may be an aspect of a more general tendency associated with auditory event perception.

Although it is conceivable that infants might not need to learn about the particulars of prosodic structure in order to detect clausal units in their native language, the situation is otherwise for subclausal units. The organization of units within clauses differs considerably from language to language. In languages like English, which use word order to indicate important grammatical relations, some prosodic marking of information that occurs together within the same phrase is likely. However, case languages like Polish use affixes to mark grammatical relations and allow much freedom in ordering words within a clause. Two words within the same phrase could be separated by words from other phrases. Any prosodic marking of phrasal units in Polish is bound to be very different from that in English. Thus, infants need to discover the nature of any prosodic marking of subclausal units in their native language.

Jusczyk, Hirsh-Pasek et al. (1992) investigated when American infants might show sensitivity to prosodic marking of major phrasal units (Subject Phrase; Predicate Phrase) in English. The stimuli were analogous to the ones with the clausal units, only this time pauses were inserted either between two phrasal groups (Coincident versions) or within a phrasal group (Noncoincident versions). At 6 months of age, the infants' listening times to the Coincident and Noncoincident versions did not differ significantly. However, by 9 months of age, the infants had significantly longer listening times for the Coincident versions of the samples. Thus, in contrast to the results for clausal units, sensitivity to prosodic markers of phrasal units in English does not appear to develop until between 6 and 9 months of age. Jusczyk, Hirsh-Pasek et al. (1992) speculated that infants may require more familiarity with native language sound structures before they can detect prosodic marking of phrasal units. In any case, the results indicate that infants are picking up information about the prosodic organization of their native language well before their first birthday.

Although the prosodic organization of the language appears to provide learners with a start toward working out the syntactic organization of the native language, it is likely that it will take them only so far. Even if the infant can detect the prosodic organization of speech input, it is not always possible to read the syntactic organization from the prosody. Indeed, mismatches in the prosodic and syntactic organization may occur even in the simple sentences that are directed to infants acquiring language. Consider the following two sentences.

(1) *LouAnn bit the apple.*
(2) *She bit the apple.*

In (1), the talker is likely to produce prosodic boundary cues after the subject NP, *LouAnn*. However, in (2), even two-year-old talkers (Gerken, 1991, in press) either produce no prosodic boundary cues or produce them between the verb and the object NP, *the apple*. This is because a weakly stressed pronoun subject tends to be phonologically joined (or "cliticized") to a following stressed verb, that is, the subject and verb form a prosodic unit. Hence, there is no prosodic marking of the syntactic boundary between the subject and the predicate phrases.

This brings up the interesting question of how infants respond to utterances in which prosodic and syntactic boundaries mismatch. Only a small percentage of the spontaneous speech samples (about 15%) used by Jusczyk, Hirsh-Pasek et al. (1992) contained potential mismatches of the sort found in (2). So, Gerken, Jusczyk, and Mandel (1994) created new materials to compare infants' responses to sentences with pronoun subjects, as in (2), to sentences with lexical NP subjects, as in (1). Nine-month-olds exposed to the sentences with lexical NP subjects behaved exactly like the infants in the Jusczyk et al. (1992) study, namely, they listened significantly longer to samples in which pauses were inserted between the subject and object NP phrases. In contrast, infants who heard the sentences with pronoun subjects did not show a significant preference for either type of segmentation. In a follow-up experiment, Gerken et al. (1995) used sentences in which there was likely to be a prosodic boundary between a pronoun subject and the verb, namely, sentences with inversions between a pronoun and an auxiliary, that is, yes–no questions. In such sentences, the pronoun and auxiliary tend to form a separate clitic group. For these sentences, 9-month-olds listened significantly longer to versions with pauses between the subject and verb phrases.

To summarize, there is some prosodic marking of syntactic units in speech directed to children, and infants are sensitive to it. Thus, prosody can provide learners with an entry to syntactic organization even though the correlation between prosodic and syntactic units is less than perfect.

Given that infants demonstrate some sensitivity to potential prosodic markers of syntactic units, when might they actually begin using this information in segmenting speech? How can we determine if infants are truly organizing the incoming speech signal into units such as clauses or phrases? The issue here is akin to one faced by early psycholinguistics when trying to convince others that units of linguistic analysis corresponded to something real in the behavior of listeners. One approach that the early psycholinguists used was to show that linguistic units tend to be natural units for encoding and remembering information conveyed in speech. For example, it was shown that adults could remember information better when the materials had a linguistic, rather than arbitrary, organization (e.g., Epstein, 1961).

Analogously, prosody could provide infants with an organization for encoding and remembering speech information. Mandel, Jusczyk, and Kemler Nelson (1993) investigated whether prosodic organization enhances 2-month-olds' memory for speech. They used the HAS procedure to determine whether words that are prosodically linked within a clause are better remembered by infants than words produced as individual items from a list. If prosody helps in perceptual organization during on-line speech processing, then memory for words should be better in a sentential context than in a list. Half of the infants heard stimuli that were produced as complete sentences; the other half heard the same sequences of words but these were taken from long lists of words spoken in isolation. The overall durations of both types of materials were matched. During the preshift phase, infants repeatedly heard either a single sentence or list sequence. Following habituation to this stimulus, the preshift phase ended and was followed by a 2-min silent interval. In the postshift phase, the infants heard either the same stimulus as during the preshift phase, one that differed by one word, or one that differed by two words. The results indicated that performance was significantly better for the sentences than for the lists. Thus, even 2-month-olds can benefit from the organization provided by sentential prosody. Not only are infants sensitive to prosodic markers in the speech stream, but these markers may play a role in what infants remember about utterances.

In conclusion, infants are attuned to prosodic features in the input right from birth. During the first few months infants apparently respond to general properties that hold across a wide variety of different languages (or perhaps even acoustic signals). Nevertheless, even the organization provided by such features may play an important role in the infant's retention of speech information. Attention to the prosodic organization characteristic of the native language appears to develop between 6 and 9 months of age.

IV. RELATING DEVELOPMENTS IN SPEECH PERCEPTION AND SPEECH PRODUCTION

Until fairly recently, research on the development of speech perception and production proceeded quite independently of one another. One reason for this had to do with the available methodology for studying perception and production. The most successful measures for studying perception generally target infants under 1 year of age, whereas most studies of speech production have relied on the utterances of children beyond their first birthday. This picture has begun to change. More data are available on how perceptual capacities are influenced by input from the native language during the first year. Furthermore, analyses of babbling infants have advanced considerably, and the relation of babbling to the production of the first words in the native language has become clearer (Elbers & Ton, 1985; Ferguson & Macken, 1983; Leonard, Schwartz, Chapman, & Morris, 1981; Vihman & Miller, 1988).

A milestone in speech production occurs around 6 months of age, when children begin to engage in reduplicative (or canonical) babbling (Oller, 1980; Roug, Landberg, & Lundberg, 1989; Stark, 1980; Vihman, 1993a). In reduplicative babbling, the infant produces sequences of syllables usually consisting of a stop consonant combined with an open central vowel (e.g., *babababa*). A small consonantal repertoire of elements that involve simple ballistic movements is present at this stage (Vihman, 1993a). Little variation occurs in either intonation or constituent consonant and vowel segments. Reduplicative babbling is observed cross-linguistically with similar tendencies noted for languages such as English (Oller, 1980; Stark, 1980), Dutch (Koopmans van Beinum & van der Stelt, 1986), and Swedish (Roug et al., 1989).

The issue of when babbling begins to take on characteristics of native language sound patterns has been much debated (Atkinson, MacWhinney, & Stoel, 1968; Brown, 1958; de Boysson-Bardies, Sagart, & Durand, 1984; Olney & Scholnick, 1974; Weir, 1966). However, most of these claims were based on measures that asked adults to judge the language backgrounds of infants from samples of babbling. More recent investigations have undertaken acoustic analyses of babbling and have compared it to adult productions in target languages. For example, de Boysson-Bardies, Halle, Sagart, and Durand (1989) found that differences in vowel production by 10-month-olds from French, Arabic, English, and Chinese backgrounds tend to parallel adult productions of vowels in these languages. Similarities have also been noted between infants' babbling and adult productions of consonants. An extensive longitudinal study (de Boysson-Bardies et al., 1992) with infants from French, Swedish, English, and Japanese backgrounds plotted the drift toward native language consonantal categories. The infants were seen from 9 months of age until they achieved vocabularies of 25 words or more. The consonants produced in infants' babbling were compared to those in adult words used as targets by the infants. Even at 10 months, there were differences in the distribution of manner and place categories in the productions of the infants from the different language backgrounds. For example, analyses of the distribution of stop consonants in adult production indicated that these were most prevalent in Swedish followed by English, then Japanese, and last, French. The production of stops by the infants showed exactly the same pattern. Thus, there are indications that the phonetic segments that appear in babbling from 10 months of age onward are influenced by the target language.

Native language influences on babbling are not limited to the repertoire of phonetic segments. There is also evidence for early language-specific prosodic influences (A. G. Levitt, 1993). In a study of five French- and five English-learning infants between 5 and 13 months, Whalen, Levitt, and Wang (1991) found intonational differences in babbling that were consistent with those in the adult target languages. Also, rhythmic properties relating to the timing of syllables in the native language may emerge even earlier than any influences on segmental properties of babbling (A. G. Levitt, Utman, & Aydelott, 1992). In addition, investigations of syllable structure in babbling reveal effects of language-specific influences toward the end of the first year. A. G. Levitt et al. (1992) found that between 11 and 13 months, their French-learning infant was less likely to produce closed syllables than was their English-learning infant. This difference is in line with the distribution of open and closed syllables in the two target languages. Vihman (1992) also found evidence for differences in syllable structures among the infants from four different language backgrounds (Swedish, Japanese, English, and French). In particular, although all the children she studied had certain phonetic tendencies in common (producing syllables such as [da], [ha], and [hə]), there were also cross-linguistic differences. For instance, Japanese infants were much more likely to produce velars in association with back vowels (e.g., [ko], [go]). In addition, Swedish infants produced syllables in which [t] and [d] were associated with a full range of vowels, rather than just front vowels as infants from the other language backgrounds tended to do.

Hence, the emerging picture of the development of speech production shows evidence of language-specific influences, especially during the latter half of the first year. These trends in the development of speech production occur within the same general time frame as the appearance of language-specific influences on perception. Although it appears that language-specific influences develop sooner in perception than in production, this cannot be ascertained without data on the development of perception and production within the same individuals.

A number of interesting issues are yet to be resolved concerning relations between perception and production during development. For example, in what ways do infants' sensitivity to distributional properties in the input affect what they produce? To understand this, we need to know more than simply the frequency with which certain features and relations appear. We also need to know which properties infants are actually attending to in the input. Are there also influences of production on perception? For example, Vihman (1993b) has discussed the notion of an "articulatory filter," a phonetic template (unique to each child) that renders similar patterns in adult speech unusually salient or memorable. Could such a filter influence perceptual processes by altering which aspects of speech input infants are most likely to attend to? For example, if the articulatory filter serves to focus attention on certain patterns in the input, might this increase the likelihood that words embodying such patterns are more apt to be added to the lexicon? At the same time, one can ask if perceptual factors, such as the density of lexical neighborhoods (Luce, Pisoni, & Goldinger, 1991), influence whether or not infants attempt to add a new item to their lexicons.

V. SUMMARY AND CONCLUSIONS

The past twenty-five years have seen a rapid growth in our knowledge of infant speech perception capacities. It is clear that even newborns possess a number of important capacities that help them to begin to categorize information in speech. Studies of speech capacities in the first few months of life indicate that infants are well positioned to discriminate and categorize speech sounds that may appear in any of the world's languages. These general capacities for perceiving speech begin to evolve into ones adapted to dealing effectively with native language sound patterns sometime during the middle of the first year. By 9 months, infants are already sensitive to regularly appearing features of native language sound patterns. The evolution of perceptual capacities with respect to the native language appears to presage changes observed in speech production capacities.

Acknowledgments

Preparation of this manuscript was facilitated by a research grant from N.I.C.H.D. (#15795). The author thanks Ann Marie Jusczyk for comments she made on the manuscript.

References

Abramson, A. S., & Lisker, L. (1970). Discriminability along the voice continuum: Cross language tests. In *Proceedings of the Sixth International Congress of Phonetic Sciences*. Prague. Academia.

Aslin, R. N., & Pisoni, D. B. (1980). Some developmental processes in speech perception. In G. H. Yeni-Komshian, J. F. Kavanagh, & C. A. Ferguson (Eds.), *Child phonology*. New York: Academic Press.

Aslin, R. N., Pisoni, D. B., Hennessy, B. L., & Perey, A. J. (1981). Discrimination of voice onset time by human infants: New findings and implications for the effects of early experience. *Child Development, 52,* 1135–1145.

Aslin, R. N., Pisoni, D. B., & Jusczyk, P. W. (1983). Auditory development and speech perception in infancy. In M. M. Haith & J. J. Campos (Eds.), *Infancy and the biology of development* (pp. 573–687). New York: Wiley.

Atkinson, K., MacWhinney, B., & Stoel, C. (1968). *An experiment on the recognition of babbling* (Working Paper No. 14). Berkeley: University of California, Language Behavior Research Laboratory.

Bahrick, L. E., & Pickens, J. N. (1988). Classification of bimodal English and Spanish language passages by infants. *Infant Behavior and Development, 11,* 277–296.

Beckman, M., & Edwards, J. (1990). Lengthening and shortenings and the nature of prosodic constituency. In J. Kingston & M. E. Beckman (Eds.), *Papers in laboratory phonology: I. Between the grammar and physics of speech* (pp. 152–178). Cambridge, UK: Cambridge University Press.

Benedict, H. (1979). Early lexical development: Comprehension and production. *Journal of Child Language, 6,* 183–201.

Bertoncini, J., Bijeljac-Babic, R., Blumstein, S. E., & Mehler, J. (1987). Discrimination in neonates of very short CV's. *Journal of the Acoustical Society of America, 82,* 31–37.

Bertoncini, J., Bijeljac-Babic, R., Jusczyk, P. W., Kennedy, L. J., & Mehler, J. (1988). An investigation of young infants' perceptual representations of speech sounds. *Journal of Experimental Psychology: General, 117,* 21–33.

Best, C. T. (1991, April). *Phonetic influences on the perception of non-native speech contrasts by 6-8 and 10-12 month olds.* Paper presented at the biennial meeting of the Society for Research in Child Development, Seattle, WA.

Best, C. T. (1993). Emergence of language-specific constraints in perception of native and non-native speech: A window on early phonological development. In B. de Boysson-Bardies, S. de Schoen, P. Jusczyk, P. McNeilage, & J. Morton (Eds.), *Developmental neurocognition: Speech and face processing during the first year of life* (pp. 289–304). Dordrecht: Kluwer.

Best, C. T., & McRoberts, G. W. (1989, April). *Phonological influences on the perception of native and non-native speech contrasts.* Paper presented at the biennial meeting of the Society for Research in Child Development, Kansas City, MO.

Best, C. T., McRoberts, G. W., & Sithole, N. M. (1988). Examination of the perceptual reorganization for speech contrasts: Zulu click discrimination by English-speaking adults and infants. *Journal of Experimental Psychology: Human Perception and Performance, 14,* 245–360.

Best, C. T., Morrongiello, B., & Robson, R. (1981). Perceptual equivalence of acoustic cues in speech and nonspeech perception. *Perception & Psychophysics, 29,* 191–211.

Bladon, R. A., Henton, C. G., & Pickering, J. B. (1984). Towards an auditory theory of speaker normalization. *Language and Communication, 4,* 59–69.

Blumstein, S. E., & Stevens, K. N. (1978). Acoustic invariance for place of articulation in stops and nasals across syllabic context. *Journal of the Acoustical Society of America, 62,* S26.

Blumstein, S. E., & Stevens, K. N. (1980). Perceptual invariance and onset spectra for stop consonants in different vowel environments. *Journal of the Acoustical Society of America, 67,* 648–662.

Brown, R. (1958). *Words and things.* Glencoe, IL: Free Press.

Brown, R., & Fraser, C. (1964). The acquisition of syntax. *Monographs of the Society for Research in Child Development, 29,* 9–34.

Carden, G., Levitt, A., Jusczyk, P. W., & Walley, A. C. (1981). Evidence for phonetic processing of cues to place of articulation: Perceived manner affects perceived place. *Perception & Psychophysics, 29,* 26–36.

Carrell, T. D., Smith, L. B., & Pisoni, D. B. (1981). Some perceptual dependencies in speeded classification of vowel color and pitch. *Perception & Psychophysics, 29,* 1–10.

Collier, R., & t'Hart, J. (1975). The role of intonation in speech perception. In A. Cohen &

S. G. Nooteboom (Eds.), *Structure and process in speech perception* (pp. 107–121). Heidelberg: Springer-Verlag.

Cooper, W. E., & Paccia-Cooper, J. (1980). *Syntax and speech.* Cambridge, MA: Harvard University Press.

Cruttenden, A. (1986). *Intonation.* Cambridge, UK: Cambridge University Press.

Crystal, D. (1969). *Prosodic systems and intonation in English.* London: Cambridge University Press.

Crystal, T. H., & House, A. S. (1988). Segmental durations in connected speech signals: Current results. *Journal of the Acoustical Society of America, 88,* 101–112.

Cutler, A. (1991). Exploiting prosodic probabilities in speech segmentation. In G. T. M. Altmann (Ed.), *Cognitive models of speech processing: Psycholinguistic and computational perspectives* (pp. 105–121). Cambridge, MA: MIT Press.

Cutler, A., & Butterfield, S. (1992). Rhythmic cues to speech segmentation: Evidence from juncture misperception. *Journal of Memory and Language, 31,* 218–236.

Cutler, A., & Carter, D. M. (1987). The predominance of strong initial syllables in the English vocabulary. *Computer Speech and Language, 2,* 133–142.

Cutler, A., & Norris, D. G. (1988). The role of strong syllables in segmentation for lexical access. *Journal of Experimental Psychology: Human Perception and Performance, 14,* 113–121.

de Boysson-Bardies, B., Halle, P., Sagart, L., & Durand, C. (1989). A cross-linguistic investigation of vowel formants in babbling. *Journal of Child Language, 16,* 1–17.

de Boysson-Bardies, B., Sagart, L., & Durand, C. (1984). Discernible differences in the babbling of infants according to target language. *Journal of Child Language, 11,* 1–15.

de Boysson-Bardies, B., Vihman, M. M., Roug-Hellichius, L., Durand, C., Landberg, I., & Arao, F. (1992). Material evidence of selection from the target language. In C. A. Ferguson, L. Menn, & C. Stoel-Gammon (Eds.), *Phonological development: Models, research, implications* (pp. 369–391). Timonium, MD: York Press.

DeCasper, A. J., & Spence, M. J. (1986). Prenatal maternal speech influences newborns' perception of speech sounds. *Infant Behavior and Development, 9,* 133–150.

Delattre, P. C., Liberman, A. M., & Cooper, F. S. (1955). Acoustic loci and transitional cues for consonants. *Journal of the Acoustical Society of America, 27,* 769–773.

Eilers, R. E. (1977). Context sensitive perception of naturally produced stop and fricative consonants by infants. *Journal of the Acoustical Society of America, 61,* 1321–1336.

Eimas, P. D. (1974). Auditory and linguistic processing of cues for place of articulation by infants. *Perception & Psychophysics, 16,* 513–521.

Eimas, P. D. (1975a). Auditory and phonetic coding of the cues for speech: Discrimination of the [r-l] distinction by young infants. *Perception & Psychophysics, 18,* 341–347.

Eimas, P. D. (1975b). Speech perception in early infancy. In L. B. Cohen & P. Salapatek (Eds.), *Infant perception: From sensation to cognition.* New York: Academic Press.

Eimas, P. D. (1985). The equivalence of cues for the perception of speech by infants. *Infant Behavior and Development, 8,* 125–138.

Eimas, P. D., & Miller, J. L. (1980a). Contextual effects in infant speech perception. *Science, 209,* 1140–1141.

Eimas, P. D., & Miller, J. L. (1980b). Discrimination of the information for manner of articulation. *Infant Behavior and Development, 3,* 367–375.

Eimas, P. D., & Miller, J. L. (1992). Organization in the perception of speech by young infants. *Psychological Science, 3,* 340–345.

Eimas, P. D., Miller, J. L., & Jusczyk, P. W. (1987). On infant speech perception and the acquisition of language. In S. Harnad (Ed.), *Categorical perception* (pp. 161–195). New York: Cambridge University Press.

Eimas, P. D., Siqueland, E. R., Jusczyk, P., & Vigorito, J. (1971). Speech perception in early infancy. *Science, 171,* 304–306.

Elbers, L., & Ton, J. (1985). Play pen monologues: The interplay of words and babbles in the first words period. *Journal of Child Language, 12,* 551–564.

Epstein, W. (1961). The influence of syntactical structure on learning. *American Journal of Psychology, 74,* 80–85.

Ferguson, C. A., & Macken, M. A. (1983). The role of play in phonological development. In K. E. Nelson (Ed.), *Children's language.* Hillsdale, NJ: Erlbaum.

Fisher, C. L. (1991, April). *Prosodic cues to phrase structure in infant directed speech.* Paper presented at the Stanford Child Language Research Forum, Stanford, CA.

Friederici, A. D., & Wessels, J. M. I. (in press). Phonotactic knowledge and its use in infant speech perception. *Perception & Psychophysics.*

Gerken, L. A. (1991). The metrical basis for children's subjectless sentences. *Journal of Memory and Language, 30,* 431–451.

Gerken, L. A. (in press). Young children's representation of prosodic phonology: Evidence from English-speakers' weak syllable omissions.

Gerken, L. A., Jusczyk, P. W., & Mandel, D. R. (1994). *When prosody fails to cue syntactic structure: Nine-month-olds sensitivity to phonological vs syntactic phrases. Cognition, 51,* 237–265.

Gerken, L. A., Landau, B., & Remez, R. E. (1989). Function morphemes in young children's speech perception and production. *Developmental Psychology, 25,* 204–216.

Gleitman, L., Gleitman, H., Landau, B., & Wanner, E. (1988). Where the learning begins: Initial representations for language learning. In F. Newmeyer (Ed.), *The Cambridge Linguistic Survey; Vol. 3. Psychological and biological aspects of language.* Cambridge, MA: Harvard University Press.

Gleitman, L., & Wanner, E. (1982). The state of the state of the art. In E. Wanner & L. Gleitman (Eds.), *Language acquisition: The state of the art* (pp. 3–48). Cambridge, UK: Cambridge University Press.

Goodsitt, J. V., Morse, P. A., Ver Hoove, J. N., & Cowan, N. (1984). Infant speech perception in multisyllabic contexts. *Child Development, 55,* 903–910.

Grieser, D., & Kuhl, P. K. (1989). The categorization of speech by infants: Support for speech-sound prototypes. *Developmental Psychology, 25,* 577–588.

Grosjean, F., & Gee, J. P. (1987). Prosodic structure and spoken word recognition. *Cognition, 25,* 135–155.

Hillenbrand, J. M., Minifie, F. D., & Edwards, T. J. (1979). Tempo of spectrum change as a cue in speech sound discrimination by infants. *Journal of Speech and Hearing Research, 22,* 147–165.

Hirsh-Pasek, K., Kemler Nelson, D. G., Jusczyk, P. W., Wright Cassidy, K., Druss, B., & Kennedy, L. (1987). Clauses are perceptual units for young infants. *Cognition, 26,* 269–286.

Holmberg, T. L., Morgan, K. A., & Kuhl, P. K. (1977, December). *Speech perception in early infancy: Discrimination of fricative consonants.* Paper presented at the meeting of the Acoustical Society of America, Miami Beach, FL.

Huttenlocher, J. (1974). The origins of language comprehension. In R. L. Solso (Ed.), *Theories in cognitive psychology* (pp. 331–368). New York: Wiley.

Jusczyk, P. W. (1985). The high amplitude sucking procedure as a methodological tool in speech perception research. In G. Gottlieb & N. A. Krasnegor (Eds.), *Measurement of audition and vision in the first year of postnatal life: A methodological overview* (pp. 195–222). Norwood, NJ: Ablex.

Jusczyk, P. W. (1989, April). *Perception of cues to clausal units in native and non-native languages.*

Paper presented at the biennial meeting of the Society for Research in Child Development, Kansas City, MO.

Jusczyk, P. W. (1992). Developing phonological categories from the speech signal. In C. A. Ferguson, L. Menn, & C. Stoel-Gammon (Eds.), *Phonological development: Models, research, implications* (pp. 17–64). Timonium, MD: York Press.

Jusczyk, P. W. (1993a). From general to language specific capacities: The WRAPSA Model of how speech perception develops. *Journal of Phonetics, 21,* 3–28.

Jusczyk, P. W. (1993b). Some reflections on developmental changes in speech perception and production. *Journal of Phonetics, 21,* 109–116.

Jusczyk, P. W. (in press). How word recognition may evolve from infant speech perception capacities. In G. Altmann & R. Shillcock (Eds.), *Cognitive models of speech. Processing: The second Sperlonga Workshop.* London: Academic Press, 27–55.

Jusczyk, P. W., & Aslin, R. N. (1995). Recognition of familiar patterns in fluent speech by 7½ month old infants. *Cognitive Psychology*

Jusczyk, P. W., Bertoncini, J., Bijeljac-Babic, R., Kennedy, L. J., & Mehler, J. (1990). The role of attention in speech perception by infants. *Cognitive Development, 5,* 265–286.

Jusczyk, P. W., Charles-Luce, J., & Luce, P. A. (1994). Infants' sensitivity to high frequency vs low frequency phonetic sequences in the native language. *Journal of Memory and Language, 33,* 630–645.

Jusczyk, P. W., Copan, H., & Thompson, E. (1978). Perception by two-month-olds of glide contrasts in multisyllabic utterances. *Perception & Psychophysics, 24,* 515–520.

Jusczyk, P. W., Cutler, A., & Redanz, N. (1993). Preference for the predominant stress patterns of English words. *Child Development, 64,* 675–687.

Jusczyk, P. W., & Derrah, C. (1987). Representation of speech sounds by young infants. *Developmental Psychology, 23,* 648–654.

Jusczyk, P. W., Friederici, A. D., Wessels, J., Svenkerud, V. Y., & Jusczyk, A. M. (1993). Infants' sensitivity to the sound patterns of native language words. *Journal of Memory and Language, 32,* 402–420.

Jusczyk, P. W., Hirsh-Pasek, K., Kemler Nelson, D. G., Kennedy, L., Woodward, A., & Piwoz, J. (1992). Perception of acoustic correlates of major phrasal units by young infants. *Cognitive Psychology, 24,* 252–293.

Jusczyk, P. W., Kennedy, L. J., & Jusczyk, A. M. (in press). Young infants' retention of information about syllables. *Infant Behavior and Development.*

Jusczyk, P. W., Kennedy, L. J., Jusczyk, A. M., Schomberg, T., & Koenig, N. (in press). Young infants' retention of information about bisyllabic utterances. *Journal of Experimental Psychology: Human Perception and Performance.*

Jusczyk, P. W., & Krumhansl, C. (1993). Pitch and rhythmic patterns affecting infants' sensitivity to musical phrase structure. *Journal of Experimental Psychology: Human Perception and Performance, 19,* 1–14.

Jusczyk, P. W., Pisoni, D. B., Fernald, A., Reed, M., & Myers, M. (1983). Infants' discrimination of the duration of a rapid spectrum change in nonspeech signals. *Science, 222,* 175–177.

Jusczyk, P. W., Pisoni, D. B., & Mullennix, J. (1992). Some consequences of stimulus variability on speech processing by 2-month-old infants. *Cognition, 43,* 253–291.

Jusczyk, P. W., & Thompson, E. J. (1978). Perception of a phonetic contrast in multisyllabic utterances by two-month-old infants. *Perception & Psychophysics, 23,* 105–109.

Karzon, R. G. (1985). Discrimination of a polysyllabic sequence by one- to four-month-old infants. *Journal of Experimental Child Psychology, 39,* 326–342.

Klatt, D. H. (1975). Vowel lengthening is syntactically determined in connected discourse. *Journal of Phonetics, 3,* 129–140.

Klatt, D. H. (1989). Review of selected models of speech perception. In W. Marslen-Wilson (Ed.), *Lexical representation and process* (pp. 169–226). Cambridge, MA: MIT Press.

Koopmans van Beinum, F. J., & van der Stelt, J. M. (1986). Early stages in the development of speech movements. In B. Lindblom & R. Zetterström (Eds.), *Precursors of early speech.* New York: Stockton.

Krumhansl, C. L., & Jusczyk, P. W. (1990). Infants' perception of phrase structure in music. *Psychological Science, 1,* 70–73.

Kuhl, P. K. (1976). Speech perception in early infancy: The acquisition of speech sound categories. In S. K. Hirsh, D. H. Eldridge, I. J. Hirsh, & S. R. Silverman (Eds.), *Hearing and Davis: Essays honoring Hallowell Davis.* St. Louis, MO: Washington University Press.

Kuhl, P. K. (1979). Speech perception in early infancy: Perceptual constancy for spectrally dissimilar vowel categories. *Journal of the Acoustical Society of America, 66,* 1668–1679.

Kuhl, P. K. (1983). Perception of auditory equivalence classes for speech in early infancy. *Infant Behavior and Development, 6,* 263–285.

Kuhl, P. K. (1991). Human adults and human infants show a "perceptual magnet effect" for the prototypes of speech categories, monkeys do not. *Perception & Psychophysics, 50,* 93–107.

Kuhl, P. K. (1993). Innate predispositions and the effects of experience in speech perception: The native language magnet theory. In B. de Boysson-Bardies, S. de Schoen, P. Jusczyk, P. McNeilage, & J. Morton (Eds.), *Developmental neurocognition: Speech and face processing in the first year of life* (pp. 259–274). Dordrecht: Kluwer.

Kuhl, P. K., & Miller, J. D. (1982). Discrimination of auditory target dimensions in the presence or absence of variation in a second dimension by infants. *Perception & Psychophysics, 31,* 279–292.

Kuhl, P. K., Williams, K. A., Lacerda, F., Stevens, K. N., & Lindblom, B. (1992). Linguistic experiences alter phonetic perception in infants by 6 months of age. *Science, 255,* 606–608.

Lacerda, F. (1992, July 23). *Does young infants' vowel perception favor high/low contrasts?* Paper presented at the 25th International Congress of Psychology, Brussels, Belgium.

Ladefoged, P. (1975). *A course in phonetics.* New York: Harcourt Brace Jovanovich.

Lasky, R. E., Syrdal-Lasky, A., & Klein, R. E. (1975). VOT discrimination by four to six and a half month old infants from Spanish environments. *Journal of Experimental Child Psychology, 20,* 215–225.

Lehiste, I., Olive, J. P., & Streeter, L. (1976). The role of duration in disambiguating syntactically ambiguous sentences. *Journal of the Acoustical Society of America, 60,* 1199–1202.

Leonard, L. B., Schwartz, R. G., Chapman, K., & Morris, B. (1981). Phonological factors influencing early lexical acquisition: Lexical orientation. *Child Development, 52,* 882–887.

Levitt, A. G., Jusczyk, P. W., Murray, J., & Carden, G. (1988). The perception of place of articulation contrasts in voiced and voiceless fricatives by two-month-old infants. *Journal of Experimental Psychology: Human Perception and Performance, 14,* 361–368.

Levitt, A. G. (1993). The acquisition of prosody: Evidence from French- and English-learning infants. In B. de Boysson-Bardies, S. de Schoen, P. Jusczyk, P. McNeilage, & J. Morton (Eds.), *Developmental neurocognition: Speech and face processing in the first year of life* (pp. 385–398). Dordrecht: Kluwer.

Levitt, A. G., Utman, J., & Aydelott, J. (1992). From babbling towards the sound systems of English and French: A longitudinal two-case study. *Journal of Child Language, 19,* 19–49.

Liberman, A. M., Cooper, F. S., Shankweiler, D. P., & Studdert-Kennedy, M. G. (1967). Perception of the speech code. *Psychological Review, 74,* 431–461.

Liberman, A. M., Harris, K. S., Hoffman, H. S., & Griffith, B. C. (1957). The discrimination of speech sounds within and across phoneme boundaries. *Journal of Experimental Psychology, 54,* 358–368.

Lisker, L. (1986). "Voicing" in English: A catalog of acoustic features signalling /b/ versus /p/ in trochees. *Language and Speech, 29,* 3–11.

Lisker, L., & Abramson, A. S. (1964). A cross language study of voicing in initial stops: Acoustical measurements. *Word, 20,* 384–422.

Lisker, L., & Abramson, A. S. (1970). The voicing dimension: Some experiments in comparative phonetics. In *Proceedings of the Sixth International Congress of Phonetic Sciences.* Prague: Academia.

Lively, S. E. (1993). An examination of the perceptual magnet effect. *Journal of the Acoustical Society of America, 93,* 2423.

Luce, P. A., & Charles-Luce, J. (1983, May). *Contextual effects on the consonant/vowel ratio in speech production.* Paper presented at the 105th meeting of the Acoustical Society of America, Cincinnati, OH.

Luce, P. A., Pisoni, D. B., & Goldinger, S. D. (1991). Similarity neighborhoods of spoken words. In G. T. M. Altman (Ed), *Cognitive models of speech perception: Psycholinguistic and computational perspectives.* Cambridge, MA: MIT Press.

Mandel, D. R., Jusczyk, P. W., & Kemler Nelson, D. G. (1993). *Does sentential prosody improve 2-month-olds' memory for speech?* Paper presented at the biennial meeting of the Society for Research in Child Development, New Orleans, LA.

Martin, C. S., Mullennix, J. W., Pisoni, D. B., & Summers, W. V. (1989). Effects of talker variability on recall of spoken word lists. *Journal of Experimental Psychology: Learning, Memory, and Cognition, 15,* 676–684.

Mehler, J., Jusczyk, P. W., Lambertz, G., Halsted, N., Bertoncini, J., & Amiel-Tison, C. (1988). A precursor of language acquisition in young infants. *Cognition, 29,* 144–178.

Miller, J. L., & Eimas, P. D. (1979). Organization in infant speech perception. *Canadian Journal of Psychology, 33,* 353–367.

Miller, J. L., & Eimas, P. D. (1983). Studies on the categorization of speech by infants. *Cognition, 13,* 135–165.

Miller, J. L., & Liberman, A. M. (1979). Some effects of later-occurring information on the perception of stop consonant and semivowel. *Perception & Psychophysics, 25,* 457–465.

Miyawaki, K., Strange, W., Verbrugge, R., Liberman, A. M., Jenkins, J. J., & Fujimura, O. (1975). An effect of linguistic experience: The discrimination of /r/ and /l/ by native speakers of Japanese and English. *Perception & Psychophysics, 18,* 331–340.

Moffitt, A. R. (1971). Consonant cue perception by twenty-to-twenty-four-week old infants. *Child Development, 42,* 717–731.

Morgan, J. L. (1986). *From simple input to complex grammar.* Cambridge, MA: MIT Press.

Morse, P. A. (1972). The discrimination of speech and nonspeech stimuli in early infancy. *Journal of Experimental Child Psychology, 13,* 477–492.

Nakatani, L., & Dukes, K. (1977). Locus of segmental cues for word juncture. *Journal of the Acoustical Society of America, 62,* 714–719.

Nozza, R. J., Rossman, R. N. F., Bond, L. C., & Miller, S. L. (1990). Infant speech sound discrimination in noise. *Journal of the Acoustical Society of America, 87,* 339–350.

Oller, D. K. (1980). The emergence of speech sounds in infancy. In G. H. Yeni-Komshian, J. F. Kavanagh, & C. A. Ferguson (Eds.), *Child phonology* (pp. 93–112). New York: Academic Press.

Olney, R. K., & Scholnick, E. K. (1974). Adult judgments of age and linguistic differences in infant vocalization. *Journal of Child Language, 3,* 145–155.

Peters, A. (1983). *The units of language acquisition.* Cambridge, UK: Cambridge University Press.

Pollock, K., & Schwartz, R. G. (1990). Phonological perception of early words in 15-20 month old children.

Price, P. J., Ostendorf, M., Shattuck-Hufnagel, S., & Fong, C. (1991). The use of prosody in syntactic disambiguation. *Journal of the Acoustical Society of America, 90,* 2956–2970.

Rand, T. C. (1971). Vocal tract size normalization in the perception of stop consonants. *Haskins Laboratories Status Report on Speech Research,* pp. 141–146.

Reitveld, A. C. M. (1988). Woordklemtoon inn spraak. In M. P. R. van der Broeke (Ed.), *Ter spraake* (pp. 132–143). Dordrecht: Foris.

Reitveld, A. C. M., & Koopmans-van Beinum, F. J. (1987). Vowel reduction and stress. *Speech Communication, 6,* 217–229.

Repp, B. H. (1982). Phonetic trading relations and context effects: New experimental evidence for a speech mode of perception. *Psychological Bulletin, 92,* 81–110.

Roug, L., Landberg, I., & Lundberg, L. (1989). Phonetic developments in early infancy: A study of four Swedish children during the first eighteen months of life. *Journal of Child Language, 16,* 19–40.

Scott, D. R. (1982). Duration as a cue to the perception of a phrase boundary. *Journal of the Acoustical Society of America, 71,* 996–1007.

Scott, D. R., & Cutler, A. (1984). Segmental phonology and the perception of syntactic structure. *Journal of Verbal Learning and Verbal Behavior, 23,* 450–466.

Searle, C. L., Jacobson, J. Z., & Rayment, S. G. (1979). Stop consonant discrimination based on human audition. *Journal of the Acoustical Society of America, 65,* 799–809.

Siqueland, E. R., & DeLucia, C. A. (1969). Visual reinforcement of non-nutritive sucking in human infants. *Science, 165,* 1144–1146.

Stark, R. E. (1980). Stages of speech development during the first year of life. In G. H. Yeni-Komshian, J. F. Kavanagh, & C. A. Ferguson (Eds.), *Child phonology* (pp. 73–92). New York: Academic Press.

Stevens, K. N., & Blumstein, S. E. (1981). The search for invariant acoustic correlates for phonetic features. In P. D. Eimas & J. L. Miller (Eds.), *Perspectives on the study of speech.* Hillsdale, NJ: Erlbaum.

Strange, W., & Broen, P. A. (1981). The relationship between perception and production of /w/, /r/, and /l/ by three-year-old children. *Journal of Experimental Child Psychology, 31,* 81–102.

Streeter, L. A. (1976). Language perception of 2-month-old infants shows effects of both innate mechanisms and experience. *Nature (London), 259,* 39–41.

Streeter, L. A. (1978). Acoustic determinants of phrase boundary perception. *Journal of the Acoustical Society of America, 64,* 1582–1592.

Studdert-Kennedy, M. G., Liberman, A. M., Harris, K. S., & Cooper, F. S. (1970). Motor theory of speech perception: A reply to Lane's critical review. *Psychological Review, 77,* 234–249.

Suomi, K. (1993). An outline of a developmental model of adult phonological organization and behavior. *Journal of Phonetics, 21,* 29–60.

Swoboda, P., Morse, P. A., & Leavitt, L. A. (1976). Continuous vowel discrimination in normal and at-risk infants. *Child Development, 47,* 459–465.

Templin, M. (1957). *Certain language skills in children* (Institute of Child Welfare Monographs). Minneapolis: University of Minnesota Press.

Trehub, S. E. (1973). Infants' sensitivity to vowel and tonal contrasts. *Developmental Psychology, 9,* 91–96.

Trehub, S. E. (1976). The discrimination of foreign speech contrasts by infants and adults. *Child Development, 47,* 466–472.

Verbrugge, R. R., Strange, W., Shankweiler, D. P., & Edman, T. R. (1976). What information enables a listener to map a talker's vowel space? *Journal of the Acoustical Society of America, 60,* 198–212.

Vihman, M. M. (1992). Early syllables and the construction of phonology. In C. A. Ferguson,

L. Menn, & C. Stoel-Gammon (Eds.), *Phonological development: Models, research, implications* (pp. 393–422). Timonium, MD: York Press.

Vihman, M. M. (1993a). The construction of a phonological system. In B. de Boysson-Bardies, S. de Schoen, P. Jusczyk, P. McNeilage, & J. Morton (Eds.), *Developmental neurocognition: Speech and face perception in the first year of life* (pp. 411–419). Dordrecht: Kluwer.

Vihman, M. M. (1993b). Variable paths to word production. *Journal of Phonetics, 21,* 61–82.

Vihman, M. M., & Miller, R. (1988). Words and babble at the threshold of language acquisition. In M. D. Smith & J. L. Locke (Eds.), *The emergent lexicon* (pp. 151–184). San Diego, CA: Academic Press.

Weir, R. (1966). Some questions on the child's learning of phonology. In F. Smith & G. A. Miller (Eds.), *The genesis of language* (pp. 153–169). Cambridge, MA: MIT Press.

Werker, J. F. (1991). The ontogeny of speech perception. In I. G. Mattingly & M. Studdert-Kennedy (Eds.), *Modularity and the motor theory of speech perception* (pp. 91–109). Hillsdale, NJ: Erlbaum.

Werker, J. F., Gilbert, J. H., Humphrey, K., & Tees, R. C. (1981). Developmental aspects of cross-language speech perception. *Child Development, 52,* 349–355.

Werker, J. F., & Lalonde, C. E. (1988). Cross-language speech perception: Initial capabilities and developmental change. *Developmental Psychology, 24,* 672–683.

Werker, J. F., Lloyd, V. L., & Pegg, J. E. (1993). *Toward explaining experiential influences on language processing.* Paper presented at the International Conference on Signal to Syntax: Bootstrapping from Speech to Grammar in Early Acquisition, Brown University, Providence, RI.

Werker, J. F., & Pegg, J. E. (1992). Infant speech perception and phonological acquisition. In C. A. Ferguson, L. Menn, & C. Stoel-Gammon (Eds.), *Phonological development: Models, research, implications* (pp. 285–311). Timonium, MD: York Press.

Werker, J. F., & Polka, L. (1993). The ontogeny and developmental significance of language-specific phonetic perception. In B. de Boysson-Bardies, S. de Schoen, P. Jusczyk, P. McNeilage, & J. Morton (Eds.), *Developmental neurocognition: Speech and face processing in the first year of life* (pp. 275–288). Dordrecht: Kluwer.

Werker, J. F., & Tees, R. C. (1984). Cross-language speech perception: Evidence for perceptual reorganization during the first year of life. *Infant Behavior and Development, 7,* 49–63.

Whalen, D. H., Levitt, A., & Wang, Q. (1991). Intonational differences between the reduplicative babbling of French- and English-learning infants. *Journal of Child Language, 18,* 501–506.

Williams, L. (1977a, October). *The effects of phonetic environment and stress placement on infant discrimination of place of stop consonant articulation.* Paper presented at the Second Boston University Conference on Language Development, Boston.

Williams, L. (1977b). The voicing contrast in Spanish. *Journal of Phonetics, 5,* 169–184.

CHAPTER 9

Language Acquisition: The Lexicon and Syntax

Eve V. Clark

I. INTRODUCTION

Speakers rely on a large stock of words when they communicate. The community of speakers agrees on the meaning or meanings assigned to each word form. For instance, speakers of English refer to a bicycle with the word *bicycle,* speakers of Dutch with the word *fiets,* and speakers of French with the word *vélo.* In each community of speakers, the relation between word form and word meaning is a conventional one, accepted or agreed on by all the speakers in that community. Speakers of each language, then, draw on a common set of forms with agreed-on meanings when they talk.

In general, words provide the building blocks for larger units. They may be combined as idioms, where the meanings of the parts do not add up to the meaning of the whole, as in *to belt up, to be in a flap, to hit the sack, to keep tabs on,* or *to blow one's own trumpet.* Idioms like these are typically restricted in syntax, so some, for instance, may not appear in the passive (compare *He blew his own trumpet* vs. **His own trumpet was blown by himself).* Words may be combined in short phrases that act as if they were single words, as in *by and large, in short, happy go lucky,* or *once upon a time.* Again, these forms are fixed: their word order is frozen, and many are used only in restricted contexts. *Once upon a time,* for example, serves to introduce fairy tales and rarely occurs outside that context. Finally, words can combine, following

Speech, Language, and Communication

the syntactic rules of a language, to form an indefinite number of noun phrases (e.g., *the lone skier, a red fox, three children*) and verb phrases (e.g., *raced down the hill, crossed the road, climbed over the gate*) in each language. Words, fixed phrases, and idioms, then, all contribute to the construction of clauses (e.g., *Justin changed gear, Rod plotted the data, Sophie is practicing her flute*). Speakers build their utterances (both clauses and combinations of clauses) from words, fixed phrases, and idioms. And these are also the lexical units identified by listeners as they parse and interpret utterances heard from others.

In short, lexical items "clothe" syntactic structure. They are what exemplify a relative clause (*Duncan pointed at the man who was running*), an adverbial clause (*Duncan went outside when he heard the car*, or a verb complement (*They wanted to climb the hill*). Without words, there is no way for the syntax of a language to be realized. Equally, without words, there is no way to exemplify the phonological system or the morphology of language, in inflections (e.g., in *jump -s, race -d, wait -ing, know -n; cup -s, toy -s, cat -'s*), derivations (e.g., *watch -er, violin -ist, construct -ion, silver -y, green -ish, palm -ate*), or compound words (e.g., *snow-plough, key-hole, pile-driver, writing desk*). In using language, children reveal what they know about it. And when children start to talk, they start with words—word forms and word meanings.

I argue in this chapter that lexical and syntactic development go hand in hand. Children learn the syntactic forms that go with specific lexical items, and gradually accumulate sets of words that can act the same way syntactically. It is unclear when (or whether) young children learn rules of syntax. Rather, I suggest, there is growing evidence that they learn syntactic properties specific to individual lexical items. As they learn more lexical items, they become more likely to act consistently in the syntactic patterns they produce. (Whether this consistency is best described in terms of rules or strategies remains an open question.) The present chapter focuses first on the acquisition of the lexicon and of individual lexical items, how children build up a vocabulary (isolating forms from the stream of speech, constructing hypotheses about possible meanings, and mapping those meanings onto forms). Children must also elaborate semantic fields, linking words whose meanings are related; analyze word structures, so they are able to identify stems and affixes and their relative contributions to meaning; and coin new words to express meanings where they lack the relevant conventional forms.

After a review of early lexical development, I turn to the acquisition of syntax, the point when children begin to combine words to convey meanings not conveyable by single words on their own. The first such combinations may not match the adult conventions on how to form relative clauses or complement structures because they often lack critical indications of structure (e.g., *who, that, to, for, after*). I therefore trace how some syntactic forms are first produced and then elaborated as children move from two-word combinations to later, more adultlike forms in their speech. In particular, I focus on relative clauses, adverbial clauses, and complements, and trace their emergence in the speech of young children acquiring syntax.

Throughout this chapter, one recurring theme is the extent to which children's acquisition of syntax is lexically based. That is, how far is production a matter of learning which constructions can occur with each lexical item, for instance, with each verb? This question is particularly important for charting the course of acquisition, assessing where children learn item by item, and at what point they make generalizations that can be applied to new cases. I end with a brief discussion of the process of acquisition, and how discrepancies between comprehension and production are vital to acquisition itself. The picture of acquisition I present here is set against a background of some consideration of the sheer size of the learning task required for the lexicon, and hence for the syntax, of one's first language.

II. THE LEXICON

How many words do children have to learn? Adult vocabulary size in English has been estimated at between 50,000 and 100,000 words. And in the period from about age 2 to age 6, children are estimated to acquire around 14,000, a rate of some nine words a day. In school, from textbooks alone, children are exposed to at least 3000 new words a year up to age 17, aside from words learnt from reading at home, from newspapers, from sports, from television or radio shows, and from other nonschool sources (Carey, 1978; Nagy & Anderson, 1984; Templin, 1957). All this, of course, applies to children learning a first language. Bilingual children must learn close to double these figures, since they have words from each language in many domains, and so can talk equally easily about certain topics in either language.

What do children have to learn? For each word, set phrase, or idiom, children have to be able to segment out the form from the stream of speech and assign some meaning to it. On subsequent occasions, they must be able to identify the form spoken by a range of speakers, then look it up in memory and so retrieve the initial meaning assigned to it. As they hear a word spoken in more contexts, they may also refine their hypotheses about its meaning and adjust any information stored in memory. In trying to convey a particular meaning, they also have recourse to memory and they use the meaning they have assigned to retrieve the pertinent form for production. In short, mastering each word is no small task. Add to this the mastery of how each word is used in combination with other words, and the task becomes even more formidable. Yet children appear to acquire vocabulary readily and rapidly throughout their childhood years. After a few weeks or months of producing just one word at a time, they begin to combine words and within a few months start to produce three-, four-, and five-word utterances on a frequent basis. In the section that follows, I review some of what we know about early word uses, about the mapping of meanings onto forms, about the building of a vocabulary in different semantic domains, and about the parallels observable across languages in early acquisition.

A. Early Word Uses in Production

When children attempt to produce their first words, these are not always readily recognized by the speakers around them. 1- and 2-year-olds have to work hard to produce the right sounds, in the right order, both in words and in combinations of words. Learning how to do this in production takes both time and extensive practice (see Ferguson, Menn, & Stoel-Gammon, 1992; Jusczyk, Chapter 8, this volume). Children usually start attempting some words in production around the end of their first year. Some start talking as early as 10 months, others not until as much as a year later. There is a similar range in what children produce in the first few months of talking. Some produce just one word at a time for several months (a one-word stage) before beginning to combine words into longer utterances; others start to combine words within weeks of the first word produced (Clark, 1993; Dromi, 1987). By age 2, children may produce anywhere from 50 to around 600 distinct words. And they typically understand many more than they produce.

Their first use of these words do not necessarily match adult usage. Some may be produced initially only in a single context, for example, *bye-bye* said only when standing by a particular door in the house. But such contextually bound uses typically last for only a short time before children extend the range of such words to something closer to adult use. Other words may be used appropriately but at first be underextended from the adult's point of view. For example, a child may say *shoe* only upon seeing shoes on someone's feet, but not upon seeing them in a closet or lying on the floor (Reich, 1976). And still others, sometimes amounting to as much as 40% of a 50 to 100-word vocabulary, are at first overextended. That is, they are used for a much larger range of referents than in adult speech: a word like *dog* may be produced to pick out not only dogs, but also cats, sheep, cows, and other four-legged mammals (Anglin, 1977; Clark, 1973; Rescorla, 1980). It is only as children master further words in production that they begin to restrict their overextensions. Once they produce *cat,* for example, they remove cats from the extension of *dog,* and so on (e.g., Barrett, 1986). Occasionally, children's early uses may fail to match adult usage altogether, with the mismatch resulting in a failure to communicate anything (e.g., Bloom, 1973). But for most word uses (including over- and underextensions), children's early uses overlap with adults' and are typically interpretable in context, even though the children do not yet know the full adult meanings (Huttenlocher & Smiley, 1987).

What do such uses tell us about children's knowledge of the lexicon? First, their attempts to produce word forms show that they focus on the conventional terms used by adults. Children do not make up sound sequences wholesale and then assign meanings to them. They aim for the adult targets, even if their articulatory skill causes them to fall far short in what they actually produce. The word *squirrel,* for example, may be produced at first as [ga],[1] the words *button, bottle,* and *spoon,* all as [ba], and the words *light, there,* and *dog,* all as [da]. Yet in comprehension, children have clearly represented the target adult forms since they respond to them and do not confuse them. As their articulatory skill improves, they differentiate their own productions and change them steadily in the direction of the adult targets.

Second, the first meanings children assign overlap with adult meanings. This suggests that children are able to select potential meanings in context with considerable success. Moreover, when they overextend words, they appear to do so for communicative reasons, because they lack other more appropriate words in their production repertoires. That is, they typically understand words appropriately when they hear them, even when they overextend them in production. For example, when asked to point to instances of *dog,* they choose pictures of dogs rather than of other animals (such as sheep) to which they themselves have extended *dog* on other occasions (Thomson & Chapman, 1977). This, I suggest, is because they are not yet able to produce the word *sheep,* or are unable to retrieve it when they need it. For the same reason, they may rely heavily on general purpose verbs like *do* for a large range of specific actions, even though they understand the relevant specific terms when they hear them. The result is that children understand verbs like *throw* or *turn on,* but in talking about throwing a ball or turning on a light, they themselves produce *do.* Children's success in early word uses, then, can be attributed perhaps more to their ability to assign relevant meanings than to their skill in matching adult pronunciations.

B. First Meanings

Children's assignments of possible meanings to their early word forms suggest that they draw heavily for their first hypotheses on their ontological categories. They have, of course, had up to a year or more to form conceptual categories of objects and actions, relations and properties, based on their own observations of consistencies in the word around them. For several months before they begin to speak themselves, they have observed the objects and activities around them, the relations they have to each other, and the range of entities that make up their everyday surroundings. They play with, manipulate, and match objects around them. They fit them into boxes, and empty them out; arrange them in heaps or towers and knock them down; they push them and throw them. They watch and participate in all kinds of activities from clapping, exchanging objects, hiding their faces, crawling, sitting, standing, walking, carrying; opening and shutting containers and doors; pouring liquids and spilling them; eating, with or without utensils, and drinking. And above all, they watch the events around them, the kinds of activities and range of participants each involves, and the relations each bears to the others. The conceptual categories children build up in their first year of life provide the basis for their first hypotheses about word meaning.

When children begin to isolate word forms and assign meanings to them, they draw on the conceptual categories they have already represented in memory. They can use such categories to create potential meanings for newly isolated word forms. In this way, they can draw on categories of objects, relations, and states, activities, and events. The consistency with which children appear to assign meaning types suggests that they make certain assumptions about what words can mean. That is, they seem to draw on certain working assumptions as they make an initial mapping between meaning and form. For example, where they have no label yet for an object, they act as if a newly identified label must pick out the whole object and not just a part of it. Yet later on, when they hear further potential labels, they readily give up such an assumption and instead assign such meanings as 'superordinate term,' 'subordinate term,' 'property,' or 'state,' depending on the circumstances. Their notional categories, then, play a central role in lexical acquisition by providing potential meanings when children first try to create a meaning to map onto some newly identified form. How such a mapping is achieved seems to depend on certain assumptions about what words can be used for, the kinds of categories they can denote.

Some candidate assumptions in the mapping of potential meanings to words for objects and activities are listed in Table 1. Some of these assumptions remain unaffected by developmental changes or additions to the lexical repertoire. For instance, the *type assumption* holds as much for adult speakers as for children. Others may be given up early, for instance, the *whole-object assumption*. Others may apply only to objects or only to activities. For instance, the *taxonomic assumption* applies only to categories of objects and hence to terms that denote objects, since it is inconsistent with the nature of categories of actions. Still other assumptions may continue to

TABLE 1   Some Assumptions in the Early Mapping of Meanings[a]

Words for categories of objects:

1. *Whole-object assumption:* Speakers use words to pick out whole objects, not just a part or property of an object.
2. *Type assumption:* Speakers use words to denote types of objects.
3. *Basic-level assumption:* Speakers use words to pick out objects in basic-level categories.
4. *Equal-detail assumption:* Speakers use words to pick out equally detailed instances of object categories from within a single domain.
5. *Taxonomic assumption:* Speakers use words to pick out coherent categories of objects.

Words for categories of actions:

1. *Whole-action assumption:* Speakers use words to pick out whole actions, not just a part of an action.
2. *Type assumption:* Speakers use words to denote types of actions.
3. *Basic-level assumption:* Speakers use words to pick out basic-level action categories.
4. *Equal-detail assumption:* Speakers use words to pick out equally detailed instances of action categories.

---

[a]From Clark (1993).

apply for adults, but only in a more restricted domain. However, the inventory of such working assumptions, and their interactions with children's existing lexicons and with more general pragmatic principles, has yet to be fully established (Clark, 1993; Markman, 1987; Mervis, 1987).

Children often appear to assign *some* meaning right away to a new word, and to then produce it with that meaning (Carey, 1978; Heibeck & Markman, 1987). Such initial assignments of meaning have been called "fast mapping." As soon as children identify a possible meaning, a word can enter their repertoire and be available for use. But it may take them years to add to and adjust that initial meaning before it corresponds to the conventional meaning in use among adults. Reliance on fast mapping and a willingness to use newly acquired words mean that children do not wait until they are sure of the adult meaning before they try to use words. They simply call on and use whatever seems appropriate from their repertoires. Since there is no overt signal to inform children that they have acquired the conventional meaning, this strategy of immediate use helps children to build an extensive vocabulary at a rapid rate.

C. Pragmatic Principles

Speakers of a language rely on a large number of tacit agreements every day, agreements about which form conventionally conveys which meaning (see Clark and Bly, Chapter 11, this volume). That is, all the speakers within a particular speech community agree, for example, that *beech* designates a particular kind of tree and that *cat* designates a particular kind of mammal.

So, in speaking to each other, they observe the principle of conventionality (Clark, 1993), namely:

"For certain meanings, there is a form that speakers expect to be used in the language community."

Different communities may have different conventions. For example, speakers of French will use *hêtre* in lieu of English *beech,* and *chat* in lieu of *cat.* In effect, each language community has its own set of conventions. The principle of conventionality captures the general nature of the agreements that hold among speakers over time, so they can count on consistency of use from one occasion to the next.

When speakers choose a form to express a particular meaning, they do so because they mean something that they would not have meant had they chosen some other expression. They rely, then, on the fact that different forms have different meanings. Along with conventionality, speakers assume the principle of contrast:

"Speakers take every difference in form to mark a difference in meaning."

In other words, speakers do not tolerate any full synonyms. But they do tolerate multiple meanings being conventionally carried by one form. These two principles, conventionality and contrast, allow speakers to maintain language as a system of communication over time, and to maximize its usefulness by excluding total overlaps in meaning (full or true synonyms). Speaker choices of forms, then, mean what they do in part because they contrast with other options in the same semantic domain and in the language at large (see Clark, 1987, 1990).

For speakers of any language, these pragmatic principles have the following general consequences:

1. Words contrast in meaning.
2. Established words have priority.
3. Innovative words fill lexical gaps.

That is, when any new form is introduced into a conversation, the meaning it carries is assumed to contrast with all other forms already in use in the language. Moreover, if some meaning is already conventionally carried by a particular form, that form/meaning combination will take precedence over any lexical innovation that might be coined to carry that very meaning. The presence, then, of a conventional term already *in* the lexicon preempts the coining of a new term with just the same meaning. But when speakers wish to convey some meaning that has no conventional expression, they can do so by coining a new word, provided they make sure their addressees will be able to interpret it as intended.

The same consequences hold for children acquiring a lexicon, but here, there is an additional dimension, since children are starting from a point where nearly every word in the lexicon is unfamiliar. As a result, they do not know, often, whether there is a conventional expression for some meaning or not. But the assumption that different forms differ in meaning allows them to focus on *how,* not *whether,* each new word they encounter differs in meaning from each of the words they already know. Contrast, then, offers considerable economy of effort, since otherwise children would have to establish, for each new expression, that it differed in meaning from all the terms already acquired. When children encounter terms new to them, unfamiliar words, they can therefore assign them to lexical gaps. Equally, when they wish to talk about something for which they lack a conventional expression, they can coin a new word, again to fill a lexical gap. This is just what adults do too, but the difference is that children may coin words for meanings that have conventional expressions. It is just that children have not yet learnt what they are. For children, then, conventionality and contrast have the following consequences:

1. Words contrast in meaning.
2. Established words have priority.
3. New (unfamiliar) words fill lexical gaps.
4. Innovative words fill lexical gaps.

Conventionality and contrast guide the process of acquisition in the sense that they guide children's uses of words. They also constrain the inferences children make about unfamiliar words and about lexical innovations (Clark, 1993). In doing this, these principles also interact with other assumptions children make about potential meanings for word forms during acquisition, but unlike many of these assumptions, conventionality and contrast continue to play a critical role for adult speakers too. Other assumptions may be given up altogether or become restricted in their application as children learn more about the structure of specific domains in the lexicon.

But in order to find the limitations on the assumptions they start out with, children must do two things: they must learn which terms belong to specific semantic domains and what semantic relations link the senses of these words. I turn next, therefore, to the elaboration of semantic domains.

D. Elaborating Semantic Domains

By the time they can produce 50 distinct words, children can talk about several different domains. They have a few words for people (e.g., *mummy, daddy, baby* [used in self-reference]), animals (*dog, cat, bird*), toys (*ball, block, doll*), household objects (*light, clock, telephone*), and utensils (*cup, spoon, bottle*); activities and states (*up, down, on, off, there* [completing an action or transferring an object]); and a number of routines also involving activities of some kind (*night-night, upsy-daisy, peek-a-boo*) (e.g., Clark, 1978, 1979; Dromi, 1987; Nelson, 1973). Children rapidly add new words to these early domains, extending and elaborating the distinctions they can make. Each early domain is essentially expanded and subdivided as children add more words.

The typical course of elaboration within a domain (here, terms for animals) is illustrated for one child in Table 2. In the first six months of production, children may accumulate several terms for domestic animals, a word like *bird, duck,* or *chicken,* typically applied to birds in general, and one or two terms for wild animals. Over the next 12–18 months, they may add many more terms for both domestic and wild animals; they add a good many terms for birds and for reptiles, and some terms for insects. By age 2, the domain for animals can be organized into several subdomains (see Clark, 1995).

E. Lexical Innovations

Children also expand their lexicon quite readily by coining new words. But for this, they need to analyze the internal structure of words they already know. They need to be able to identify the roots present in compound

TABLE 2   Animal Terms in One Child's Speech[a]

The first six months of production (1;0,29–1;6,0)
    1;0,29 doggie, 1;1,15 dog, 1;1,26 bear 1;3,3 mouse, 1;3,23 cat, 1;4,28 horse
    1;2,0 bird, 1;3,0 duck, −1;4 chicken
    1;5,6 turtle

The next six months of production (1;6,1–1;11,30)
    1;6,13 cow, 1;6,28 rabbit, 1;11,30 goat
    1;7,19 lion, 1;8,8 alligator, 1;11,16 gorilla, 1;10,24 seal
    1;7,2 goose
    1;6,4 fish, 1;8,7 frog, 1;8,8 snake, 1;8,22 crab, 1;10,19 ladybug
    1;7,20 animal

Elaborations in the second year of production (2;0–3;0)
    2;0,8 puppy-dog <toy>, 2;2,24 baby-rabbit, 2;5,21 mummy-bunny <toy>, 2;7,27 sheep, 2;11,1 cattle, 2;11,1 baby-cattle, 2;11,1 daddy-cattles, 2;11,3 bronco-horse, 2;11,10 bucking-horse
    2;0,6 gorilla, 2;0,11 hippo, 2;1,7 camel, 2;4,10 baboon, 2;4,16 tiger, 2;5,21 monkey, 2;7,15 wolf, 2;7,15 raccoon, 2;8,8 armadillo, 2;8,8 fox, 2;8,17 beaver
    2;3,21 stork, 2;3,21 ostrich, 2;4,6 robin, 2;4,17 sparrow, 2;4,19 flamingo, 2;4,20 dove, 2;5,10 grouse, 2;5,14 woodpecker, 2;8,6 owl
    2;5,1 trout, 2;5,4 flounder, 2;5,6 spider, 2;5,6 grasshopper, 2;7,2 fly, 2;7,2 bee, 2;8,14 butterfly, 2;9,21 lizard-animal <live>, 2;9,21 frog-animal <live>

[a]From E. V. Clark (unpublished diary data). This table includes only terms for animals, and not terms for parts or properties, or verbs for animal activities also acquired during this period.

nouns like *head-light* or *push-chair*, for example, and the root–affix combinations in words like *walker* (*walk, -er*) or *moving-van* (*move, -ing, van*). In fact, children make spontaneous analyses of complex words from an early age, and can pick out roots inside such words, as shown in Table 3. Once they have a repertoire of roots and affixes, and some knowledge of how these are combined in conventional lexical items, children are in a position to coin new words when the need arises.

They coin new nouns, new verbs, and new adjectives. The earliest nouns they coin in English appear around age 2 and are compound in form, usually constructed from two noun roots, as in *crow-bird* (picture of a bird, 1;7), *oil-spoon* (spoon for cod-liver oil, 1;11), *coffee-churn* (coffee grinder, 2;0), or *butterfly-shirt* (T-shirt with butterflies on it, 2;5,14). Between age 2 and 3, they also begin to produce a few derivational suffixes in new nouns, as in *You're the sworder* (role in pretend play, 2;4) or *That is a climber against the wall* (a ladder, 2;5,24). Their new verbs are all formed through conversion or

TABLE 3   Some Spontaneous Analyses of Word Forms[a]

---

(1) Mother, pointing at a picture of a ladybug: What's that?
    D (2;4,13): *A lady-bug! That like 'lady.'*
(2) D (2;6,20, to his father, about a stick): *This is a running-stick.*
    Father: A running-stick?
    D: *Yes, because I run with it.*
(3) D (2;9,10): *You know why this is a HIGH-chair? Because it is high.*
(4) Mo: We're going to a place called Sundance.
    D (2;11,0): *And you dance there. If there is music, we will dance there.*
(5) D (2;11,28, looking at flowering ice-plants): *What's that called?*
    Mo: That's ice-plant.
    D: *Does it grow ice?*
(6) D (3;0,4, playing with toy motor-boat; Mo touches the small hatch over the rear locker)
    Mo: D'you remember what that little closet is called?
    D: *No.*
    Mo: A locker.
    D: *And what does it lock up inside it?*
(7) D (3;1,10, on the way home, after Fa mentioned the word 'campus'): *A campus is where you go camping!*
(8) D (3;2,15): *Hey, 'golden' begins with 'Goldilocks,' in one of my books!*
(9) D (3;2,16): *Egg-nog comes from egg!*
(10) D (3;2,20, as he climbed into the car, holding both index fingers up to his head):
     Do you know what head-lights are?
     Mo: No.
     D: *They're lights that go on in your head!*
(11) D (3;3,3, while dressing): *If you put my underpants on OVER these, they'd be over-pants! Wouldn't that be funny?!*
(12) D (3;4,8 adding Lego blocks to a wall round a 'field' containing a Lego donkey): *These are lockers which lock the donkey up in the farmyard.*

---

[a]From E.V. Clark (unpublished diary data).

zero derivation (with no suffix), generally from nouns, as in *Don't hair me* (don't brush my hair, 2;4), *I'm lawning* (mowing the lawn, 2;9), or *Make it bell* (make the bell ring, 3;0). And their new adjectives are formed with the suffix *-y*, as in *Too dampy* (too damp, wet, 2;2), *It's bumpy* (describing a door banging, 2;6), or *That looks growly, doesn't it?* (describing a dinosaur drawing, 3;5). Some typical examples of early coinages from English-speaking children are given in Table 4.

In each case, children appear to favor devices that are common in the language and therefore well represented in the conventional words they already know. They also favor options that offer transparent combinations of roots or roots and affixes. That is, familiar roots remain readily recognizable in the new combination. Their earliest coinages make minimal changes in the elements used: new compounds and new verbs both build on bare roots, with no affixes at all. As they get older, they appear to favor those devices that adults also prefer in their coinages. These tendencies, which are also attested for other languages, suggest that children rely on some general principles for constructing new words. First, they make use of transparency of meaning in their construction of new words, building them from elements they already know. Second, they rely on simplicity of form, initially making the least adjustment possible in the forms of their new words. And third, they are sensitive to and track the productivity of each option for forming new words. Simplicity appears particularly important in the earlier stages of acquisition, while productivity mainly affects children's choices later on. Transparency remains important throughout (Clark, 1993; Clark & Berman, 1984; Clark & Cohen, 1984; Clark & Hecht, 1982).

F. Cross-Linguistic Parallels

Children appear to follow a similar course in lexical acquisition, regardless of the language being acquired. Early vocabularies for children acquiring very different languages show extensive overlap in the kinds of things children first acquire words for, and there has been relatively little change over the last century in early vocabularies (Clark, 1979). At the same time, children must become sensitive to the typology of the language being learnt at an early stage. They need to know, in identifying word forms, whether they are acquiring a polysynthetic language like West Greenlandic, where noun and verb bases form the core, modified by affixes, of whole utterances; a synthetic language like Hebrew, with word forms consisting of sequences of consonants, versus one like Spanish, where both vowels and consonants serve to identify word forms, yet where, for both languages, base word forms are modified by inflections expressing multiple meanings simultaneously; an agglutinative language like Turkish or Hungarian, where each derivational or inflectional morpheme adds a single meaning to

TABLE 4   Typical Early Coinages in English[a]

Innovative nouns

 (1) D (1;10,10, looking at a man with very curly fair hair: *Bubble-hair.*
 (2) D (1;11,28 wanting to be read "Lion in the Meadow"): *read ∂ lion-book.*[b]
 (3) D (2;0,5, told that a friend was getting ready to leave): *Christiane packing ∂..∂..∂ pack-case.*
 (4) D (2;0,11, pointing out a loose piece of tape on a box serving as a 'kennel' for toy puppy-dog): *Eve buy ∂ tape, mend puppydog-house.*
 (5) D (2;1,9, sitting inside an orange crate): *I reading ∂ book in ∂ orange-box.*
 (6) D (2;2,0, describing small and large sieves in the sink): *That ∂ tea-sieve.* (then pointing at the large one for vegetables): *That ∂ water-sieve.*
 (7) D (2;3,17, having constructed a Lego house with two trees inside)
     Father: What kind of house is that?
     D: *A Christmas-tree-house.*
 (8) D (2;5,26, as he reached across the kitchen counter): *I'm a big reacher.*

Innovative verbs

 (9) D (2;4,13, grinding pepper onto the counter): *I'm sanding.* [= making x into sand]
 (10) D (2;6,23, showing Fa two pencils): *I sharped them.* [= sharpen]
 (11) D (2;8,4, with some sleep in one eye): *I have my window open so that sleep can wind away.* [= blow away, via the wind]
 (12) D (2;8,20, to Mo holding hose in the garden): *an' water the dirt off my stick.* [= wash off with water]
 (13) D (2;10,23, holding hand extended, palm down): *Straight your hand out like this and let me hit it.* [= straighten]
 (14) D (2;11,29, pretending to be in a canoe): *I'm going to lie down under the blanket and then I'll oar.* [= row]
 (15) D (3;1,6, taking stick Mo has been carrying): *Let me stick it hard.* [= touch firmly, hit, with the stick]
 (16) D (3;2,9, picking up Cuisinart blade from the sink)
     Mother: You shouldn't take that. It's very sharp.
     D: *But I didn't blade myself.* [= cut with the blade]

Innovative adjectives

 (17) D (2;5,23, as Fa closed the car trunk): *It makes me windy.* [= blown by the wind]
 (18) D (2;6,13, watching Mo cook strips of veal): *These are floured.* [= covered in flour]
 (19) D (2;6,22, describing wet newspaper): *It's all soaky. The paper is soaky.* [= soaked]
 (20) D (2;7,5, driving home in the dark): *It's very nighty.* [= dark]
 (21) D (2;10,23, looking at remains of a house wall built of stone): *There's a rocky house.* [= made/built of rocks]
 (22) D (3;1,1, objecting as Mo removed a dieffenbachia stem): *No, it's not poisony.* [= poisonous]
 (23) D (3;2,23, describing a sandwich): *I want it all crusty.* [= with crusts on]
 (24) D (3;6,22, looking at a rabbit-stamp on the back of his hand): *Hey, d'you know what happens if you rub this? It'll get . . .*
     Mo: Faint?
     D: *Fainted.* [= faint, faded]

[a]From Clark (1993, unpublished diary data).

[b]The schwa (∂) represents the indeterminate vowel D used as a filler at this stage for various grammatical morphemes. He later replaced it by *the* or *a*, as appropriate.

the base word; or an analytic language like Mandarin Chinese, with no inflections, only distinct words, to mark particular modulations of meanings.

How children analyze existing words and build paradigms of forms related in meaning depends critically on their being able to identify candidate words. This in turn depends on their becoming sensitive to the characteristic structures at word- and sentence-level in their language. Evidence that they begin to take account of typological features at an early age (around 2 onwards) comes from their use of novel word formation. Children appear to be sensitive both to general structural features such as prefixing versus suffixing and to the relative productivity of options for new word formation. This sensitivity to distributional properties shows up in their propensity to pick up the more widespread and more frequent options first. In word formation, in their earliest coinages, children consistently favor options that are among the most productive and hence the most frequent in adult speech. This is apparent, for instance, in children's reliance initially on single suffixes to express such meanings as agentivity (e.g., Polish -*acz*), state (e.g., Russian -*ost'*), or activity (e.g., English zero derivation of verbs from nouns) (e.g., Chmura-Klekotowa, 1971; Clark, 1993; MacWhinney, 1976). Moreover, children acquiring languages such as French or Hebrew, where compounding is not productive, do not use it at all in early coinages. This is in marked contrast to children acquiring English or German, for example, who produce novel compound nouns from age 2 or younger (Clark, 1993).

Other factors also play an important role as children identify and begin to construct word forms to convey new meanings. For example, in the earlier stages of acquiring a language, children attend to the simplicity of the form required and prefer forms that require few or no changes over forms that require more extensive adjustments. They are also attentive to transparency of meaning in that they depend only on those resources that are already known to them, and hence transparent. Where only stems are transparent but not yet any suffixes, they will rely only on stems, provided the language in question has compounding as an option. Once children acquire the meanings of some affixes, they will begin to use those too. But mapping the meanings of affixes takes time, so for languages that depend on derivation rather than compounding, children may only begin to construct new words in any numbers from age 3 to 4 onwards (Clark, 1993). These factors, together with productivity, conventionality, and contrast, play a major role in children's acquisition and use of word formation.

G. Input and Lexical Acquisition

In attending to the typology of the language they are learning, children necessarily attend to their major source of information, the language input they receive from the adults around them. This input not only provides typological information, but also information about contexts of use for different forms. For example, events that involve motion may receive rather different packaging in different languages. In English, verbs of motion often include information about manner or cause (as in *walk, stroll, stagger, run*) and add information about path by means of particles and prepositional phrases (e.g., *run away, walk up the hill, stroll across the road*). In Spanish, motion verbs include path information (as in *salir* 'go–out,' *subir* 'go–up,' *poner* 'put–on,' *juntar* 'put–together,' or *meter* 'put–in') and add information about manner through adverbs, adverbial phrases, or participles, as in *la botella entró en la cueva flotando* 'the bottle went-into the cave floating = the bottle floated into the cave' (Talmy, 1985). English and Spanish exhibit the same typological patterns in both transitive and intransitive actions, that is, caused motion and spontaneous motion. Some languages do make a distinction here. Korean, for example, combines motion and path within one word, just as Spanish does, for caused motion (transitive verbs), but for spontaneous motion (intransitive verbs), it relies on separate elements for motion, path, and manner.

In talking about motion events, children appear to be sensitive to differences across languages in whether path is combined with motion or not, and also, to whether a motion is caused or spontaneous. That is, in English, children aged 14–28 months make extensive use of particles and prepositional phrases to mark the path of caused motion, while in Korean, children the same age rely on verbs alone. In English, children rely on the same patterns for spontaneous motion too, while in Korean, they use different verbs for spontaneous versus caused motion. As a result, Korean children distinguish linguistically, from an early age, between transitive and intransitive motion events (Choi & Bowerman, 1991).

Some research has suggested that children learn nouns before verbs. That is, in their early production vocabularies, they often have more nouns than verbs (Gentner, 1982). The explanation offered is that the relational nature of verbs and their linkage to one or more nouns makes them more complex for acquisition. But when other relational terms (e.g., English particles like *up* or *off*) and words for routines (e.g., *peek-a-boo, upsy-daisy,* or *uh-oh*) are counted along with lexical verbs, the asymmetry becomes less striking (e.g., Bloom, Tinker, & Margulis, 1993). In fact, the proportions probably depend largely on the input children hear. For example, Korean-speaking children may acquire proportionately more verbs at an early age than English-speakers (Choi & Gopnik, 1993), but still learn more nouns than verbs early on (Au, Dapretto, & Song, 1994).

Input also plays a role with respect to the argument structure and complement types first exemplified by children for specific verbs. De Villiers (1985) found high correlations between the range of constructions used with verbs in the input and the range each child produced, but lower correlations across the three children she studied. That is, individual parental input played an important role in exposing each child to the possible constructions associated with different verbs. If verbs and their associated constructions are so closely linked in acquisition, this would suggest that the line between what is lexical and what is syntactic or constructional is not always an easy one to draw. Moreover, it is important to remember that what children understand and therefore have stored in memory often far surpasses what they produce, both in the earlier stages of acquisition (e.g., Goldin-Meadow, Seligman, & Gelman, 1976) and later, even in adulthood (e.g., Clark & Hecht, 1983).

In summary, building up a repertoire of words is critical to the task of acquiring a language. Children produce their first words at 12–18 months, and may have a vocabulary of up to 600 words by the age of 2. But what they can produce may lag far behind what they understand, especially during the earlier stages of acquisition. Children rely both on their ontological categories and on input as they assign meanings to new words. Conceptual categories and organization offer a base onto which they can map words, and the input that they hear shapes and constrains the precise mapping made for each word. But words are rarely used by adults in isolation, on their own. They are combined with other words to express additional meanings, meanings that, together, are more than the sum of the parts.

III. EARLY SYNTAX

When do children start to combine words in production? The answer varies with the child. Some appear to go through a distinct one-word stage lasting several months, while others begin to combine words within weeks of producing their first single word utterance (Clark, 1993; Dromi, 1987; Peters & Menn, 1993). This variation across children, along with marked individual differences in articulatory skill in the first year of talking, suggest that motor skill in producing words may be a major factor in determining when children start to produce more than one word at a time. Some children also go through a distinct two-word stage before attempting longer combinations. Once children combine words, though, we can attribute to them some knowledge of syntactic structure, and hence of the meanings contributed by specific patterns of combination. It is only with the emergence of systematic word combinations, together with reliance on such factors as word order and morphological marking of case and agreement for person and number, that they can be credited with some mastery of the syntactic constructions of their first language.

Children's earliest word combinations typically consist of two words, though most quickly move on to produce longer sequences as well. Some may take time to build up a repertoire of two-word combinations, relying at first on a small number of fixed patterns. For example, they may combine a variety of terms with *more,* as in *More milk* (glossable as 'I'd like some milk' or 'I'd like some more milk'), *More shoe* ('there's another shoe'), *More read* ('read me another book'), and so on. Many children appear to rely on certain fixed patterns such as this alongside combinations that appear much freer. What is striking, though, is that the kinds of relations expressed in early combinations appear very similar in meaning across languages. Children learning English, Finish, Hebrew, and Samoan appear to express the same kinds of meanings with their earliest word combinations (see Braine, 1976; Slobin, 1970). Some typical early combination types are illustrated for English in Table 5. From these it can be seen that children talk about the names and places for objects, about possessors, about properties, about events, and about what they do and do not want.

But any analysis of early combinations must depend heavily on the context of each utterance. An utterance like *Mommy sock* may be used to indicate possession on one occasion ('That's Mommy's sock') and agency on another ('Mommy's putting on a/my sock') (see Bloom, 1971). In a language like English, early combinations lack all grammatical information in the shape of case marking (e.g., *I* vs. *me*) or agreement between subject and verb (e.g., *He runs* vs. *They run*). Moreover, word order is often determined pragmatically rather than grammatically.[2] It often marks information as "given" versus "new" and so depends on what has just been talked about by the preceding speaker (e.g., Bates, 1976). Word order and inflections to mark agreement typically emerge in English only after children have begun to combine words, and it is only then that one can with certainty identify particular noun phrases as the subjects or objects of verbs (Bowerman, 1973).

In English, children begin to add noun and verb inflections between 1;6 and 2;0, although their general use may not meet adult criteria for many months (Brown, 1973).[3] In adding inflections, children appear attentive to the inherent meanings of the relevant terms, whether nouns (e.g., Mervis &

TABLE 5 Common Early Word-Combination Types[a]

Locate:	baby high chair	Desire:	more milk
	there book		want ball
Label:	that car	Negate:	no wet
	see doggie		allgone milk
Possess:	baby shoe	Question:	where ball?
	mama dress		
Event:	hit ball	Quality:	big boat
	block fall		

[a]From Slobin (1970).

Johnson, 1991) or verbs (e.g., Bloom, Lifter, & Hafitz, 1980; Clark, 1993). Their patterns of acquisition offer further evidence that children begin with a certain amount of word-by-word learning before they generalize to whole syntactic classes and hence to unfamiliar members of the syntactic class 'noun' or 'proper noun,' say. But in the course of learning, children also make certain generalizations, and, as a result, make consistent errors on irregular forms. They produce *mans* for plural *men*, *feets* or *foots*[4] for plural *feet*, and past tense forms like *comed*, *bringed*, *seed*, and *throwed* in place of (irregular) *came*, *brought*, *saw*, and *threw* (Kuczaj, 1977, 1978).

In short, as children elaborate their utterances by combining words, they also elaborate them by adding inflections to their nouns and verbs, and by inserting other grammatical morphemes such as articles and prepositions. Some children may go through a distinct two-word stage,[5] while others quickly move from one word at a time to longer combinations.

A. Semantic Bootstrapping

Adding the appropriate inflections, though, requires that children have already identified the syntactic category of the word in question, as a noun or a verb, for example. Children presumably do this well before they begin to produce inflections. And they do it, it has been suggested, through semantic bootstrapping. That is, although grammatical categories like 'noun' and 'verb' are not defined semantically, nouns and verbs typically refer to distinct semantic types in parental speech. People and objects are picked out by nouns; activities and changes of state by verbs; and properties of objects by adjectives. And adults talk about objects, actions, and properties when they talk to small children. When they use a verb, therefore, they do so with the relevant elements that belong with that word class. Verbs are accompanied by verb inflections (e.g., *he climbs, they are climbing, you climbed*) and nouns by noun inflections (e.g., *a kitten, three kittens, the kitten's tail*). Adult input is therefore consistent with a correlation of conceptual category (object, action, property) and word class (noun, verb, adjective), and thereby offers children a way in to the syntax of their first language.

If children assume different word classes on the basis of their meaning-to-form mappings of ontological types, they should be able to bootstrap their way into the syntactic categories needed for organizing words at the level of the clause. Once they have a basic framework of meaning-based information about possible word classes and the words that belong to them, they can learn more about what else belongs in each class by observing their distribution and identifying other properties. Such semantic bootstrapping, it has been argued, is critical to the acquisition of syntax (Grimshaw, 1981; Macnamara, 1972; Maratsos, 1990; Pinker, 1984, 1989).

To identify all the properties of a syntactic category may take time. With verbs, for example, children need to learn which inflections mark distinctions of aspect, tense, number, person, and gender, as well as any markers for such features as transitivity, finiteness, and specificity. The number of such distinctions varies with different languages. With nouns, children will need to identify inflections for such categories as case, number, and gender.

Children appear to attend to and exploit clues to word class quite early. Before age 2, English-speaking children attend to the difference between common and proper nouns (e.g., Gelman & Taylor, 1984; Katz, Baker, & Macnamara, 1974). Also around 2, they distinguish nouns and adjectives (Taylor & Gelman, 1988), and begin to attend to the difference between count and mass nouns (Gordon, 1985; Soja, Carey, & Spelke, 1991). They are also able to distinguish verbs and nouns. Here, their knowledge of specific inflections and inflectional paradigms presumably plays a role in assigning unfamiliar terms to the categories of 'noun' or 'verb,' thereby endowing them with some initial meaning (see Brown, 1957; Dockrell & McShane, 1990; Gleitman, 1990).

In summary, once children discover the correlation between their conceptual categories of objects, actions, and categories, and the relevant syntactic word classes, they can use properties of those word classes to increase their repertoires. New verbs will have the same inflectional properties as familiar ones, and new nouns the inflectional properties of familiar nouns. Once children have bootstrapped their way into the system, they can use both semantic and syntactic information to advance further along the road to mastering syntax.

B. Clause Structure

Children must go beyond identifying words as nouns or verbs if they are to learn the syntax of their language. They must learn which verbs occur with which configurations of arguments: whether a verb requires a subject and an object (e.g., *hit,* as in *Jan hit the ball* but not **Jan hit* or **The ball hit*), or only a subject (e.g., *skip,* as in *Jan skipped,* but **Jan skipped the road*). They must learn which kind of argument belongs in each slot (an agent, instrument, place, etc.). And they must learn the meaning conveyed by each verb frame or construction, that is, by the set of argument types. In fact, children appear to monitor the patterns of use associated with individual verbs in the input they hear. Maternal variety of use, the range of constructions used with each verb, is the best predictor of young children's own verb uses (de Villiers, 1985). This in turn suggests that children learn verbs one by one, perhaps in relative isolation from each other. That is, they do not initially make generalizations about structure or argument configurations, but rather gradually add to the structures associated with each separate verb (Tomasello, 1992; see also Kuczaj, 1982; Maratsos, 1983).

At some point, though, children must be able to make certain generalizations about possible argument structures. First, even where they have received little or no direct information about argument structure, children are willing to use a newly heard verb with an intransitive or transitive frame, depending on the prior discourse context (Braine, Brody, Fisch, Weisberger, & Blum, 1990). Second, children coin new verbs from nouns and adjectives from as young as 2 to 2½ years. And in doing so, they assign argument frames consistent with the meaning intended (Bowerman, 1974; Clark, 1982; Maratsos, Gudeman, Gerard-Ngo, & DeHart, 1987). To do this, they must have set up some representation of the relevant verb frames for the expression of specific meaning types.

Some verbs are used with two distinct frames or configurations of arguments. They alternate, depending on which perspective the speaker chooses in representing an event. Compare the uses of a verb like *load* in *They loaded the cart with hay* and *They loaded hay into the cart*. While this locative verb alternates, others allow only one perspective. Children take some time to learn, for each verb, which configuration of arguments is the conventional one, and whether each verb can alternate. They make such errors as *I'm going to cover a screen over me* (4;5, for 'cover myself with a screen'), *Can I fill some salt into the bear?* (a bear-shaped salt-shaker, 5;0, for 'fill the bear with salt'), and *Feel your hand to that* (6;10, for 'feel that with your hand') (Bowerman, 1982, 1988; Gropen, Pinker, Hollander, & Goldberg, 1991; see also Brinkmann, 1993). Mastering such alternations takes a long time and, for some verbs, is only complete at around age 10 to 12.

Other verbs can appear in either active or passive form, again offering alternative perspectives on the same event. Compare *Ken lit the fire* and *The fire was lit by Ken*. Not all verbs allow the passive alternation. Children learn the passive first for physical action verbs, like *hold*, and only later for mental activity verbs, like *like*. When they produce passives, they construct them with *be* and with *get*, as in *He got hit from his sister*, from around age 2;6 to 3;0, but they may take some time to learn how to mark the Agent of the action, with *by* (e.g., Budwig, 1990; Clark & Carpenter, 1989a, 1989b; Horgan, 1978; Maratsos, Fox, Becker, & Chalkley, 1985). Again, full mastery of the passive and where it can be used takes time, and depends, in the earlier stages, on knowledge about the meanings of specific verbs.

To produce more elaborate utterances, children must master a variety of devices and construction types in order to express different meanings within a clause. For example, to express negation or disagreement, they need to use forms like *not, never, no one, nothing,* and *nowhere*. To ask questions, they need *wh*-words like *what, where, who, when,* and *why*. But these lexical items alone are not enough. Children must also learn how to use them, how to choose both the form that conveys the relevant meaning and the construction that that form demands. In English, for example, the construction of negative and interrogative utterances depends critically on the acquisition of auxiliary verbs. Negatives depend on auxiliaries (e.g., *has* in *Justin hasn't finished lunch*) as do questions (e.g., *did* in *Where did Rod go?*) (e.g., Johnson, 1983; Klima & Bellugi, 1966).

Children also start to use adjuncts to mark present versus nonpresent time quite early on. For example, many 2-year-olds adopt a term like *tomorrow* or *yesterday* to refer to nonpresent times, but do not yet distinguish past from future with adverbs. For sequence in time, 2- and 3-year-olds rely on *and* and *and then*, or bare adverbs like *first* or *before*. Later on, they start to use conjunctions like *before, while, when,* and *after* with a full clause (Clark, 1970, 1971; Coker, 1978; Decroly & Degand, 1913; Harner, 1975, 1976). These forms complement children's emerging mastery of tense marking on verbs (Brown, 1973; see also Gerhardt, 1988).

Children also elaborate the noun phrases they use. They begin to distinguish definite from indefinite (with *the, this,* or *that,* vs. *a*) (Warden, 1976). They use quantifiers like *all, some,* and *every* (Donaldson & Lloyd, 1974; Hanlon, 1988); and they add qualifying adjectives (e.g., *the big dog, the red car*) and prepositional phrases (e.g., *the man with a hat*) to distinguish particular individuals (e.g., Tager-Flusberg, 1982). In short, once children begin to combine words, they steadily elaborate on the meanings they express. And they do this by adding words and constructions to their initial repertoires.

C. Embedding

Children also begin very early to combine what for adults would be separate clauses. Such clause combinations may be hard to detect prior to production of the relevant conjunctions or complementizers. Take an utterance like *Get down, cart* (1;8,12). This was produced on an occasion when the child wanted to climb down from his highchair in order to go and fetch his toy cart from the next room. Had he said, *I'm getting down to fetch my cart*, we would have no hesitation in crediting him with a complete utterance consisting of a main clause ('I'm getting down') and an embedded complement ('to get my cart'). But without the pertinent grammatical markers, complementizers (*to, for, that*), relative pronouns (*who, that, which*), or conjunctions (*when, before, if, because*), it may be hard to discern the antecedents to such constructions in children's early combinations of two or more predicates.

Relative clauses appear first with no relative pronoun, and may be used first only with empty nouns such as *thing, ones,* or *kind,* as in *Look the ones Mommy got* (2;9). Only after this, according to Limber (1973), do children produce relative clauses attached to full nouns like *book* or *ball,* as in *Here the ball that I got* (2;11) (see also Hamburger & Crain, 1982). But even the earliest spontaneous relative clauses may be attached to nouns with some content, as in the early examples shown in Table 6. Relative pronouns like *that, who,* or *which,* though, rarely appear before age 2½ or even 3.

Children also begin to talk about sequences of events, often well before

TABLE 6   Some Early Relative Clauses[a]

(1) D (1;11,22, showing off a cookie he'd been given): *Look I got!*
(2) D (2;0,0): *I see ə building Eve go.*
(3) D (2;0,1, picking up his doll): *Here ə doll Shelli give Damon.*
(4) D (2;0,6, reading Jersey Zoo book, at the page with a map): *That ə map gorilla live.*
(5) D (2;0,9): *Herb work ə big building have ə elevator 'n it.*
(6) D (2;0,14, looking at a picture in a book): *That ə birdhouse ə bird lives.*
(7) D (2;0,9, after discussion of his birthday a month earlier, but no mention of Shelli): *Where Shelli gave ə doll ə Damon?*
(8) D (2;1,30; after talking about the dark, D brought up something he'd seen the evening before): *I see swimmingpool have lights on.*
(9) D (2;2,5, after deciding he'd heard a truck, not a car, outside): *I go outside see ə truck may have dirt in it.*
(10) D (2;2,16, D looking for his thimble that he'd mislaid) Mother: Where did you have your thimble? D: *I leave it over there where I eat supper.*
(11) D (2;4,19, speaking of a toy): *I'm going to show you where Mr Lion is.*
(12) D (2;5,16, touching a wet spot on the front of the newspaper): *That paper what Eve got fell into a tiny puddle.*

[a]From D.V. Clark (unpublished diary data).

age 2. At first, they indicate sequence linguistically by order of mention alone. That is, they describe successive actions with no explicit links between them. Then, between age 2 and 3, after starting to use terms like *and* and *and then* to link sequences of events, they begin to use a variety of conjunctions to mark the relevant sequential relations. These include *when, before, after, if,* and *because.* (Conjunctions marking simultaneity, such as *while* or *as,* tend to emerge only later.)

In producing a conjunction to mark temporal sequence, children must take account of the actual sequence in time, the meaning of the conjunction, and the prior discourse. Children and adults alike tend to reflect actual time order in their descriptions of sequence, and the meaning of the conjunction will then affect its placement, whether it introduces the first or second clause of the utterance. The structure of the preceding discourse determines which event is talked about first, independent of its actual place in the sequence (Clark, 1970). The first temporal conjunction to be produced is *when.* It can indicate general location in time ('time at which') or sequence ('when/after event-1'), and is often indeterminate between the two. Some typical examples of early utterances that mark sequence in time, mostly with *when,* are listed in Table 7. Notice that although the conjunction is omitted in utterances (1)–(5) of Table 7, the child's order of mention reflects the actual order of the events. Sequences can also be indicated by terms like *once,* as in (10), *first . . . then,* or *next.*

Young children also talk from early on about events that are contingent on each other, linked not only in time but also by causality or condi-

TABLE 7   Some Early Temporal Clauses*a*

---

(1) D (1;11,16, alluding to the morning before when his Fa had gone running very early): *Damon sad Herb go ∂ walk, say byebye.*

(2) D (2;0,18, to Fa who had just been picked up in the car): *I get out Eve stops.*

(3) D (2;1,11): *I get bigger, I have tea.*

(4) D (2;1,23, sitting in his car seat): *I get out!*
Mother: Not yet!
D: *Get home, get out.*
Mo: Yes. Then you'll get out.

(5) D (2;2,19, fantasizing): *You get a tiny baby, and I get bigger, I carry you back home.*

(6) D (2;4,26, at breakfast, to Fa): *The toast make a noise when you put butter on.*

(7) D (2;4,26, playing with the light switch on the door of the lower oven): *When I press this button, the light goes off.*

(8) D (2;5,3, as he was being put down for a nap): *When you close the door, then I can kick all my blankets off.*

(9) D (2;5,17, shaking a rattle Mo had bought as a present): *When I was a little baby, I used ∂ do that. And then I drop it down.*

(10) D (2;6,18, after putting the book *Henny Penny* on the table): *Once I get up, I'm going to show you Foxy Loxy an' ∂ crown.*

(11) D (2;6,20, picking up a stick he used for drumming): *This makes my knuckle don't hurt when I run.*

(12) D (2;6,22): *I going ∂ bring this pile of books to the table, after I aten my supper, then I can read them.*

(13) D (2;6,27): *You wear gloves when it's snowy-time.*

---

*a*From E.V. Clark (unpublished diary data).

tionality. And the relevant conjunctions, *because* and *if,* emerge at about the same time as the various temporal connectives. Just as for temporal relations, children first imply contingency by simple juxtaposition, as when K (2;4) was climbing into her crib; *Climb in. Be fun.* She then toppled in, laughing. The same child, on top of the jungle gym with a sheet draped over it, pointed to the sheet and said: *Sit here. Fall down* (2;4).[6] Children then begin to mark sequence with subordinate clauses, and in particular to use predictive *when* clauses, as when L (2;6) said *When I go to Grammy's, I'll eat with my fingers.* They soon go on to produce an early form of generic utterance, as in the generalization in (1):

(1)   Adult: What are umbrellas for?
L (2;7): *When rain comes, we put an umbrella on top of us.*

This is followed shortly by production of *if,* as in (2) and (3):

(2)   Adult: Laurie, what if your baby cries?
L (2;8, putting doll in cradle): *Wants Mommy if her cry.*
Adult: What sweetheart?
L: *Cries. Want Mamma.*
(two turns later)
L: *Her cry if her want me.*

(3)   K (2;10, has hurt her eye)
       Adult: How does your eye feel?
       K (with her finger in her eye): *If I touch it, it hurts.*

Only after this do children produce hypothetical conditionals, as in the following utterances:

(4)   R (2;10): *If Bulldozer-man saw a fire, he would call the fire depart-
       ment.*
(5)   Adult: Molly, what if you ate three chocolate cakes?
       M (3;6): *You would have a tummy ache.*

And by this point too, children appear to be aware that *if*, but not *when*, is the appropriate choice for hypothetical situations, as indicated by the first repair in G's utterance (3;10): *When I was <repair> if I was a tiger, I would cook pa <repair> popcorn* (Reilly, 1986). English-speaking children produce future predictives with *when* before those with *if*. The choice between the two conjunctions depends on the certainty of the antecedent event: certain events take *when*, uncertain ones *if*. In an analysis of three children's uses, Bowerman (1986) noted that English-speaking children appear to appreciate the relevance of certainty to conjunction choice from their first uses on. Where they have no basis for projecting how certain the event is, they always choose *if*, as in the following utterance from D:

(6)   D (2;8,5, sitting in the bath): *If I get my graham cracker in the wa-
       ter, it'll get all soapy.*

Children go through several stages in the production of conditional clauses as they learn where *when* and *if* do and do not overlap, and as they come to understand hypothetical conditionals (Bowerman, 1986; Reilly, 1986).

   Children also begin to use infinitival complement structures between age 2 and 3. When they learn *to* in such constructions as *He wants to go out*, they do not learn it as a general infinitive marker for *go out*, the verb in the complement. Rather, they learn that it can go with certain main or matrix verbs such as *want* or *go*. The earliest matrix verbs acquired are *want, go, get/got*, and *have*. Children typically omit the *to* altogether at first and then begin to use [ə] (the neutral vowel, schwa) as a place-holder for it, as in an utterance like *She wants ə get it*. The schwa is gradually replaced by *to* with the first matrix verbs acquired, *want* and *go*. From then on, *to* is used from the start with each newly acquired matrix verb, *like, be supposed, need, start, show how*, and so on (Bloom, Tackeff, & Lahey, 1984). Here, then, each specific lexical item being learnt, the matrix verb, becomes associated in turn with the *to* that introduces the complement.

   Finally, complements generally take as their subject the nearest preceding noun phrase. In *Rod wanted Kate to read the book, Kate* is the subject of *read;* in

Rod would like to read the book, Rod is the subject of *read.* But the nearest noun phrase is not always the subject of the verb in the complement. Consider the verb *to promise.* In *Justin promised Ned to turn a somersault,* the person turning the somersault is Justin, not Ned, even though *Ned* appears in the noun phrase nearest the complement. The meanings of complement verbs like *promise* take children many years to master (Chomsky, 1969; Kessel, 1970).

D. Form and Function

As children acquire the meanings of words and constructions, they must also learn how each element is used. But because they do not begin with full adult knowledge of the conventions, they may assign nonconventional meanings and also use terms in ways that diverge considerably from adult usage. Knowing the meaning of an expression does not automatically reveal how it should be used. For example, in choosing *statesman* versus *politician,* a speaker can convey regard and respect with the former that are absent with the latter. In using *tassie* versus *cup,* the speaker would show knowledge of the dialects most familiar to addressees from southern Scotland in the first case, and other English-speaking areas in the second. Or in using *policeman* versus *cop,* a speaker would mark the reference as neutral or formal in the first case, and as informal in the second. Each choice is appropriate to different circumstances and different addressees. The lexical choices differ in connotation, in dialect, and in formality. Some constructions also differ along such dimensions. For example, when a speaker makes a request, it may be marked as formal by the construction used, as in the formal *Would you by any chance mind helping me get this gate open?* versus the less formal *Open the gate,* or *Open the gate, will you?*

Learning the distinct functions of forms closely related in meaning is a difficult task. Children may come up with inappropriate hypotheses on the way. For example, some English-speaking children may link forms of the first person pronoun to the notion of agency. *Me* is taken to indicate agency and control on the part of the child, as in *Me throw ball,* said when the ball was in the child's possession, and *I* or *my* to indicate absence of control, as in *I like peas* (Budwig, 1989). Eventually, these children must revise their initial analysis and arrive at the pertinent grammatical distinction, with *I* marking the subject of the verb, and *me* the object. Or to take another example, when children wish to talk about events that have not actually occurred, they often start out by choosing the past tense. That is, they contrast the hypothetical with the actual or present, and then pick the major nonpresent option they have mastered. It is common to hear 3- and 4-year-olds describing what they are going to do in pretend play, for example, in past-tense form, as when a 4-year-old plans some play with a friend and first assigns roles by saying, *I was the mother and you were the baby* (e.g., Kaper, 1980; Lodge, 1979).

In short, children have to work out the conventional meanings of all the forms they hear. They are not given these already analyzed, nor are they presented with any set of relevant grammatical distinctions a priori. Those must be worked out for each word and each construction. Some grammatical paradigms children encounter are much more complex than others, and presumably take longer to acquire. In addition, children should entertain more alternative hypotheses about the members of these paradigms en route to the adult system (Clark, 1990). Constructional idioms also have conventions on their use. Consider the circumstances under which one might use *Mind your head, Break a leg!, Can you pass the salt?*, or *You must have some more cake.* These too have to be learnt.

Children must learn which forms are counted as appropriate on different occasions, to different addressees, to achieve different aims. They clearly realize, from a young age, that not all addressees should receive the same kind of speech. Children as young as 2, for example, use a small, high-pitched voice and very short sentences in talking to and talking for dolls, as well as in talking to babies (Sachs & Devin, 1976). By age 4, children give instructions on how to play with a toy Noah's Ark in very different form to 2-year-olds, other 4-year-olds, and adults. Their choices reflect the knowledge they assume their addressees have, as well as the relative status conferred by age. Requests to 2-year-olds, for instance, are typically imperative in form (e.g., *Put the lamb here*), while those to adults are much less direct (e.g., *D'you think you could put the lamb here?*). In the first case, the 4-year-old speaker has higher status, and in the second, lower status, than the addressee (Shatz & Gelman, 1973). By age 5 or so, children are sensitive not only to the age and status of many addressees, but also to how these are linked to power and sex. In role-playing with puppets, they differentiate request forms, for example, using politer ones to the person with greater power, independent of age. Child-puppets address politer requests to fathers than to mothers (e.g., *Ice cream tastes nice, doesn't it?* versus *I want some ice cream*); nurse-puppets address doctors with politer forms than doctor-puppets use to nurses or patients; and student-puppets use politer forms to teacher-puppets than to fellow students (Andersen, 1990). By age seven, children are well on their way in learning which forms have which functions, and to differentiating some of their usage on the basis of who their addressees are and what they know.

In summary, as children add more complex structures to their repertoires, they often tie new structures to specific lexical items. Complement structures, for example, at first are produced with only or two verbs. Children then add to this repertoire, consistently marking new matrix verbs by a following *to*. With adverbial clauses, children must learn the meanings of particular conjunctions, *when, after, until, if, because,* and learn how their meanings contrast. The same holds for relative clauses where they must distinguish *that, who,* and *which,* in addition to learning the relevant structure for each embedded clause-type. And for each of the forms and constructions learnt, children must also learn the functions. Learning forms, meanings, and functions takes time.

IV. THE PROCESS OF ACQUISITION

Production of language is only part of what is involved in any language use. So data from production alone may give a rather biased picture of what goes on during acquisition. In conversations, we both speak and listen. It may be tempting, therefore, to assume that production and comprehension are symmetrical, and that both rely on the same representations of linguistic information in memory. But in fact, differences between the two processes show up from the first in acquisition and continue to exist for adult speakers. The asymmetry between them, with comprehension leading production, in fact plays a critical role in the acquisition process itself (see also Bock, Chapter 6, this volume).

How are production and comprehension related in acquisition? Comprehension leads production and offers children a critical guide when they come to talk. For example, children typically understand words before they produce them. Young 1-year-olds understand words for up to three or four months before they try to say them; older children understand comparative constructions before they use them themselves; they can also interpret novel word forms before they are able to produce those same forms to coin words. In short, comprehension surpasses production, and does so in both children and adults (Clark, 1993; Clark & Hecht, 1983). Because of this, reliance on production data alone may lead researchers to seriously underestimate what children know. Production data must be supplemented, wherever possible, by comprehension data as well.

For children, the asymmetry between comprehension and production is important to acquisition itself. It allows children to work at their own pace without having to depend on adult speakers producing examples of target forms at just the right moment. The process seems to work as follows. Take the word *cup.* Children first set up a representation for comprehension, a C-representation, of the word form in memory, together with whatever meaning they have attached to it. This C-representation contains auditory information, the sound segments and their ordering, needed for identifying the word *cup.* When children next hear this sequence, they can recognize it as having been heard before and also access their meaning for it. Without a C-representation for comprehension, they would not know whether they had heard *cup* before, nor could they track successive uses in order to refine the meaning attached to it. As children hear further input, of course, they add further C-representations to memory.

Once a form has been stored for comprehension, children can also start trying to produce it. But producing a word so it is recognizable takes a lot of practice, much like any other motor skill. And to produce a word, children have to set up a P-representation, a representation for production. This will contain all the articulatory information needed to produce each word, information about the articulation of sound segments, their sequencing within words, and their relation to syllables and to stress, as well as to neighboring words. In addition, when children try to say a word, they need a target to measure their own effort against. They need some way to check on the adequacy of their P-representation, and hence on how recognizable their utterance is. Children's pronunciations must eventually match those of other speakers in the community.

One way of achieving this is to check their own productions against adult productions of the relevant words. But adults may not be around, or, even if they are, are unlikely to produce the right word just when it is needed. An alternative option for children is to make use of their own C-representations. Although, under this view, these contain no articulatory information, they offer a target against which to check children's productions. The closer the match between the output in production and the C-representation, the better aligned the two are. By checking what they say against their C-representations, children can detect any mismatch between their production and their comprehension.

To do this, children, like adults, must monitor what they say (Levelt, 1983, 1989). That is, they monitor the form they produce and compare it against the relevant C-representation. If it does not match, they identify the parts that do not match and make another attempt. The general process of aligning production with comprehension, then, involves the following steps (Clark, 1993):

1. Children create a C-representation for a word form, x.
2. Children try to create a P-representation for x.
3. Children execute the P-representation and, monitoring their word form, compare the form heard with their own existing C-representation for x.
4. Children then correct the P-representation for x.

The evidence for this general process is extensive. First, children make repairs to their own speech, spontaneously, from a very early age. Their repairs typically move them closer to the adult forms. In recognition tasks, children consistently reject imitations of their own defective pronunciations in favor of the conventional adult versions. Given two forms that they fail to distinguish in production, children nonetheless reliably distinguish them in comprehension. And once they master the pronunciation of a new segment, children add it only to those words where it was omitted previously. These findings strongly support the role of C-representations in the gradual refining of children's productions.

Once children can adjust their P-representations for forms where there was an initial mismatch, they can be said to have aligned their production with the relevant C-representation. The asymmetry between comprehension and production is central to this process of change that is integral to acquisition. Children rely on already-established C-representations when they check on their P-representations. With mismatches, they try to adjust their P-representations. This adjustment may take longer with some forms than others, so interim repairs may be only partly successful. But with constant monitoring, children eventually come to produce adultlike forms. This holds for both words and larger constructions. Such a model offers a general means of accounting for the myriad changes that take place during acquisition.

V. CONCLUSION

In acquisition, the lexicon and syntax are intertwined. Syntax in children's language emerges as part and parcel of their lexical knowledge. Each word carries with it a specification not only of its meaning (or meanings) but also its syntax, the range of constructions in which it can occur. For a noun like *horse*, the range consists of occurrence in noun phrases, typically preceded by an article or demonstrative (*the horse, that horse*), plus an adjective (*that roan horse,*) a quantifier (*two bay horses*), or a combination of these elements (*two of those piebald horses*). For a verb like *want*, the range of syntactic constructions includes occurrence with a direct object noun phrase (*want the cup*), an infinitival complement, with or without a direct object (*want to play chess, want to swim*), and with a *for–to* complement (*want to Jan to stay*). And for adjectives like *uneven* or *erstwhile,* the range of syntactic constructions may include both attributive and predicative uses (as in *the uneven road, the road was uneven*), or only attributive ones (as in *his erstwhile friend*). Children learn not only the meanings of words, but also their syntactic range, along with their internal morphological structure (in the case of complex words), and their phonological shape. To know a word, children need to have represented all four kinds of information about it. This representation may be only for comprehension, as is most likely for terms like *erstwhile, ilk, whilom,* or *distaff.* Or they may have one representation for comprehension and one for production, as is the case for the majority of terms in everyday use.

The importance of the lexicon stems in part from the conventional meanings it expresses, and in part from its role in the combinations of lexical items used to express further meanings. In the latter, the lexicon exemplifies the structure of a language and makes syntax audible, in the same way that words themselves make morphological structure and phonological shape audible. When one tries to separate out any one of these dimensions, meaning, syntax, morphology, or phonology, it is clear that lexical acquisition provides the crux for language acquisition. Words are central. Word form (morphological structure and phonological shape) emerges early but only in combination with word meaning. Children do not learn forms just for the sake of it. They learn words to use them, to convey their own interests and desires, and to respond to those of others. But words used singly offer only limited options in this regard, and children soon learn how to combine them to convey more complex meanings. In doing this, they add to the basic lexical meanings the meanings conveyed by specific combinatorial options. And in doing so, they learn which options, which syntactic structures, go with each lexical item, and add this information to what they already know about meaning and form. In short, lexical knowledge and syntactic knowledge are interdependent, so they necessarily emerge together in the process of acquiring a language.

Acknowledgment

Preparation of this chapter was supported in part by the Center for the Study of Language and Information, Stanford University.

Endnotes

1. This form would result from (i) inability to produce liquids like /l/ and /r/; (ii) inability to produce consonant clusters like /sk-/ or clusters combined with a glide /skw-/, with a resultant simplification to the stop alone /k/; and (iii) voicing of the initial stop, /g-/ (or nonaspiration to reflect its form in the target cluster), combined with (iv) the common prototypical vowel, with no obstruction of the vocal tract, /a/, to result in the production [ga].

2. There are probably individual differences in which children recognize each of these factors as having a grammatical role. Some children give evidence of not recognizing the grammatical role of word order, for example, until well after the onset of quite elaborate combinations, and after the acquisition of noun and verb inflections. But there has been little detailed study of word order, perhaps because given-new based orders often parallel grammatical (subject-verb-object) ones (see also Braunwald, 1993).

3. In more highly inflected languages, children begin to make use of inflections for case, number, person, and tense rather earlier. See, for example, Aksu-Koç and Slobin (1985), Berman (1985), MacWhinney (1978), and Smoczyńska (1985).

4. The plural form children construct depends, of course, on which stem children pick up on (*foot* or *feet,* say) to begin with. Stem choice also seems to be at work when children choose either *break* or *broke* for the stem of the verb *break,* or *think* or *thought* for the verb *think* (see Clark, 1993, for further discussion).

5. This may also be a reflection of articulatory skill, with these children needing to perfect two-word sequences before they attempt longer ones (but see Gerken, 1991).

6. These utterances from K, as well as the examples from G, L, M, and R, are taken from Reilly (1986).

References

Aksu-Koç, A., & Slobin, D. I. (1985). The acquisition of Turkish. In D. I. Slobin (Ed.), *The crosslinguistic study of language acquisition* (Vol. 1, pp. 839–878). Hillsdale, NJ: Erlbaum.

Andersen, E. S. (1990). *Speaking with style: The sociolinguistic skills of children.* London: Routledge.

Anglin, J. M. (1977). *Word, object, and conceptual development.* New York: Norton.

Au, T. K.-F., Dapretto, M., & Song, Y.-K. (1994). Input vs. constraints: Early word acquisition in Korean and English. *Journal of Memory and Language, 33,* 567–592.

Barrett, M. D. (1986). Early semantic representations and early word usage. In S. A. Kuczaj, II & M. D. Barrett (Eds.), *The development of word meaning: Progress in cognitive development research* (pp. 39-67). Berlin & New York: Springer-Verlag.

Bates, E. (1976). *Language and context.* New York: Academic Press.

Berman, R. A. (1985). The acquisition of Hebrew. In D. I. Slobin (Ed.), *The crosslinguistic study of language acquisition* (Vol. 1, pp. 255–371). Hillsdale, NJ: Erlbaum.

Bloom, L. (1971). Why not pivot grammar? *Journal of Speech and Hearing Disorders, 36,* 40–50.

Bloom, L. (1973). *One word at a time.* The Hague: Mouton.

Bloom, L., Lifter, K., & Hafitz, J. (1980). Semantics of verbs and the development of verb inflections in child language. *Language, 56,* 387–412.

Bloom, L., Tackeff, J., & Lahey, M. (1984). Learning *to* in complement constructions. *Journal of Child Language, 11,* 391–406.

Bloom, L., Tinker, E., & Margulis, C. (1993). The words children learn: Evidence against a noun bias in early vocabularies. *Cognitive Development, 8,* 431–450.

Bowerman, M. (1973). *Early syntactic development: A cross-linguistic study with special reference to Finnish.* Cambridge, UK: Cambridge University Press.

Bowerman, M. (1974). Learning the structure of causative verbs: A study in the relationship of cognitive, semantic, and syntactic development. *Papers & Reports on Child Language Development* (Stanford University), *8,* 142–179.

Bowerman, M. (1982). Reorganizational processes in lexical and syntactic development. In E. Wanner & L. R. Gleitman (Eds.), *Language acquisition: The state of the art* (pp. 319–346). Cambridge, UK: Cambridge University Press.

Bowerman, M. (1986). First steps in acquiring conditionals. In E. C. Traugott, A. ter Meulen, J. S. Reilly, & C. A. Ferguson (Eds.), *On conditionals* (pp. 285–307). Cambridge, UK: Cambridge University Press.

Bowerman, M. (1988). The 'no negative evidence' problem: How do children avoid constructing an overly general grammar? In J. A. Hawkins (Ed.), *Explaining language universals* (pp. 73–101). Oxford: Blackwell.

Braine, M. D. S. (1976). Children's first word combinations. *Monographs of the Society for Research in Child Development, 41* (Serial No. 164).

Braine, M. D. S., Brody, R. E., Fisch, S. M., Weisberger, M. J., & Blum, M. (1990). Can children use a verb without exposure to its argument structure? *Journal of Child Language, 17,* 313–342.

Braunwald, S. (1993, March). *Differences in two sisters' acquisition of first verbs.* Paper presented at the biennial meeting of the Society for Research in Child Development, New Orleans, LA.

Brinkmann, U. (1993). Non-individuation versus affectedness: What licenses the promotion of the prepositional object? In E. V. Clark (Ed.), *Proceedings of the 25th annual Child Language Research Forum* (pp. 158–170). Stanford, CA: CSLI.

Brown, R. (1957). Linguistic determinism and the part of speech. *Journal of Abnormal and Social Psychology, 55,* 1–5.

Brown, R. (1973). *A first language: The early stages.* Cambridge, MA: Harvard University Press.

Budwig, N. (1989). The linguistic marking of agentivity and control in child language. *Journal of Child Language, 16,* 263–284.

Budwig, N. (1990). The linguistic marking of nonprototypical agency: An exploration into children's use of passives. *Linguistics, 28,* 1221–1252.

Carey, S. (1978). The child as word learner. In M. Halle, J. Bresnan, & G. A. Miller (Eds.), *Linguistic theory and psychological reality* (pp. 264–293). Cambridge, MA: MIT Press.

Chmura-Klekotowa, M. (1971). *Neologizmy slowotwórcze w mowie dzieci* [Derivational neologisms in children's speech]. *Prace Filologiczne* (Warsaw), *21,* 99–235.

Choi, S., & Bowerman, M. (1991). Learning to express motion events in English and Korean: The influence of language-specific lexicalization patterns. *Cognition, 41,* 83–121.

Choi, S., & Gopnik, A. (1993). Nouns are not always learned before verbs: An early verb spurt in Korean. In E. V. Clark (Ed.), *Proceedings of the 25th annual meeting of the Child Language Research Forum* (pp. 96–105.) Stanford, CA: CSLI.

Chomsky, C. S. (1969). *The acquisition of syntax in children from 5 to 10.* Cambridge, MA: MIT Press.

Clark, E. V. (1970). How young children describe events in time. In G. B. Flores d'Arcais & W. J. M. Levelt (Eds.), *Advances in psycholinguistics* (pp. 275–284). Amsterdam: North-Holland.

Clark, E. V. (1971). On the acquisition of the meaning of *before* and *after*. *Journal of Verbal Learning and Verbal Behavior, 10,* 266–275.

Clark, E. V. (1973). What's in a word? On the child's acquisition of semantics in his first language. In T. E. Moore (Ed.), *Cognitive development and the acquisition of language* (pp. 65–110). New York: Academic Press.

Clark, E. V. (1978). Discovering what words can do. In D. Farkas, W. M. Jacobsen, & K. W. Todrys (Eds.), *Papers from parasession on the lexicon* (pp. 34–57). Chicago: Chicago Linguistic Society.

Clark, E. V. (1979). Building a vocabulary: Words for objects, actions, and relations. In P. Fletcher & M. Garman (Eds.), *Language acquisition: Studies in first language development* (pp. 149–160). Cambridge, UK: Cambridge University Press.

Clark, E. V. (1982). The young word-maker: A case study of innovation in the child's lexicon. In E. Wanner & L. R. Gleitman (Eds.), *Language acquisition: The state of the art* (pp. 390–425). Cambridge, UK: Cambridge University Press.

Clark, E. V. (1987). The principle of Contrast: A constraint on language acquisition. In B. MacWhinney (Ed.), *Mechanisms of language acquisition* (pp. 1–33). Hillsdale, NJ: Erlbaum.

Clark, E. V. (1990). On the pragmatics of contrast. *Journal of Child Language, 17,* 417–432.

Clark, E. V. (1993). *The lexicon in acquisition.* Cambridge, UK: Cambridge University Press.

Clark, E. V. (1995). Later lexical development. In P. Fletcher & B. MacWhinney (Eds.), *Handbook on child language* (pp. 393–412). Oxford: Blackwell.

Clark, E. V., & Berman, R. A. (1984). Structure and use in the acquisition of word-formation. *Language, 60,* 547–590.

Clark, E. V., & Carpenter, K. L. (1989a). The notion of source in language acquisition. *Language, 65,* 1–32.

Clark, E. V., & Carpenter, K. L. (1989b). On children's uses of *from, by,* and *with* in oblique noun phrases. *Journal of Child Language, 16,* 349–364.

Clark, E. V., & Cohen, S. R. (1984). Productivity and memory for newly-formed words. *Journal of Child Language, 11,* 611–625.

Clark, E. V., & Hecht, B. F. (1982). Learning to coin agent and instrument nouns. *Cognition, 12,* 1–24.

Clark, E. V., & Hecht, B. F. (1983). Comprehension, production, and language acquisition. *Annual Review of Psychology, 34,* 325–349.

Coker, P. L. (1978). Syntactic and semantic factors in the acquisition of *before* and *after*. *Journal of Child Language, 5*, 261–277.

Decroly, O., & Degand, J. (1913). Observations relatives au développement de la notion du temps chez une petite fille. *Archives de Psychologie, 13*, 113–161.

de Villiers, J. G. (1985). Learning how to use verbs: Lexical learning and the influence of input. *Journal of Child Language, 12*, 587–595.

Dockrell, J., & McShane, J. (1990). Young children's use of phrase structure and inflectional information in form-class assignments of novel nouns and verbs. *First Language, 10*, 127–140.

Donaldson, M., & Lloyd, P. (1974). Sentences and situations: Children's judgments of match and mismatch. In *Problèmes actuels en psycholinguistique/Current problems in psycholinguistics* (pp. 73–87). Paris: Editions du Centre National de la Recherche Scientifique (Colloques internationaux No. 206).

Dromi, E. (1987). *Early lexical development.* Cambridge, UK: Cambridge University Press.

Ferguson, C. A., Menn, L., & Stoel-Gammon, C. (Eds.). (1992). *Phonological development: Models, research, implications.* Timonium, MD: York Press.

Gelman, S. A., & Taylor, M. (1984). How two-year-old children interpret proper and common names for unfamiliar objects. *Child Development, 55*, 1535–1540.

Gentner, D. (1982). Why nouns are learned before verbs: Linguistic relativity versus natural partitioning. In S. A. Kuczaj, II (Ed.), *Language development: Vol. 2. Language, culture, and cognition* (pp. 301–334). Hillsdale, NJ: Erlbaum.

Gerhardt, J. [Gee]. (1988). From discourse to semantics: The development of verb morphology and forms of self-reference in the speech of a 2-year-old child. *Journal of Child Language, 15*, 337–393.

Gerken, L. (1991). The metrical basis for children's subjectless sentences. *Journal of Memory and Language, 30*, 431–451.

Gleitman, L. R. (1990). The structural sources of verb meanings. *Language Acquisition, 1*, 3–55.

Goldin-Meadow, S., Seligman, M. E. P., & Gelman, R. (1976). Language in the two-year-old. *Cognition, 4*, 189–202.

Gordon, P. (1985). Evaluating the semantic categories hypothesis: The case of the count/mass distinction. *Cognition, 20*, 209–242.

Grimshaw, J. (1981). Form, function, and the language acquisition device. In C. L. Baker & J. J. McCarthy (Eds.), *The logical problem of language acquisition* (pp. 165–182). Cambridge, MA: MIT Press.

Gropen, J., Pinker, S., Hollander, M., & Goldberg, R. (1991). Syntax and semantics in the acquisition of locative verbs. *Journal of Child Language, 18*, 115–151.

Hamburger, H., & Crain, S. (1982). Relative acquisition. In S. A. Kuczaj, II (Ed.), *Language development: Vol. 1. Syntax and semantics* (pp. 245–273). Hillsdale, NJ: Erlbaum.

Hanlon, C. (1988). The emergence of set-relational quantifiers in early childhood. In F. S. Kessel (Ed.), *The development of language and language researchers* (pp. 65–78). Hillsdale, NJ: Erlbaum.

Harner, L. (1975). *Yesterday and tomorrow:* Development of early understanding of the terms. *Developmental Psychology, 11*, 864–865.

Harner, L. (1976). Children's understanding of linguistic reference to past and future. *Journal of Psycholinguistic Research, 5*, 65–84.

Heibeck, T. H., & Markman, E. M. (1987). Word learning in children: An examination of fast mapping. *Child Development, 58*, 1021–1034.

Horgan, D. (1978). The development of the full passive. *Journal of Child Language, 5*, 65–80.

Huttenlocher, J., & Smiley, P. (1987). Early word meanings: The case of object names. *Cognitive Psychology, 19*, 63–89.

Johnson, C. E. (1983). The development of children's interrogatives: From formulas to rules. *Papers and Reports on Child Language Development* (Stanford University), *22*, 108–115.

Kaper, W. (1980). The use of the past tense in games of pretend. *Journal of Child Language, 7*, 213–215.

Katz, N., Baker, E., & Macnamara, J. (1974). What's in a name? A study of how children learn common and proper names. *Child Development, 45*, 469–473.

Kessel, F. S. (1970). The role of syntax in children's comprehension from ages six to twelve. *Monographs of the Society for Research in Child Development, 35*(Serial No. 139).

Klima, E. S., & Bellugi, U. (1966). Syntactic regularities in the speech of children. In J. Lyons & R. J. Wales (Eds.), *Psycholinguistics papers: Proceedings of the 1966 Edinburgh Conference* (pp. 183–208). Edinburgh: Edinburgh University Press.

Kuczaj, S. A., II. (1977). The acquisition of regular and irregular past tense forms. *Journal of Verbal Learning and Verbal Behavior, 16*, 589–600.

Kuczaj, S. A., II. (1978). Children's judgments of grammatical and ungrammatical irregular past-tense verbs. *Child Development, 49*, 319–326.

Kuczaj, S. A., II. (1982). On the nature of syntactic development. In S. A. Kuczaj, II (Ed.), *Language development: Vol. 1. Syntax and Semantics* (pp. 37–71). Hillsdale, NJ: Erlbaum.

Levelt, W. J. M. (1983). Monitoring and self-repair in speech. *Cognition, 14*, 41–104.

Levelt, W. J. M. (1989). *Speaking: From intention to articulation.* Cambridge, MA: MIT Press/Bradford.

Limber, J. (1973). The genesis of complex sentences. In T. E. Moore (Ed.), *Cognitive development and the acquisition of language* (pp. 169–185). New York: Academic Press.

Lodge, K. R. (1979). The use of the past tense in games of pretend. *Journal of Child Language, 6*, 365–369.

Macnamara, J. (1972). Cognitive basis of language learning in infants. *Psychological Review, 79*, 1–13.

MacWhinney, B. (1976). Hungarian research on the acquisition of morphology and syntax. *Journal of Child Language, 3*, 397–410.

MacWhinney, B. (1978). The acquisition of morphophonology. *Monographs of the Society for Research in Child Development, 43*(Serial No. 174).

Maratsos, M. P. (1983). Some current issues in the study of the acquisition of grammar. In J. H. Flavell & E. M. Markman (Eds.), *Handbook of child psychology: Vol. 3. Cognitive development* (pp. 707–786). New York: Wiley.

Maratsos, M. P. (1990). Are actions to verbs as objects are to nouns? On the differential semantic bases of form, class, category. *Linguistics, 28*, 1351–1379.

Maratsos, M. P., Fox, D. E. C., Becker, J. A., & Chalkley, M. A. (1985). Semantic restrictions on children's passives. *Cognition, 19*, 167–191.

Maratsos, M. P., Gudeman, R., Gerard-Ngo, P., & DeHart, G. (1987). A study in novel word learning: The productivity of the causative. In B. MacWhinney (Ed.), *Mechanisms of language acquisition* (pp. 89–113). Hillsdale, NJ: Erlbaum.

Markman, E. M. (1987). How children constrain the possible meanings of words. In U. Neisser (Ed.), *Concepts and conceptual knowledge: Ecological and intellectual factors in categorization* (pp. 255–287). Cambridge, UK: Cambridge University Press.

Mervis, C. B. (1987). Child-basic object categories and early lexical development. In U. Neisser (Ed.), *Concepts and conceptual knowledge: Ecological and intellectual factors in categorization* (pp. 201–233). Cambridge, UK: Cambridge University Press.

Mervis, C. B., & Johnson, K. E. (1991). Acquisition of the plural morpheme: A case study. *Developmental Psychology, 27*, 222–235.

Nagy, W. E., & Anderson, R. C. (1984). The number of words in printed school English. *Reading Research Quarterly, 19*, 304–330.

Nelson, K. (1973). Structure and strategy in learning to talk. *Monographs of the Society for Research in Child Development, 38*(Serial No. 149).

Peters, A. M., & Menn, L. (1993). False starts and filler syllables: Ways to learn grammatical morphemes. *Language, 69,* 742–777.

Pinker, S. (1984). *Language learnability and language development.* Cambridge, MA: Harvard University Press.

Pinker, S. (1989). *Learnability and cognition: The acquisition of argument structure.* Cambridge, MA: MIT/Bradford.

Reich, P. (1976). The early acquisition of word meaning. *Journal of Child Language, 3,* 117–123.

Reilly, J. S. (1986). The acquisition of temporals and conditionals. In E. C. Traugott, A. ter Meulen, J. S. Reilly, & C. A. Ferguson (Eds.), *On conditionals* (pp. 309–331). Cambridge, UK: Cambridge University Press.

Rescorla, L. (1980). Overextension in early language development. *Journal of Child Language, 7,* 321–335.

Sachs, J., & Devin, J. (1976). Young children's use of age appropriate speech styles in social interaction and role-playing. *Journal of Child Language, 3,* 81–98.

Shatz, M., & Gelman, R. (1973). The development of communication skills: Modifications in the speech of young children as a function of listener. *Monographs of the Society for Research in Child Development, 38*(Serial No. 152).

Slobin, D. I. (1970). Universals of grammatical development in children. In G. B. Flores d'Arcais & W. J. M. Levelt (Eds.), *Advances in psycholinguistics* (pp. 174–186). Amsterdam: North-Holland.

Smoczyńska, M. (1985). The acquisition of Polish. In D. I. Slobin (Ed.), *The crosslinguistic study of language acquisition* (Vol. 1, pp. 595–686). Hillsdale, NJ: Erlbaum.

Soja, N. N., Carey, S., & Spelke, E. S. (1991). Ontological categories guide young children's inductions of word meaning: Object terms and substance terms. *Cognition, 38,* 179–211.

Tager-Flusberg, H. (1982). The development of relative clauses in child speech. *Papers & Reports on Child Language Development* (Stanford University), *21,* 104–111.

Talmy, L. (1985). Lexicalization patterns: Semantic structure in lexical form. In T. E. Shopen (Ed.), *Language typology and syntactic description: Vol. 3. Grammatical categories and the lexicon* (pp. 57–149). Cambridge, UK: Cambridge University Press.

Taylor, M., & Gelman, S. A. (1988). Adjectives and nouns: Children's strategies for learning new words. *Child Development, 59,* 411–419.

Templin, M. C. (1957). *Certain language skills in children: Their development and interrelationships.* Minneapolis: University of Minnesota Press.

Thomson, J. R., & Chapman, R. S. (1977). Who is 'Daddy' revisited: The status of two-year-olds' over-extended words in use and comprehension. *Journal of Child Language, 4,* 359–375.

Tomasello, M. (1992). *First verbs: A case study of early grammatical development.* Cambridge, UK: Cambridge University Press.

Warden, D. A. (1976). The influence of context on children's use of identifying expressions and references. *British Journal of Psychology, 67,* 101–112.

CHAPTER 10

The Neurobiology of Language

Sheila E. Blumstein

I. INTRODUCTION

One of the most challenging issues related to human language is understanding how it is organized and processed in the brain. Such study is
described under the broad rubric of the neurobiology of language and defines the field of neurolinguistics. The domain of inquiry has largely focused
on investigations of aphasic patients, exploring the clinical and behavioral
manifestations of their disorder and the accompanying lesion localization.
These "experiments in nature" provide the traditional approach to the study
of language/brain relations, and without question, they have provided the
major insights to date. Nevertheless, in more recent years, the increased
sophistication of electrophysiological and metabolic techniques has provided a new and exciting approach to the study of the neurobiology of
language. These latter studies allow investigation of neural activity in normal subjects in addition to the study of brain-damaged patients. Taken
together, these three approaches: clinical/lesion investigations using imaging techniques such as computerized axial tomography (CAT scan) and
magnetic resonance imaging (MRI); electrophysiological studies using
evoked related potentials (ERP); and metabolic techniques using positron
emission tomography (PET), provide converging data on the nature of the
representation of language, the processes involved in language use, and
ultimately its underlying neural organization.

It is the object of this chapter to review the current state of knowledge of
the neurobiology of language. Particular emphasis will be on studies of

Speech, Language, and Communication

adult aphasia. Studies involving ERP and PET are also reviewed as they speak to issues concerning language organization and language processing.

A. Research Methodologies

All experimental methodologies have both strengths and weaknesses. Clinical/lesion investigations of adult patients provide a view of language breakdown subsequent to brain damage. As such, they serve as a window into the fractionation of language in individuals who had normal language and cognitive functions prior to the damage. Charting the relation between patterns of language breakdown and underlying neuropathology provides the closest analogy to lesion mapping in animal investigations. Unlike lesion mapping studies in animals, however, it is impossible to control for the site and size of the lesion. Grouping patients by lesion site then is quite difficult and usually involves gross localization schemas making it difficult to determine the precise relation between language behavior and underlying lesion. In addition, it is problematic to assume a one-to-one relation between brain structure and language function. As John Hughlings Jackson stated ". . . to locate the damage which destroys speech and to localise [sic] speech are two different things" (quoted in Henry Head, 1963, p. 50). It is possible that a lesion may affect pathways leading to a particular functional area without damaging that area. Moreover, the processing components ultimately contributing to language are complex and are usually inferred from investigations of patients' behavior on different language tasks, such as naming and comprehension, behaviors that in themselves may require different processing components. Finally, studies with aphasic patients typically rely on behavioral measures and aphasic patients typically show increased variability compared to neurologically intact control patients on these measures. As a result, it is often difficult to titrate out statistically reliable effects. Nonetheless, studies with aphasic patients have provided the basis for the major hypotheses generated and tested to date in metabolic studies with neurologically intact subjects.

The advantages of metabolic studies such as PET are that they provide a potential means of mapping brain function in neurologically intact subjects and of investigating specific aspects of language without the complicating factors of lesions, which potentially affect more than one component of language. PET is a technique that examines changes in cerebral blood flow in localized brain areas during cognitive activities. The time frame over which blood flow is measured is about 40 s. The assumption underlying this methodology is that the greater the involvement of a particular area of the brain in a particular cognitive activity, the greater will be the metabolic activity, hence cerebral blood flow, to that area. Nevertheless, this technique has its own weaknesses and potential problems. Perhaps the biggest challenge is determining whether and how much neuronal activity relates to a functional activity. Typically, PET studies use complex statistical algorithms for determining the significance of the metabolic activity obtained. To determine the localization of particular functions, PET studies use the subtraction technique. This technique assumes that particular cognitive and language tasks or functions can be broken down into discrete components or processes contributing to that function, and that these functions are additive. To focus on the particular function of interest, the metabolic activity contributing to the other functions or processes is subtracted out, leaving the isolated function and its proposed neurological site. For example, in determining the metabolic activity in understanding the meaning of a word, the metabolic activity related to auditory perception and the perception of the sound-shape of the word is subtracted. The neuronal activity remaining is assumed to reflect cerebral activity specifically related to the meaning of the word. What is not clear is whether the processes of language can be assumed to be additive in this simple way. Nevertheless, the PET technique provides an exciting new way of exploring the neurobiology of language.

Finally, electrophysiological studies have recently provided some interesting correlates of language function. To date, however, they do not provide information on localization since the exact origin of the electrical activity cannot be determined by current techniques. ERPs do provide a means of exploring patterns of electrical potentials that correlate with various aspects of language including speech or phonological processing, word meaning, and syntactic processing. The ERP methodology measures brain activity at the scalp in synchrony with the presentation of a stimulus. Variations in electrical brain potentials are assumed to serve as electrophysiological markers of the particular activity under investigation. As with PET studies, analytic techniques must be developed to identify significant patterns from the underlying random electrical activity of the brain. Identifying these patterns from background noise is indeed a major challenge. Moreover, it is unclear whether this technique is sensitive enough to measure and distinguish the more subtle aspects of language and its underlying processing components.

B. Theoretical Framework

As a preliminary step in the discussion of the neurobiology of language, it may be useful to consider some broad theoretical issues that have guided research in this field. Much as linguistic research has been guided by considerations of the structural levels of the linguistic grammar, such as phonology, lexicon/semantics, and syntax, so have linguistic investigations of aphasia (see Frazier, Chapter 1, this volume). The major question has been whether language deficits in aphasia reflect selective impairments to these components and to their representations, that is, the primitive units or structural properties of the components, or alternatively, the processes involved in accessing these components. Consideration of aphasia as a deficit in the components of the grammar, or in the processes involved in accessing the components, speaks directly to the issue of the modularity of language. Throughout the history of the study of aphasia, various forms of modularity theories have been postulated (for a review, see Fodor, 1983; Head, 1963).

Broadly speaking, evidence clearly supports the view that language is modular, in that it is an autonomous system that is (within limits) functionally and neurologically distinct from other higher cortical functions. Dissociations have been found in which language is impaired and cognitive abilities are spared and vice versa (Irigary, 1967; Tissot, Lhermitte, & Ducarne, 1963; Zangwill, 1964). Studies of brain-damaged patients also suggest that mathematical, musical, and artistic abilities may be dissociated from language (Gardner, 1983). Nevertheless, considerably stronger claims have been made about the modularity of language. In particular, in some versions of the modularity theory, it has been hypothesized that language consists of submodules such as lexical, syntactic, and semantic, which are functionally autonomous, with a restricted domain of analysis and processing (Fodor, 1983; Garrett, 1979). Evidence from the neurobiology of language may speak to the broad claims of the theory of modularity and to the particular form that such a modular theory may take. Consideration of the components of the grammar (phonology, lexicon/semantics, and syntax) provides an organizational framework from which to explore the neurobiology of language.

Before reviewing the major components of the grammar in relation to the neurobiology of language, it is worthwhile to briefly review some of the major clinical and neuroanatomical manifestations underlying the aphasias. For approximately 90% of right-handers, the left hemisphere is dominant for language. Brain damage within the left hemisphere has different effects on language and speech depending on the site and extent of the lesion. Although there have been recent challenges to the reliability of classification schemas in aphasia, and more important, concern about whether such schemas provide the bases from which language impairments may be studied (Caramazza, 1984; Schwartz, 1984), it goes without saying that a broad array of language behaviors is impaired in particular ways as a function of different areas of brain damage. The clinical syndromes that characterize these aphasias are based on a constellation of language abilities and disabilities defined in terms of language faculties or functions such as speaking, understanding, reading, and writing (Goodglass & Kaplan, 1972).

Classical approaches to the clinical/neurological basis of language disorders in adult aphasics have typically characterized the aphasia syndromes in broad anatomical (anterior and posterior) and functional (expressive and receptive) dichotomies (see Geschwind, 1965). The two aphasia syndromes that best characterize the anterior/posterior and expressive/receptive dichotomy are, respectively, Broca's and Wernicke's aphasia. Patients with Broca's aphasia show a profound expressive deficit in the face of relatively good auditory language comprehension. Speech output is typically nonfluent in that it is slow, labored, and often dysarthric, and the melody pattern seems flat. Furthermore, speech output is often agrammatic, characterized by the omission of grammatical words such as *the* and *is,* as well as the incorrect usage of grammatical endings. Syntactic structures are generally limited to simple sentences with few embeddings and dependent clauses. As to other language abilities, naming an object on presentation is generally fair to good, and repetition of language is usually good or better than spontaneous speech output. The underlying neuropathology includes the frontal operculum as well as premotor and motor regions posterior and superior to the frontal operculum, extending to the white matter below and including the basal ganglia and insula (Damasio, 1991).

The syndrome of Wernicke's aphasia is characterized by both language input and language output impairments. Auditory language comprehension is severely impaired. Speech output is fluent and well articulated. Grammatical structures seem relatively intact, although syntactic phrases may be inappropriately juxtaposed. Most characteristically, the semantic content of the output is severely compromised. Language is empty of semantic content, often difficult to understand, with the overuse of high-frequency, low-content words such as *thing, be, have, this.* In addition, literal paraphasias (sound substitution errors) and verbal paraphasias (word substitution errors) occur in speech output. There are some Wernicke's aphasia patients who also produce neologisms or "jargon." Another frequent characteristic of this disorder is "logorrhea" or 'press' for speech, whereby patients, even in a conversational setting, talk on and on without stopping. Other associated language impairments include a moderate to severe naming deficit and a severe repetition disorder. The neuropathology associated with Wernicke's aphasia involves the posterior region of the left superior temporal gyrus, often extending to the supramarginal and angular gyrus (Damasio, 1991).

II. THE SOUND STRUCTURE OF LANGUAGE: PHONOLOGY

It is generally assumed that in the case of both language production and language reception words or lexical entries ultimately contact a common representation, specified in terms of segments, phonetic features, and rules for their combination that are specific to the sound structure of language. Nonetheless, to effect encoding and decoding of speech requires different mechanisms relating to the speech apparatus in the former and to the auditory system in the latter, and for that reason the interface of these two systems with the lexicon for speech production and speech perception requires a unique set of operations (see Fowler, Chapter 2, and Nygaard and Pisoni, Chapter 3, this volume). For this reason, it is useful to consider the neurobiology of speech production and speech perception separately.

A. Speech Production

Linguistic theory makes a clear distinction between phonology and phonetics, and the facts of aphasia support such a distinction, particularly in the investigation of speech production deficits. In some cases, patients may produce a wrong sound segment, but its phonetic implementation is correct, that is, for *teams* the patient says *keams*. In other cases, patients may produce the correct sound segments but their phonetic implementation is distorted, that is, for *teams* the patient produces an initial /t/ that is overly aspirated.

Research investigations have focused on the patterns of speech production errors of aphasic patients. A number of different methodologies have been used to elicit productions from patients including conversational speech, naming, and repetition. Despite the different methodologies used, a consistent finding is that nearly all aphasic patients, regardless of the aphasia syndrome, display impairments implicating a deficit at the phonological level. Critically, the patterns of impairment are similar, suggesting that despite the different underlying neuropathology, a common mechanism is impaired. The similar patterns of performance are particularly striking given the different clinical characteristics and neuropathology of the patients investigated. The mechanism impaired in the phonological output impairment of all of these patients relates to the selection and/or organization of the features comprising the candidate lexical entries. Selection impairments reflect the inappropriate choice of a feature and hence the appearance of an inappropriate segment in a particular position. Planning impairments reflect the inappropriate ordering of the segments or alternatively the inappropriate influence of phonetic context on the ultimate feature or segment selected. The patterns of sound substitutions indicate that it is indeed the selection of an inappropriate feature and not the selection of an inappropriate segment that underlies these types of errors.

The types of errors produced by aphasic patients can be categorized in terms of four descriptive categories. Together they suggest that the basis of the errors reflects a selection as well as a planning deficit (Blumstein, 1973). These errors include: phoneme substitution errors in which a segment is substituted for another (e.g., *teams* → *keams*); simplification errors in which a phoneme or syllable is deleted (e.g., *green* → *geen*); addition errors in which an extra phoneme or syllable is added to a word (e.g., *see* → *stee*); and environment errors in which the occurrence of a particular phoneme is influenced by the surrounding phonetic context; these errors include metathesis (*e.g., degree → gedree*), and progressive and regressive assimilation errors (e.g., *Crete → kreke,* and *→ trete,* respectively). The stability of these patterns is evidenced by their occurrence across languages: French (Bouman & Grunbaum, 1925; Lecours & Lhermitte, 1969); German (Bouman & Grunbaum, 1925; Goldstein, 1948); English (Blumstein, 1973; Green, 1969); Turkish (Peuser & Fittschen, 1977); Russian (Luria, 1966); and Finnish (Niemi, Koivuselka-Sallinen, & Hanninen, 1985).

The pattern of sound substitutions is consistent with the view that the incorrect features have been selected or activated but have been correctly implemented by the articulatory system. Thus, most substitution errors involve a change in value of a single feature. For example, the production of *doy* for *toy* reflects a change in the feature of voicing. Similarly, the production of *dut* for *nut* represents a change in the feature of nasality. Relatively few substitution errors produced by aphasic patients involve changes in more than one feature.

Phonological errors also suggest that the nature of the syllable structure (i.e., the organization of consonants and vowels) of the lexical candidate constrains the type and extent of errors made during the selection process (Blumstein, 1973, 1990). In particular, the occurrence of phoneme substitution errors is more likely to occur when the syllable contains a single consonant than when it is part of a consonant cluster, for example, /f/ is more likely to undergo a phoneme substitution error in the word *feet* than in the word *fleet*. Simplification and addition errors are more likely to result in the canonical syllable structure Consonant-Vowel, for example, consonants are more likely to be deleted in a word beginning with two consonants, *sky →* *ky,* and consonants are more likely to be added in a word beginning with a vowel, *army → jarmy*. And finally, assimilation errors across word boundaries preserve the syllable structure relations of the lexical candidates. That is, if the influencing phoneme is at the beginning of the target word, so is the assimilated phoneme, for example, *history books → bistory books*. If the influencing phoneme is at the end of the target word, so is the assimilated phoneme, for example, *roast beef → roaf beef*. These results show that information about the syllable structure of a word is represented in the lexicon, and this information is used in the planning buffer for sentence production. If this were not the case, the syllable constraints shown in the assimilation errors would not occur across word boundaries.

Despite the systematicity and regularity of the phonological errors just described, the particular occurrence of such an error cannot be predicted. That is, sometimes patients may make an error on a particular word, and other times they will produce it correctly. Nor are the errors unidirectional (Blumstein, 1973; Hatfield & Walton, 1975). A voiced stop consonant may become voiceless (e.g., /d/ → /t/), and a voiceless stop consonant may become voiced (e.g., /t/ → /d/). Thus, the patterns of errors reflect statistical tendencies. Because patients are able to produce the correct utterance and because their errors are systematic (although not predictable), it suggests that the underlying phonological representations are intact, but that either the level of activation of the features has been changed or there has been a failure to select the appropriate phonological representation from the lexicon. Even though virtually all aphasic patients regardless of lesion site display similar patterns of phonological impairment, they vary in the severity of the impairment. Patients with Broca's aphasia and damage to anterior brain structures produce many more such errors than do patients with Wernicke's aphasia (Blumstein, 1973).

While the phonological patterns are similar across patients, phonetic deficits seem to be more selective. A long-held observation is that patients with anterior aphasia produce phonetic errors. The implied basis for these errors is one of articulatory implementation; that is, the commands to the articulators to encode the word are incorrect, poorly timed, and so forth. A number of studies have explored these phonetic patterns of speech by investigating the acoustic properties or the articulatory parameters underlying the production of particular phonetic dimensions. The dimensions investigated include voicing in stop consonants (e.g., /p t k/ vs. /b d g/) and fricatives (e.g., /f s/ vs. /v z/), place of articulation in stop consonants (e.g., /b/ vs. /d/ vs. /g/) and fricatives (e.g., /f/ vs. /s/), and the nasal and stop manner of articulation (e.g., /n m/ vs. /d b/). Studies of speech production in aphasia patients with damage to anterior brain structures (including patients with Broca's aphasia) have shown that these patients have difficulty producing phonetic dimensions that require the timing of two independent articulators. These findings have emerged in the analysis of two phonetic dimensions, voicing and nasality. In the case of the feature voicing, the dimension studied is voice-onset time, that is, the timing relation between the release of a stop consonant and the onset of vocal cord vibration. The production of nasal consonants also requires appropriate timing between two articulators, in this case, the release of the closure in the oral cavity and the velum opening.

Results of analyses of the production of the voicing and nasal phonetic dimensions have shown that aphasic patients with anterior brain-damage (including patients with Broca's aphasia) evidence significant deficits (Blumstein, Cooper, Goodglass, Statlender, & Gottlieb, 1980; Blumstein, Cooper, Zurif, & Caramazza, 1977; Freeman, Sands, & Harris, 1978; Gandour & Dardarananda, 1984a; Itoh, Sasanuma, Hirose, Yoshioka, & Ushijima, 1980; Itoh et al., 1982; Itoh, Sasanuma, & Ushijima, 1979; Shewan, Leeper, & Booth, 1984). These same patterns emerge across different languages. They occur not only in English and Japanese, for which voice-onset time serves to distinguish two categories of voicing, voiced and voiceless, but also in Thai, for which voice-onset time serves to distinguish three categories of voicing in stop consonants, prevoiced, voiced, and voiceless aspirated.

Nevertheless, these patients also show normal patterns of production. The constellation of spared and impaired patterns of articulation suggests that their disorder affects impairments, in particular articulatory maneuvers rather than the articulatory implementation of given phonetic features. The evidence comes from studies of voicing in stop consonants. In English, the feature voicing in stop consonants can be cued in several ways. As discussed earlier, voice-onset time provides one measure of voicing for stop consonants occurring in initial position. A second measure is the duration of the vowel preceding a stop consonant. Vowels are short before voiceless stops (e.g., *write*) and long before voiced stops (e.g. *ride*). If patients have a deficit related to the implementation of the feature voicing, then they should display impairments in the production of vowel length preceding voiced and voiceless stop consonants as well as voice-onset time. In contrast, if they have a deficit related to particular articulatory maneuvers, such as the timing of two independent articulators, the production of voice-onset time may be impaired, while the production of vowel length may be normal. Results indicate that although these patients show an impairment in the implementation of the voicing phonetic dimension via voice-onset time, they are able to maintain the distinction between voiced and voiceless stops on the basis of the duration of the preceding vowel (Baum, Blumstein, Naeser, & Palumbo, 1990; Duffy & Gawle, 1984). Moreover, there is no systematic relation within the same patient between the ability to realize the voicing dimension by means of voice-onset time and vowel duration (Tuller, 1984). Thus, these patients do not have a disorder affecting the articulatory production of the feature voicing, but a disorder affecting particular articulatory maneuvers, namely the timing or integration of movements of two independent articulators.

Although patients with anterior aphasia show a disorder in temporal coordination, their disorder does not reflect a pervasive timing impairment. Fricative durations do not differ significantly from those of nonaphasic patients (Harmes et al., 1984), and the patients maintain the intrinsic duration differences characteristic of fricatives varying in place of articulation; for example, /s/ and /š/ are longer in duration than /f/ and /θ/ (Baum et al., 1990). English-speaking patients with anterior aphasia maintain differences in the intrinsic durations of vowels; for example, tense vowels such as /i/ and /e/ are longer than their lax vowel equivalents, /I/ and /E/. In addition, Thai-speaking patients with anterior aphasia maintain the contrast between short vowels and long vowels, a contrast that is phonemic in this language (Gandour & Dardarananda, 1984b).

In addition to the impairment in the timing of independent articulators, difficulties for aphasic patients with anterior brain-damage (including Broca's aphasia) have also emerged with laryngeal control. They have shown impairments in voicing in the production of voiced fricatives (Baum et al., 1990; Harmes et al., 1984; Kent & Rosenbek, 1983), and impairments in the production of intonation (Cooper, Soares, Nicol, Michelow, & Goloskie, 1984; Ryalls, 1982).

Finally, recent investigations of coarticulation effects in patients with anterior brain-damage show that they produce relatively normal anticipatory coarticulation. For example, in producing the syllable /su/, they anticipate the rounded vowel /u/ in the production of the preceding /s/ (Katz, 1988). Nevertheless, they seem to show a delay in the time it takes to produce these effects (Ziegler & von Cramon, 1985, 1986), and they may show some deficiencies in their productions (Tuller & Story, 1986; but see Katz, 1987, for discussion). What these results suggest is that phonological planning is relatively intact, but it is the ultimate timing or coordination of the implementation of the articulatory movements that is impaired (cf. Kent & Rosenbek, 1983).

Of interest is the point that, although clearly distinguished from patients with anterior aphasia, posterior aphasia patients also display a subtle phonetic deficit. Most typically, they show increased variability in the implementation of a number of phonetic parameters (Kent & McNeill, 1987; Ryalls, 1986), including vowel formant frequencies (Ryalls, 1986) and vowel duration (Gandour et al., 1992; Ryalls, 1986; Tuller, 1984). Because these phonetic impairments are not clinically perceptible but emerge only upon acoustic analysis, they are considered to be subclinical. Nevertheless, they indicate that both anterior and posterior brain structures ultimately contribute to the speech production process.

On the basis of the findings just reviewed, several conclusions can be made concerning the nature of the phonetic disorders for patients with anterior aphasia and their ultimate underlying mechanisms. In particular, the impairment is not a linguistic one, in the sense that the patient is unable to implement a particular phonetic feature. Moreover, the patients have not lost the representation for implementation nor the knowledge base for how to implement sounds in context. Rather, particular maneuvers relating to the timing of articulators seem to be impaired, ultimately affecting the phonetic realization of some sound segments and some aspects of speech prosody.

Investigations exploring the potential neuroanatomical structures contributing to the phonetic implementation of speech suggest that there are specific neuroanatomical substrates relating to such phonetic implementation patterns. These investigations include neuroimaging (CAT scan) studies of aphasic patients, attempting to relate the behavioral characteristics outlined above with particular areas of brain damage, and PET and ERP data with neurologically intact subjects. In particular, CAT scan correlations with patterns of speech production deficits suggest the involvement of Broca's area, lower motor cortex regions for larynx, tongue, and face, and some white matter structures as well in the phonetic implementation of speech (Baum et al., 1990). PET studies with neurologically intact subjects determining regions of cerebral blood flow activity during speech production also show the importance of these areas as well as the precentral gyrus and premotor areas surrounding Broca's area (Petersen, Fox, Posner, Mintun, & Raichle, 1989). It is interesting that ERP studies with these subjects suggest that these areas seem to be involved in the production of articulatory maneuvers related specifically to the production of speech sounds and not more generally to vocal tract maneuvers that do not relate to speech (McAdam & Whitaker, 1971).

B. Speech Perception

Similar to production studies with aphasic patients, most studies exploring the role of speech perception deficits in auditory comprehension impairments have focused on the ability of aphasic patients to perceive phonemic or segmental contrasts. Studies on segmental perception have indeed shown that aphasic patients evidence deficits in processing segmental contrasts. These studies have explored patients' abilities to discriminate pairs of words or nonwords (e.g. *pear* vs. *bear, pa* vs. *ba*) or they have asked subjects to point to the appropriate word or consonant from an array of names or syllables that are phonologically confusable. Results show that patients with both anterior and posterior aphasia display some problems in discriminating phonological contrasts (Blumstein, Baker, & Goodglass, 1977; Jauhiainen & Nuutila, 1977; Miceli, Calatgirone, Gainotti, & Payer-Rego, 1978; Miceli, Gainotti, Caltagirone, & Masullo, 1980) or in labeling or identifying consonants presented in a consonant-vowel context (Basso, Casati, & Vignolo, 1977; Blumstein, Cooper et al., 1977; cf. also Boatman, Lesser, & Gordon, 1994). These problems emerge in the perception of both real words and nonsense syllables. Although there are more errors in the perception of nonsense syllables than in the perception of real words, the overall patterns of performance are similar, and essentially mirror the patterns found in the analysis of phonological errors in speech production. Namely, subjects are more likely to make speech perception errors when the test stimuli contrast by a single feature than when they contrast by two or more features (Baker, Blumstein, & Goodglass, 1981; Blumstein, Baker, & Goodglass, 1977; Miceli et al., 1978; Sasanuma, Tatsumi, & Fujisaki, 1976). Among the various types of feature contrasts, the perception of place of articulation is particularly vulnerable (Baker et al., 1981; Blumstein, Baker, & Goodglass, 1977;

Miceli et al., 1978). It is interesting that similar patterns emerge in non-brain-damaged subjects when perceiving speech under difficult listening conditions (cf. Miller & Nicely, 1955).

What is not clear from many of the studies exploring the perception of segmental contrasts is whether the failure to perceive such contrasts reflects an impairment in the perception of abstract phonetic features or alternatively an impairment relating to the extraction of the acoustic patterns associated with these features. To explore this issue, several studies have investigated categorical perception of the acoustic parameters associated with phonetic features. Categorical perception relates to the way neurologically intact subjects perceive the phonetic categories of speech. In particular, continuous changes in an acoustic parameter such as voice-onset time associated with a phonetic contrast, in this case voicing, give rise to discontinuous changes in perception; when asked to label or identify the stimuli on an acoustic continuum, listeners perceive them as belonging to discrete categories corresponding to the end-point, exemplar stimuli, and they show a sharp change in the identification of the categories usually at a particular stimulus along the continuum; when asked to discriminate the stimuli, they accurately discriminate only those stimuli that they labeled as belonging to two different categories, and fail to discriminate those stimuli that they labeled as the same phonetic category, even though all of the discrimination pairs vary along the same physical dimension. The studies exploring categorical perception in aphasia have investigated two phonetic dimensions, voicing (Basso et al., 1977; Blumstein, Cooper, et al., 1977; Gandour & Dardarananda, 1982) and place of articulation in stop consonants (Blumstein, Tartter, Nigro, & Statlender, 1984). For voicing, the acoustic dimension varied was voice-onset time, and for place of articulation, the dimension varied was the frequency of the formant transitions appropriate for /b d g/, and the presence or absence of a burst preceding the transitions. Results showed that if aphasic patients could perform only one of the two tasks (labeling or discrimination), it was the discrimination task. Most important, the discrimination functions were generally similar in shape and the locus of the phonetic boundary was comparable to that of neurologically intact subjects, even in those patients who could only discriminate the stimuli.

The fact that no perceptual shifts in boundary location were obtained for the discrimination and labeling functions for aphasic patients, that the discrimination functions remained stable even in those patients who could not label the stimuli, and that the patients perceived the acoustic dimensions relating to phonetic categories in a fashion similar to neurologically intact subjects suggest that aphasic patients do not have a deficit specific to the extraction of the spectral or temporal patterns corresponding to the phonetic categories of speech. Rather, their deficit seems to relate to the activation of the phonetic/phonological representation itself or to its ultimate contact with the lexicon. Consistent with this view is the finding that although patients may show speech perception impairments, their performance is variable; they do not show selective impairments relating to a particular phonetic feature; and the pattern of errors is bidirectional, for example, voiced consonants may be perceived as voiceless, and voiceless consonants may be perceived as voiced. This pattern of results mirrors that found in speech production studies with aphasic patients.

In contrast to the segmental features of speech, the prosodic cues (i.e., intonation and stress) are consistently less affected in aphasia. Severely impaired aphasic patients have been shown to retain some ability to recognize and distinguish the syntactic forms of commands, yes–no questions, and information questions when marked only by intonation cues (Green & Boller, 1974), even when they are unable to do so when syntactic forms are marked by lexical and syntactic cues. Nonetheless, as with intonation cues, patients' performance is not completely normal. A number of studies have revealed impairments in the comprehension of lexical/phrasal stress contrasts (e.g., *hótdog* vs. *hotdóg*) (Baum, Kelsch Daniloff, & Daniloff, 1982; Emmorey, 1987), as well as sentential contrasts (e.g., *he fed her dóg biscuits* vs. *he fed her dog bíscuits*) (Baum et al., 1982). Similar findings emerged for the perception of tone contrasts serving as lexical cues in Thai (Gandour & Daradarananda, 1983) and Chinese (Naeser & Chan, 1980). No differences have emerged in any studies between the performance of patients with anterior and posterior aphasia, an important finding consistent with the results for the perception of phonemic contrasts.

That speech perception deficits emerge in patients with both anterior and posterior aphasia suggests that the neural basis for speech perception and the auditory processing of speech is neurally complex, and includes far greater neural involvement than simply the primary auditory areas and auditory association areas in the temporal lobe. While the number of neurophysiological and electrophysiological studies focusing particularly on speech reception are few, these results provide converging evidence consistent with this view. PET studies have shown that the primary auditory cortex is activated in the processing of simple auditory stimuli (Lauter, Herscovitch, Formby, & Raichle, 1985), and both the primary auditory cortex and the superior temporal gyrus are activated in passive word recognition (Petersen, Fox, Posner, Mintun, & Raichle, 1988, 1989). These results are of no surprise. What is of interest, however, is that other cortical areas seem to be activated as well. For example, Zatorre, Evans, Meyer, and Gjedde (1992) showed increased activity in Broca's area near the junction with premotor cortex as well as the superior parietal area near the supramarginal gyrus when subjects were required to make a phonetic decision or phonetic judgment about auditorily presented CVC stimuli. Further, Ojemann (1983) has shown impairments in the ability of patients to identify auditorily presented sound segments embedded in a phonetic context /a___ma/ during electrical stimulation to a wide range of cortical areas including the inferior frontal cortex.

C. Speech Perception and Lexical Access

While results of speech perception experiments suggest that aphasic patients do not seem to have a selective impairment in processing the segmental structure underlying the auditory properties of speech, several recent studies have suggested that aphasic patients display impairments in the intersection of the sound properties of speech with lexical access. These studies have shown some interesting dichotomies in the performance of patients with Broca's and Wernicke's aphasia, which suggest that patients' impairments do not reflect speech perception deficits per se but rather deficits in the intersection of sound structure with the lexicon (cf. also Baker et al., 1981; Martin, Wasserman, Gilden, & West, 1975).

Milberg, Blumstein, and Dworetzky (1988) explored the extent to which phonological distortions affect semantic facilitation in a lexical decision task. They investigated whether a phonologically distorted prime word such as *gat* or *wat* would affect the amount of semantic facilitation for target words semantically related to the undistorted prime, for example, *cat*. Subjects were asked to make a lexical decision on the second item of stimulus pairs in which the first stimulus was semantically related to the second (e.g., *cat–dog*), or alternatively, it was systematically changed by one or more features (e.g., *gat–dog*, *wat–dog*). Neurologically intact control subjects showed a monotonic function with less semantic facilitation as phonetic distortion increased, that is, less semantic facilitation for *wat–dog* than for *gat–dog*. In contrast, Wernicke's aphasia patients showed priming in all phonologically distorted conditions (e.g., *gat–dog*, *wat–dog*), suggesting a reduced threshold compared to the control subjects for lexical access, and patients with anterior aphasia showed priming only in the undistorted semantically related condition (e.g., *cat–dog*), suggesting an increased threshold for lexical access. These results suggest that impairments in the use of phonological information to access the lexicon can manifest themselves in different ways in aphasic patients in the absence of a deficit in processing the phonological properties of speech themselves.

Similarly, the lexical status of a word affects differentially how aphasic patients perform phonetic categorization. Neurologically intact subjects typically show a *lexical effect*. For example, the locus of a phonetic boundary on an acoustic continuum varying in voice-onset time changes as a function of the lexical status of the end-point stimuli. When the end-point /d/ stimulus is a word (e.g., *dash*), and the end-point /t/ stimulus is a nonword (e.g., *tash*), there are more *d* responses along the continuum; in contrast, when the end-point /t/ stimulus is a word (e.g., *task*), and the end-point /d/ stimulus is a nonword (e.g., *dask*), there are more *t* responses along the continuum (Ganong, 1980). Patients with Broca's aphasia show a larger than normal lexical effect, placing a greater reliance on the lexical status of the stimulus in making their phonetic decisions than on the perceptual information in the stimulus. In contrast, patients with Wernicke's aphasia do not show a lexical effect at all, suggesting that top-down information does not influence phonetic categorization, and perhaps such top-down processing may even fail to guide their language performance (Blumstein, Burton, Baum, Waldstein, & Katz, 1994).

III. THE LEXICON

One of the most common clinical attributes in aphasia is a naming deficit. Such a deficit is operationally defined as an inability or inconsistency in giving the appropriate name for an object, the depiction of an action, and so on. This deficit may also manifest itself in word-finding difficulty (i.e., groping for the appropriate word), semantic paraphasias (i.e., word substitutions), or empty speech (i.e., the use of nonspecific words, as *thing, be*) in the patient's spontaneous speech output. A number of attributes contribute to the evocation of a name and can influence a subject's overall performance, including word frequency (Howes, 1964; Rochford & Williams, 1962) and its concreteness or picturability (Goodglass, Hyde, & Blumstein, 1969). In fact, some patients have been identified with selective impairments in naming particular semantic categories or classes of words (cf. Hart, Berndt, & Caramazza, 1985). Nonetheless, most aphasic patients do not have such selective deficits, but rather have a naming deficit cutting across semantic categories and word classes. The question remains as to what is the basis for these nonspecific and pervasive naming deficits. Two possibilities have been proposed. One possibility is that the patients have a lexical access impairment. In this case, the underlying lexical representation and organizational properties are intact, but the processes required to access this information are impaired. A second possibility is that the patients have an impairment in the lexical representation or semantic structure of the words themselves. Whether the deficit is one of access or representation, such lexical impairments would not only influence naming but could also affect the comprehension of language (see Cutler, Chapter 4, and Seidenberg, Chapter 5, this volume).

There is a fair amount of clinical evidence suggesting that the basis of naming impairments reflects a retrieval or access problem. A patient who is unable to name a particular object in one context or at one time may be able to do so at another. This inconsistency in object naming suggests that the representation of the lexical item is intact, but the patient may be unable to evoke its name. In support of this interpretation is the fact that the patient who has failed to name or has misnamed an object may recognize the appropriate name of the object when it is offered by the examiner. Further, having failed to name an object, patients can often say what it is used for (e.g., for *cup* they may say *drink*). In addition, they may be able to provide the generic properties of the word such as the letter it begins with and the number of syllables it contains (Goodglass, Kaplan, Weintraub, & Acker- man, 1976). Presumably, the representation of the word must be in the internal lexicon in order for the patient to be able to recall these properties.

Further insight into naming deficits can be provided by analyzing the types of misnaming errors a patient may make. When patients cannot name a particular stimulus, they may often substitute a word in the same semantic field or produce a word that is a semantic associate to the target (Rinnert & Whitaker, 1973) (e.g., for *chair*, they may say *sofa;* for *mother, father*). Nev- ertheless, although consistent with an access deficit, these results could also reflect a representation impairment. That is, if patients were operating with a restricted semantic field or a modified conceptual framework for lexical items, they could well access the appropriate semantic category without having a full sense of the word and its appropriate name. Semantically associated verbal paraphasias would then be a natural consequence of such a deficit.

Consistent with the view that patients' deficit reflects a representation impairment are results from a study by Zurif, Caramazza, Myerson, and Galvin (1974) who investigated patients' judgments about semantic related- ness. In particular, they asked subjects to group the two words of three that best went together. The words (mother, father, partner, knight, husband, shark, trout, dog, tiger, turtle, crocodile) varied along several semantic dimensions (human–nonhuman, gender, functional attribute). Results showed that neurologically intact control subjects grouped the words along these semantic dimensions; patients with Broca's aphasia did so, too, with only one minor exception. In contrast, patients with Wernicke's aphasia showed no specific pattern—they were as likely to group *mother* with *father* as *mother* with *trout*. These results were used as evidence supporting the view that patients with Wernicke's aphasia have an impairment in the underlying organization of the lexicon, hence a deficit in lexical representation (cf. Goodglass & Baker, 1976).

More recently, however, a series of studies have been conducted that challenge this view. These studies have explored on-line lexical processing by exploring semantic priming in a lexical decision task. Using an adapta- tion of a procedure developed by Meyer and Schvaneveldt (1971), the ex- perimenters asked aphasic patients to make a lexical decision about words and nonwords presented either visually (Milberg & Blumstein, 1981) or auditorily (Blumstein, Milberg, & Shrier, 1982). The target word to be judged (e.g., *dog*) was preceded by a prime that was semantically related (e.g., *cat*), semantically unrelated (e.g., *table*), or neutral that is, a nonword (e.g., *glub*) with respect to the prime. In both studies, patients with Wernicke's aphasia showed, as do control subjects, semantic facilitation, that is, they responded faster to a real-word target preceded by a semantically related prime than to one preceded by a semantically unrelated or nonword prime. Surprisingly, patients with Broca's aphasia did not show this semantic facilitation as consistently as did patients with Wernicke's aphasia. When the prime–target pairs included highly associated words, patients with Broca's aphasia showed evidence of priming (Blumstein et al., 1982). When the semantic relationships were more subtle, that is, ambiguous words (Milberg, Blumstein, & Dworetzky, 1987), or when the lexical decision target word was not temporally paired with the preceding prime (i.e., the subject was required to make a lexical decision response to each stimulus presented) (Milberg & Blumstein, 1981), they did not as a group show evidence of semantic priming. In contrast, when the same patients were asked to make judgments about the semantic relatedness of the word pairs, patients with Wernicke's aphasia performed randomly, and patients with Broca's aphasia performed well.

To account for the dichotomy between the performance of patients with Broca's and Wernicke's aphasia on these tasks, it was proposed that lexical deficits in aphasia are better characterized in terms of the processing operations required for lexical access, rather than on the integrity of the stored lexical knowledge base. In particular, it has been suggested that there are two distinct processes involved in lexical access, one called *automatic processing* that is fast acting, of short duration, not under voluntary control, and thus largely automatic, and a second called *controlled processing* that is slower acting, under a subject's voluntary control, and thus influenced by a subject's expectancies or attentional demands (Posner & Snyder, 1975; Shiffrin & Schneider, 1977). Subjects with Wernicke's aphasia show consistent evidence of semantic facilitation in the lexical decision tasks, but do not appear to be able to analyze word meaning in a simple semantic judgment task. Therefore, they seem to be able to automatically access words, and yet are unable to use the knowledge about semantic features or semantic relations in making decisions about the meanings of words. For subjects with Broca's aphasia, results are less clear-cut. The lack of consistent priming effects suggests that the automatic activation of lexical candidates may be impaired. However, these patients appear to have little difficulty analyzing word meaning using controlled processing. In fact, recent debate in the literature has centered on whether the impairment of subjects with Broca's aphasia reflects slowed access to lexical representations (Hagoort, 1993), or alternatively, a diminished activation of word candidates (Milberg, Blumstein, Katz, & Gershberg, 1995). Whatever the correct interpretation, it is worth noting that in both cases the explanation turns on the processing routines used for lexical access.

Similar results emerged in studying the time course of lexical access in sentences. Swinney, Zurif, and Nicol (1989) explored the extent to which aphasic patients use sentence context in accessing the meanings of ambiguous words. In a cross-modal lexical decision task in which the sentence is presented auditorily and the lexical target is presented visually, neurologically intact subjects show access to all meanings of an ambiguous word at its initial presentation even with a preceding biasing context toward one interpretation. Only further downstream is the meaning appropriate to the context uniquely retained. For example, in the sentence, *the man saw several spiders, roaches, and other bugs* (1) *in the corner* (2) *of the room,* subjects show semantic facilitation to all meanings of the word *bugs* (i.e., *ant* and *spy*) at time (1), but at time (2) show semantic facilitation only to *ant* (Onifer & Swinney, 1981). Swinney and his colleagues (1989) explored semantic facilitation in aphasic patients investigating whether they showed semantic facilitation to both meanings of an ambiguous word at time (1) [they did not investigate semantic facilitation downstream at time (2)]. They showed that similar to neurologically intact subjects, Wernicke's aphasia patients showed priming for both meanings of the ambiguous words at time (1), irrespective of the biasing context. In contrast, patients with Broca's aphasia showed semantic facilitation only to the most frequent meaning of the ambiguous word regardless of the biasing context. Thus, while patients with Broca's aphasia clearly show an impairment in accessing word meanings from the lexicon, similar to control subjects and Wernicke's aphasia patients, such access is *not* affected by the sentence context in which the word appears.

Evidence consistent with the observation that the emergence of word meaning is influenced by contextual factors and is not all-or-none comes from ERP studies, beginning with the seminal work of Kutas and Hillyard (1980). In a series of studies, they showed that while there are no ERP "signatures" tied to either a specific word such as *dog* or a semantic category such as *fruit,* there is a marker, the N400, which is sensitive to semantic anomaly and semantic expectations (e.g., *I take my coffee with cream and dog*). The N400 is a time-locked component that occurs between 350 and 800 ms after stimulus presentation. The N400 emerges whether the anomaly occurs in sentence-final or sentence-medial position, and whether the anomaly is in a sentence or in a more natural prose context (Kutas & Hillyard, 1980, 1983).

Of critical importance, the N400 "marker" relates specifically to semantics; it does not emerge for syntactic anomalies (i.e., tense or number errors) nor for physical changes to the stimulus (i.e., unexpected differences such as change of letter size) (Kutas & Hillyard, 1983). Moreover, lexical processing is dependent on the activation level of candidate lexical items. In particular, ERP studies have shown that the amplitude of the N400 varies as a function of the likelihood that a word will appear in a context. The N400 significantly decreases if an anomalous word is semantically related to an appropriate completion; for example, in *the game was called off because it started to umbrella, umbrella* is semantically related to the word *rain,* the natural completion of the sentence, and thus shows a significantly smaller N400 than for *coffee,* which bears no semantic relationships between *coffee* and the natural completion of the sentence. These results suggest that lexical access is graded, changing as a function of the level of activation of a word candidate (Kutas & Hillyard, 1984) and the extent to which the word candidate activates a semantic network (Kutas, Lindamood, & Hillyard, 1984). These priming effects also emerge for single words; the N400 is larger to weakly primed versus strongly primed lexical associates and is larger to unrelated than to related words (Kutas & Hillyard, 1988).

PET studies also provide important converging evidence concerning the processing components involved in lexical access (Petersen, et al., 1988, 1989; Posner, Petersen, Fox, & Raichle, 1988). These studies have shown the involvement of anterior brain structures in the semantic processing of single words in non-brain-damaged subjects, a result consistent with the impairments shown in lexical priming for Broca's aphasia subjects described above. They also showed the role of different brain areas in the perception of visually and auditorily presented words, even though each share access to a common output (articulatory) and meaning (semantic) system. Thus, the PET studies show that the performance of cognitive tasks requires the integration of a large number of component computations and in this sense such tasks seem not to be performed in a single area of the brain.

Taken together, the results of studies with aphasic patients and with neurologically intact subjects using both ERP and PET suggest that the neural basis of lexical processing is indeed complex. Both anterior and posterior brain structures seem to be involved in lexical access, although to date it is not clear what the contributions of these various structures are to lexical access and lexical processing. What does seem to be the case is that there are neurophysiological markers related to access of meaning. Moreover, lexical impairments seem to reflect deficits in lexical access and not lexical representation. A point of interest is that the processing components contributing to lexical access may be affected differently as a function of the type of aphasia and presumably as a function of the different neural structures involved.

IV. SYNTAX

Nearly all aphasic patients display syntactic impairments in their speech output. Nevertheless, the hallmark of syntactic production deficits is characterized by patients with Broca's aphasia, who clinically are often described as *agrammatic* or *telegrammatic* in their speech production. The speech output of these patients is typically nonfluent and syntactically sparse in terms of both the array of grammatical structures produced and the absence of grammatical endings such as plurals, tense markers, and free-standing grammatical words such as *the* and *have*. One critical issue is determining the basis of this agrammatic deficit. Three hypotheses have been proposed. The first suggests that the deficit reflects an economizing effort on the part of the patient to compensate for expressive difficulties and effortful speech production (Lenneberg, 1973). The second proposes that the grammatical deficit is secondary to a phonological impairment related to phonological stress (Kean, 1977). The third considers the deficit to reflect a fundamental impairment in syntax related to either the representation or processing of syntactic structures (Caplan, Baker, & Dehaut, 1985; Grodzinsky, 1990; and see Bock, Chapter 6, and Tanenhaus and Trueswell, Chapter 7, this volume). Let us explore the evidence that bears on this issue.

Analysis of data from agrammatic patients across different languages provides a first window into the possible basis of the syntactic deficit. Languages of the world implement syntactic structure in quite different ways; English depends highly on word order to implement syntactic functions such as subject or object of the verb (e.g., *John kissed Mary* vs. *Mary kissed John*); other languages are highly inflected, such as Russian or German, and use inflectional endings to mark the functions of subject and direct object; languages such as Japanese are agglutinative and mark such syntactic functions by using particles appended to word stems; still others such as Hebrew or Arabic are infixing languages and mark syntactic structures by changes on vowels within the word stem itself. It is interesting that agrammatic aphasia patients display syntactic deficits regardless of the language they speak and the way the language instantiates syntax (Menn & Obler, 1990). Thus, all of these patients display impairments with syntactic structures whether they are realized in terms of word order, inflectional endings, particles, or infixes. These results suggest that the agrammatic deficit may more likely reflect either a compensatory production mechanism or alternatively a syntactic deficit. The explanation that the deficit is a phonological one is less likely because of the very different phonetic/phonological manifestations of the syntactic properties relating to phonological stress across these different languages.

Perhaps more important, these results suggest that there are particular neural structures that are dedicated to the instantiation of a linguistic *function*, namely syntax, and these neural structures lie in Broca's area and the surrounding cortical and subcortical neural structures. Thus, syntactic deficits emerge with damage to similar neural structures irrespective of the different ways syntax may be realized in language, whether by word order, inflection, agglutination, or infixing. In this sense, syntax is marked neurologically. Additional support for this view comes from the language patterns of congenitally deaf signers who sustain brain damage to these same neural structures. These patients also display agrammatic deficits, in this case relating to the syntactic properties of sign (Corina, Vaid, & Bellugi, 1992). In American Sign Language (ASL), syntax is marked by certain hand-shape and movement configurations. The only common attribute between hand-shape and movement configurations in ASL and word order, infixing, and agglutination in aural/oral language is the syntactic function these attributes play in language.

Further analysis of productive agrammatism also reveals that it is characterized by the substitution of syntactic particles or endings for each other rather than the "loss" of these endings. For example, in English the singular form for a word is characterized phonologically by a zero marker [i.e., boy + $\emptyset$ (singular)], whereas the plural is determined by the addition of the plural form /s/ to the word stem [i.e., boy + /s/ (plural)]; thus, for English it is impossible to ascertain whether the production of the singular *boy* for the plural *boys* reflects the *loss* of the plural form or alternatively the *substitution* of the singular (zero) morphological ending for the plural. However, in other languages such as Russian, German, Japanese, Hebrew, and Arabic, the stem itself does not appear alone and all words must be marked with a morphological ending. Thus, it is possible to determine whether the agrammatic patient's production reflects the loss or substitution of a morphological marker. Results show that in these languages, agrammatic patients always use a syntactic marker, albeit from time to time, the wrong marker (Menn & Obler, 1990); thus, the syntactic markers are not lost but rather are substituted for each other. These results lend credence to the view that the basis of the agrammatic deficit is primarily a syntactic one and not an economizing effort by the patient to reduce the amount of language output.

Additional evidence supports the view that agrammatism is primarily a syntactic deficit. In addition to the deficit with morphology described above, agrammatic patients also display a reduction in the variety of syntactic structures that they use, as well as a failure to concatenate phrases that constitute a sentence. Thus, patients have great difficulty in juxtaposing the noun phrase (NP) and verb phrase (VP) of a sentence, while they may still be able to maintain the internal cohesion of the NP itself by using adjectives and the VP itself by concatenating the verb with a following object. Moreover, the occurrence of more complex sentences and phrases containing embeddings and compound nouns and verbs is rare. The failure to produce these syntactic structures, however, does not seem to reflect a loss of the "knowledge" of these structures. Goodglass, Gleason, Bernholtz, and Hyde (1972) have shown that patients may use alternative strategies to convey a meaning that they seem to be unable to express using a given syntactic structure. For example, given a structured story completion test designed to elicit a broad array of syntactic structures, patients may use reduplication to connote *very* (i.e., *hot hot* for *very hot*), use an adverbial to connote verb tense (i.e., *yesterday he go* for *he went*), or use descriptive adjectives instead of comparatives (i.e., *Mary weak, Bob strong* for *Bob is stronger than Mary*) (Gleason, Goodglass, Green, Ackerman, & Hyde, 1975; Goodglass et al., 1972).

Perhaps one of the strongest pieces of evidence suggesting that agrammatic deficits reflect an underlying syntactic impairment comes from a study by Zurif, Caramazza, and Myerson (1972) who explored whether agrammatic patients could use syntactic structures properly if given the opportunity and time. They provided the first evidence that patients with Broca's aphasia have a syntactic comprehension impairment as well as a syntactic production deficit. Specifically, they asked patients to judge how words in a written sentence "go best together." Subjects were required to cluster or put together the two words of an array of three taken from a presented sentence. Neurologically intact subjects group words very much as linguists, organizing them in terms of the syntactic relations that they hold in the sentence; thus, given the sentence, *the dog chases a cat,* a control subject clusters the determiner *the* with the noun *dog,* and clusters the verb *chases* with the direct object *a cat.* In contrast, patients with agrammatic aphasia do not seem to know what to do with the "little words." They are as likely to cluster *the* with *a* or *chases* as they are with *dog.* Thus, they show not only a failure to produce and use the grammatical words in speech production, but they also fail to use them appropriately when asked to identify the relationships among the words in a sentence.

Further studies have supported this observation that agrammatic patients have difficulty in using syntactic structures in language comprehension as well as production. In particular, these studies have examined the processing and comprehension of grammatical words and syntactic structures by patients with Broca's aphasia. One study explored the processing of the definite and indefinite articles *a* and *the* in English. If neurologically intact are presented with a square and two circles and are required to press either a square or round button, they show a shorter reaction time to the command, "press a round one" than to the command "press the round one," presumably because reference to one of the two circles requires the use of an indefinite article. In contrast, agrammatic aphasia patients show no differences in reaction time to the two commands "press a round one" and "press the round one," suggesting that they do not appropriately process the meaning difference between the two articles (Goodenough, Zurif, & Weintraub, 1977). In other research (Caramazza & Zurif, 1976), patients with Broca's aphasia showed comprehension deficits in understanding subject–object relations in embedded sentences in a picture-pointing task. It is interesting that these deficits emerged only when the test sentences were stripped of other potential semantic cues that could be used by the subjects. That is, their deficit emerged in the context of semantically reversible sentences such as *the clown chases the midget,* and not when the meaning of the sentence was constrained by semantic and real-world probabilities such as *the man patted the dog.*

The fact that most agrammatic aphasia patients display a syntactic comprehension deficit as well as a syntactic production deficit (but cf. Miceli, Mazzucchi, Menn, & Goodglass, 1983) suggests that a single impairment, namely, a central syntactic impairment, underlies their language difficulty. The deficit is considered "central" because it affects syntax independent of its language modality—speaking, comprehending, reading, and writing. As to the specific nature of this syntactic deficit, recent research has suggested that the impairment is more likely a deficit in syntactic processing than it is a deficit in syntactic representation. Several lines of research contribute to this view (although cf. Caplan et al., 1985, and Caplan & Futter, 1986, Grodzinsky, 1984, 1986, for alternative points of view). Patients who are agrammatic in both production and comprehension, nonetheless are able to make grammaticality judgments (Linebarger, Schwartz, & Saffran, 1983). Thus, these patients are able to judge the grammaticality of sentences that violate different types of syntactic structures, for example, *he shut the window that the door was open* (gapless relatives), *the girls laughed the clown* (subcategorization), and *my father knew they would give the job to* (empty elements). This relatively spared ability to make syntactic judgments in the face of grammatical comprehension and production deficits for the same type of syntactic structures suggests that syntactic representations are intact. The comprehension and production impairments probably reflect the fact that these patients have a processing deficit affecting the "mapping" of syntactic structures onto their appropriate semantic representations.

Consistent with this view are the results of several on-line syntactic processing experiments. These studies have shown that agrammatic aphasia patients do not show a sensitivity to morphological constraints that non-brain-damaged control subjects show. In particular, unlike control subjects, they fail to show faster reaction times in a lexical decision task to verbs when preceded by a grammatically appropriate modal (e.g., *is–going*) than when preceded by a grammatically inappropriate modal (e.g., *could–going*) (Blumstein, Milberg, Dworetzky, Rosen, & Gershberg, 1991). Nonetheless, these same patients show an ability to make correct syntactic judgments of these same verb phrases in an off-line grammaticality judgment task. Similarly, Friederici and Kilborn (1989) showed a delay in accessing syntactic information specified by morphological endings in subjects with Broca's aphasia compared to syntactic information provided by individual lexical items.

That the syntactic processing impairment extends beyond the processing of morphological constraints has also been shown. In particular, Baum (1988) showed that subjects with Broca's aphasia did not show sensitivity to the types of syntactic violations explored by Linebarger et al. in an on-line processing lexical decision task even though they were still able to make correct grammaticality judgments (cf. also Tyler, 1985). An interesting point is that the processing impairment does not seem to affect all of syntactic processing. Some syntactic processes seem to be normal, in particular, the processing of filler-gap constructions. In particular, it has been shown in neurologically intact subjects that processing and ultimately the comprehension of syntactically complex sentences such as relative clauses require that the syntactic processor identify the underlying syntactic structure and syntactic relations of the words in the sentence. In the case of relative clause sentences such as *this is the girl that John hit, girl* has been moved from its underlying syntactic position as object of the verb *hit,* leaving a gap or empty element after the verb *hit.* To process the sentence and to determine the correct syntactic relations, the listener must identify the gap, and the filler, in this case *girl,* associated with it, and assign it to its correct syntactic position (as object of the verb). For example, in the sentence *the car that the old lady was selling __ needed many repairs, the car* has been moved from its position as object of the verb leaving a gap (_) following *selling.* If subjects are reactivating the filler *car* at the gap site, then they should show semantic facilitation for the filler *car* even if the semantically related word is presented in the position of the gap site (after *selling*), some eight syllables downstream from the actual occurrence of *car.* Both neurologically intact subjects (Tanenhaus, Carlson, & Seidenberg, 1985) and subjects with Broca's aphasia (Blumstein, Byma, Hourihan, & Brown, in preparation) show evidence of reactivation of the filler at the gap site. Thus, impairment in comprehending *Wh*-constructions is more likely due to an access deficit than an impairment in the syntactic representations themselves.

While the major focus on syntactic deficits in aphasia has been on agrammatism in Broca's aphasia, grammatical deficits in both production and comprehension are also common in Wernicke's aphasia. Investigations of the speech production of patients with Wernicke's aphasia indicate that these patients often show paragrammatic speech exemplified by the juxtaposition of inappropriate grammatical phrases (e.g., *I saw him to the boy*). Moreover, they also show a restricted range of syntactic structure in their speech output (Gleason et al., 1980). With respect to auditory language comprehension, patients with Wernicke's aphasia also show syntactic impairments, and in fact, show similar patterns of performance to that of patients with Broca's aphasia in their comprehension of a number of critical dimensions including morphological endings, syntactic structures, syntactic complexity, and real-world plausibility (Caplan et al., 1985; Goodglass, 1968; Goodglass & Menn, 1985; Lesser, 1978; Parisi and Pizzamiglio, 1970).

What remains unclear is whether these similar patterns of performance between patients with Broca's and Wernicke's aphasia reflect different underlying impairments. Several researchers (Caplan et al., 1985; Goodglass & Menn, 1985) have suggested that the syntactic deficit of Wernicke's aphasia is similar to that of Broca's aphasia. Nevertheless, these conclusions may be premature. Several researchers have shown dissociations in patterns of performance between patients with Broca's and Wernicke's aphasia (Blumstein, Goodglass, Statlender, & Biber, 1983; Goodglass et al., 1979; von Stockert, 1972; Zurif & Caramazza, 1976), and more recent on-line experiments suggest that the nature of the processing impairments between these two groups may indeed by different (cf. Blumstein et al., 1991). Nonetheless, on-line syntactic processing research in aphasia is in its infancy and much more research will be needed before the nature of these processing deficits can be elaborated.

That there are particular processing operations related to filler-gap constructions is supported by recent ERP investigations. Garnsey, Tanenhaus, and Chapman (1989) used the emergence of an N400 for semantic anomalies to explore syntactic processing of filler-gap constructions. They showed that the filler in *Wh*-constructions is attached at the first possible gap site immediately after the verb. Thus, syntactic processing operations also leave electrophysiological markers, although they are not the same as those shown in lexical/semantic processing (Rosleer, Putz, Friederici, & Hahne, 1993).

The exploration of such syntactic markers has just begun. There is some preliminary evidence to suggest that there may be different electrophysiological patterns to types of syntactic anomalies relating to violations of phrase structure, *wh*-extraction, and subjacency rules (Neville, Nicol, Barss, Forster, & Garrett, 1991). Whether there is a particular marker for syntactic anomalies as was shown in the N400 for semantic anomalies is less clear. A potential component termed P600 has recently been identified, which emerges in the processing of certain types of syntactic anomalies (Osterhut & Holcomb, 1994). Clearly, more work needs to be done, but this research direction shows great potential for providing important insights into the processing mechanisms underlying syntax.

In sum, results from studies with aphasic patients suggest that syntactic representations are intact and that these patients display deficits in accessing these structures. Although most attention has been payed to the syntactic deficit accompanying agrammatism in patients with Broca's aphasia, patients with Wernicke's aphasia also display syntactic production and comprehension deficits. With respect to agrammatic aphasia patients, syntactic output disorders emerge with damage to anterior brain structures and these deficits occur irrespective of the grammatical structure of the particular language. Nonetheless, for both Broca's and Wernicke's aphasia patients, syntactic impairments typically affect language production as well as language comprehension. In the case of language production, patients often produce agrammatic or paragrammatic speech. In the case of language comprehension, the impairment seems to reflect a processing deficit affecting the ability to map syntactic structures onto semantic representations, presumably contributing to the language comprehension deficit of these patients. Consistent with this view are the results of recent ERP studies showing electrophysiological markers for syntactic processing and perhaps also for particular syntactic structures.

V. SUMMARY

Investigation of the neurobiology of language provides support for the view that the organization of the language system is indeed complex. All aphasic patients display phonological, lexical, and syntactic deficits regardless of aphasia type and lesion localization, suggesting that the neural instantiation of these linguistic components requires complex neural structures that are represented throughout the left hemisphere. Consideration of the neurobiology of the sound structure of language and, especially, the studies of aphasic patients suggest that the organization and ultimate implementation of the phonological sound structure is broadly represented in the left dominant hemisphere and deficits relate to selection and planning in speech production and access in speech perception. In contrast, as shown by studies of patients with aphasia and results of PET and ERP investigations, the phonetic implementation of speech seems to be subserved by specific neural substrates, and phonetic deficits reflect impairments in particular articulatory movements rather than in underlying linguistic features. With respect to the neurobiology of the lexicon and syntax, ERP and PET studies provide support for electrophysiological markers for lexical meaning and syntactic structures, and, in conjunction with data from aphasic patients, suggest that with the possible exception of productive agrammatism, the neural basis of the lexicon and syntax is broadly represented. Studies of both lexical and syntactic impairments show that these deficits emerge in both production and comprehension, and they reflect impairments to the processing mechanisms accessing lexical and/or syntactic structures rather than deficits to the representations or structures themselves.

Although this chapter has used a modular approach to language as a theoretical framework by studying separately phonology, the lexicon, and syntax, the results of this research suggest that there is little evidence to support the view that the organization of the language system itself is modular. In particular, language impairments in aphasia reflect processing disorders that cut across the linguistic components of the grammar including phonology, the lexicon, and syntax. Language impairments in aphasia are not selective with respect to a particular component of the grammar nor do they reflect impairments to particular linguistic representations. More specifically they reflect impairments to those processing routines used to access this information. This view is consistent with clinical and experimental findings showing similar patterns of linguistic impairment across different aphasia groups, and also accounts for the fact that nearly all aphasic patients show some degree of deficit in phonological, lexical, and syntactic processing, although the constellation of abilities and disabilities that these patients display is nevertheless quite different.

Future work requires greater integration of clinical and experimental findings with results from electrophysiological, metabolic, and neuroimaging studies with both neurologically intact and brain-damaged patients. Together, they will provide a window into one of the most challenging areas in cognitive neuroscience—the understanding of the neurobiology of human language.

Acknowledgment

This research was supported in part by NIH Grant DC00314 to Brown University.

References

Baker, E., Blumstein, S. E., & Goodglass, H. (1981). Interaction between phonological and semantic factors in auditory comprehension. *Neuropsychologia, 19*, 1–16.

Basso, A., Casati, G., & Vignolo, L. A. (1977). Phonemic identification defects in aphasia. *Cortex, 13*, 84–95.

Baum, S. R. (1988). Syntactic processing in agrammatism: Evidence from lexical decision and grammaticality judgement tasks. *Aphasiology, 2*, 117–135.

Baum, S. R., Blumstein, S. E., Naeser, M. A., & Palumbo, C. L. (1990). Temporal dimensions of consonant and vowel production: An acoustic and CT scan analysis of aphasic speech. *Brain and Language, 39*, 33–56.

Baum, S. R., Kelsch Daniloff, J., & Daniloff, R. (1982). Sentence comprehension by Broca's aphasics: Effects of some suprasegmental variables. *Brain and Language, 17*, 261–271.

Blumstein, S. E. (1973). *A phonological investigation of aphasic speech*. The Hague: Mouton.

Blumstein, S. E. (1990). Phonological deficits in aphasia: Theoretical perspectives. In A. Caramazza (Ed.), *Cognitive neuropsychology and neurolinguistics: Advances in models of cognitive function and impairment*. Hillsdale: Erlbaum.

Blumstein, S. E., Baker, E., & Goodglass, H. (1977). Phonological factors in auditory comprehension in aphasia. *Neuropsychologia, 15*, 19–30.

Blumstein, S. E., Burton, M., Baum, S., Waldstein, R., & Katz, D. (1994). The role of lexical status on the phonetic categorization of speech in aphasia. *Brain and Language, 46*, 181–197.

Blumstein, S. E., Byma, G., Hourihan, J., & Brown, T. (1994). On-line processing of filler-gap constructions in aphasia, manuscript in preparation, Brown University.

Blumstein, S. E., Cooper, W. E., Goodglass, H., Statlender, S., & Gottlieb, J. (1980). Production deficits in aphasia: A voice-onset time analysis. *Brain and Language, 9*, 153–170.

Blumstein, S. E., Cooper, W. E., Zurif, E. B., & Caramazza, A. (1977). The perception and production of voice-onset time in aphasia. *Neuropsychologia, 15*, 371–383.

Blumstein, S. E., Goodglass, H., Statlender, S., & Biber, C. (1983). Comprehension strategies determining reference in aphasia: A study of reflexivization. *Brain and Language, 18,* 115–127.

Blumstein, S. E., Milberg, W. P., Dworetzky, B., Rosen, A., & Gershberg, F. (1991). Syntactic priming effects in aphasia: An investigation of local syntactic dependencies. *Brain and Language, 40,* 393–421.

Blumstein, S., Milberg, W., & Shrier, R. (1982). Semantic processing in aphasia: Evidence from an auditory lexical decision task. *Brain and Language, 17,* 301–315.

Blumstein, S. E., Tartter, V. C., Nigro, G., & Statlender, S. (1984). Acoustic cues for the perception of place of articulation in aphasia. *Brain and Language, 22,* 128–149.

Boatman, D., Lesser, P. R., & Gordon, B. (1994). The functional organization of auditory speech processing as revealed by direct cortical electrical interference. *Journal of the Acoustical Society of America,* in press.

Bouman, L., & Grunbaum, A. (1925). Experimentell-psychologische Untersuchungen sur Aphasie und Paraphasie. *Zeitschrift für die Gesamte Neurologie und Psychiatrie, 96,* 481–538.

Caplan, D., Baker, C., & Dehaut, F. (1985). Syntactic determinants of sentence comprehension in aphasia. *Cognition, 21,* 117–175.

Caplan, D., & Futter, C. (1986). Assignment of thematic roles to nouns in sentence comprehension in an agrammatic patient. *Brain and Language, 27,* 117–134.

Caramazza, A. (1984). The logic of neuropsychological research and the problem of patient classification in aphasia. *Brain and Language, 21,* 9–20.

Caramazza, A., & Zurif, E. B. (1976). Dissociation of algorithmic and heuristic processes in language comprehension: Evidence from aphasia. *Brain and Language, 3,* 572–582.

Cooper, W. E., Soares, C., Nicol, J., Michelow, D., & Goloskie, S. (1984). Clausal intonation after unilateral brain damage. *Language & Speech, 27,* 17–24.

Corina, D. P., Vaid, J., & Bellugi, U. (1992). The linguistic basis of left hemisphere specialization. *Science, 255,* 1258.

Damasio, H. (1991). Neuroanatomical correlates of the aphasia. In M. T. Sarno (Ed.), *Acquired aphasia* (2nd ed.). San Diego, CA: Academic Press.

Duffy, J., & Gawle, C. (1984). Apraxic speakers' vowel duration in consonant-vowel-consonant syllables. In J. Rosenbek, M. McNeil, & A. Aronson (Eds.), *Apraxia of speech.* San Diego, CA: College-Hill Press.

Emmorey, K. D. (1987). The neurological substrates for prosodic aspects of speech. *Brain and Language, 30,* 305–320.

Fodor, J. A. (1983). *The modularity of mind.* Cambridge, MA: MIT Press.

Freeman, F. J., Sands, E. S., & Harris, K. S. (1978). Temporal coordination of phonation and articulation in a case of verbal apraxia: A voice-onset time analysis. *Brain and Language, 6,* 106–111.

Friederici, A. D., & Kilborn, K. (1989). Temporal constraints on language processing: Syntactic priming in Broca's aphasia. *Journal of Cognitive Neuroscience, 1,* 262–272.

Gandour, J., & Dardarananda, R. (1982). Voice onset time in aphasia: Thai. I. Perception. *Brain and Language, 17,* 24–33.

Gandour, J., & Dardarananda, R. (1983). Identification of tonal contrasts in Thai aphasic patients. *Brain and Language, 17,* 24–33.

Gandour, J., & Dardarananda, R. (1984a). Voice-onset time in aphasia: Thai. II: Production. *Brain and Language, 18,* 389–410.

Gandour, J., & Dardarananda, R. (1984b). Prosodic disturbances in aphasia: Vowel length in Thai. *Brain and Language, 23,* 177–205.

Gandour, J., Ponglorpisit, S., Khunadorn, F., Dechongkit, S., Boongird, P., & Boonklam, R. (1992). Timing characteristics of speech after brain damage: Vowel length in Thai. *Brain and Language, 42,* 337–345.

Ganong, W. F. (1980). Phonetic categorization in auditory word perception. *Journal of Experimental Psychology: Human Perception and Performance, 6,* 110–125.

Gardner, H. (1983). *Frames of mind: The theory of multiple intelligences.* New York: Basic Books.

Garnsey, S. M., Tanenhaus, M., & Chapman, R. (1989). Evoked potentials and the study of sentence comprehension. *Journal of Psycholinguistic Research, 18,* 51–60.

Garrett, M. (1979). Levels of processing in sentence production. In B. Butterworth (Ed.), *Language production.* London: Academic Press.

Geschwind, N. (1965). Disconnexion syndromes in animals and man. *Brain, 88,* 237–294, 585–644.

Gleason, J. B., Goodglass, H., Green, E., Ackerman, N., & Hyde, M. (1975). The retrieval of syntax in Broca's aphasia. *Brain and Language, 2,* 451–471.

Gleason, J. B., Goodglass, H., Obler, L., Green, E., Hyde, M., & Weintraub, S. (1980). Narrative strategies of aphasic and normal speaking subjects. *Journal of Speech and Hearing Research, 23,* 370–383.

Goldstein, K. (1948). *Language and language disturbances.* New York: Grune & Stratton.

Goodenough, C., Zurif, E., & Weintraub, S. (1977). Aphasics' attention to grammatical morphemes. *Language & Speech, 20,* 11–19.

Goodglass, H. (1968). Studies on the grammar of aphasics. In S. Rosenberg & J. H. Koplin (Eds.), *Developments in applied psycholinguistic research.* New York: Macmillan.

Goodglass, H., & Baker, E. (1976). Semantic field, naming, and auditory comprehension in aphasia. *Brain and Language, 3,* 359–374.

Goodglass, H., Blumstein, S. E., Gleason, J. B., Hyde, M. R., Green, E., & Statlender, S. (1979). The effect of syntactic encoding on sentence comprehension in aphasia. *Brain and Language, 7,* 201–209.

Goodglass, H., Gleason, J., Bernholtz, N. A., & Hyde, M. R. (1972). Some linguistic structures in the speech of a Broca's aphasic. *Cortex, 8,* 191–212.

Goodglass, H., Hyde, M. R., & Blumstein, S. (1969). Frequency, picturability and the availability of nouns in aphasia. *Cortex, 5,* 104–119.

Goodglass, H., & Kaplan, E. (1972). *The assessment of aphasia and related disorders.* Philadelphia: Lea & Febiger.

Goodglass, H., Kaplan, E., Weintraub, S., & Ackerman, N. (1976). The 'tip-of-the-tongue' phenomenon in aphasia. *Cortex, 12,* 145–153.

Goodglass, H., & Menn, L. (1985). Is agrammatism a unitary phenomenon? In M. L. Kean (Ed.), *Agrammatism.* New York: Academic Press.

Green, E. (1969). Phonological and grammatical aspects of jargon in an aphasic patient: A case study. *Language & Speech, 12,* 103–118.

Green, E., & Boller, F. (1974). Features of auditory comprehension in severely impaired aphasics. *Cortex, 10,* 133–145.

Grodzinsky, Y. (1984). The syntactic characterization of agrammatism. *Cognition, 16,* 99–120.

Grodzinsky, Y. (1986). Language deficits and the theory of syntax. *Brain and Language, 27,* 135–159.

Grodzinsky, Y. (1990). *Theoretical perspectives on language deficits.* Cambridge, MA: MIT Press.

Hagoort, P. (1993). Impairments of lexical-semantic processing in aphasia: Evidence from the processing of lexical ambiguities. *Brain and Language, 45,* 189–232.

Harmes, S., Daniloff, R., Hoffman, P., Lewis, J., Kramer, M., & Absher, R. (1984). Temporal and articulatory control of fricative articulation by speakers with Broca's aphasia. *Journal of Phonetics, 12,* 367–385.

Hart, J., Berndt, R. S., & Caramazza, A. (1985). Category-specific naming deficit following cerebral infraction. *Nature (London), 316,* 439–440.

Hatfield, F. M., & Walton, K. (1975). Phonological patterns in a case of aphasia. *Language & Speech, 18,* 341–357.

Head, H. (1963). *Aphasia and kindred disorders of speech* (Vol. 1). New York: Hafner.

Howes, D. (1964). Application of the word frequency concept to aphasia. In A. V. S. de Reuck & M. O'Connor (Eds.), *Disorders of language*. London: Churchill.

Irigary, L. (1967). Approche psycholinguistique de langage des dements. *Neuropsychologia, 5,* 25–32.

Itoh, M., Sasanuma, S., Hirose, H., Yoshioka, H., & Ushijima, T. (1980). Abnormal articulatory dynamics in a patient with apraxia of speech. *Brain and Language, 11,* 66–75.

Itoh, M., Sasanuma, S., Tatsumi, I., Murakami, S., Fukusako, Y., & Suzuki, T. (1982). Voice onset time characteristics in apraxia of speech. *Brain and Language, 17,* 193–210.

Itoh, M., Sasanuma, S., & Ushijima, T. (1979). Velar movements during speech in a patient with apraxia of speech. *Brain and Language, 7,* 227–239.

Jauhiainen, T., & Nuutila, A. (1977). Auditory perception of speech and speech sounds in recent and recovered aphasia. *Brain and Language, 4,* 572–579.

Katz, W. F. (1987). Anticipatory labial and lingual coarticulation in aphasia. In J. Ryalls (Ed.), *Phonetic approaches in speech production in aphasia and related disorders*. Boston: College-Hill Press.

Katz, W. F. (1988). Anticipatory coarticulatory in aphasia: Acoustic and perceptual data. *Brain and Language, 35,* 340–368.

Kean, M. L. (1977). The linguistic interpretation of aphasia syndromes: Agrammatism in Broca's aphasia. *Cognition, 5,* 9–46.

Kent, R., & McNeill, M. (1987). Relative timing of sentence repetition in apraxia of speech and conduction aphasia. In J. Ryalls (Ed.), *Phonetic approaches to speech production in aphasia and related disorders*. Boston: College-Hill Press.

Kent, R., & Rosenbek, J. (1983). Acoustic patterns of apraxia of speech. *Journal of Speech and Hearing Research, 26,* 231–248.

Kutas, M., & Hillyard, S. A. (1980). Reading senseless sentences: Brain potentials reflect semantic incongruity. *Science, 207,* 203–205.

Kutas, M., & Hillyard, S. A. (1983). Event-related potentials to grammatical errors and semantic anomalies. *Memory & Cognition, 11,* 539–550.

Kutas, M., & Hillyard, S. A. (1984). Brain potentials during reading reflect word expectancy and semantic association. *Nature (London), 307,* 161–163.

Kutas, M., & Hillyard, S. (1988). An electrophysiological probe of incidental semantic association. *Journal of Cognitive Neuroscience, 1,* 38–49.

Kutas, M., Lindamood, T., & Hillyard, S. (1984). Word expectancy and event-related brain potentials during sentence processing. In S. Kornblum & J. Requin (Eds.), *Preparatory states and processes*. Hillsdale, NJ: Erlbaum.

Lauter, J., Herscovitch, P., Formby, C., & Raichle, M. E. (1985). Tonotopic organization in human auditory cortex revealed by positron emission tomography. *Hearing Research, 20,* 199–205.

Lecours, A. R., & Lhermitte, F. (1969). Phonemic paraphasias: Linguistic structures and tentative hypotheses. *Cortex, 5,* 193–228.

Lenneberg, E. (1973). The neurology of language. *Daedalus, 102,* 115–133.

Lesser, R. (1978). *Linguistic investigations of aphasia*. London: Arnold.

Linebarger, M., Schwartz, M., & Saffran, E. (1983). Sensitivity to grammatical structure in so-called agrammatic aphasics. *Cognition, 13,* 361–392.

Luria, A. R. (1966). *Higher cortical functions in man*. New York: Basic Books.

Martin, A. D., Wasserman, N. H., Gilden, L., & West, J. (1975). A process model of repetition in aphasia: An investigation of phonological and morphological interactions in aphasic error performance. *Brain and Language, 2,* 434–450.

McAdam, D. W., & Whitaker, H. A. (1971). Language production: Electroencephalographic localization in the normal human brain. *Science, 172,* 499–502.

Menn, L., & Obler, L. (1990). *Agrammatic aphasia* (Vols. 1–3). Amsterdam: John Benjamins.

Meyer, D. E., & Schvaneveldt, R. W. (1971). Facilitation in recognizing pairs of words; Evidence of a dependence between retrieval operations. *Journal of Experimental Psychology, 90,* 227–234.

Miceli, G., Caltagirone, C., Gainotti, G., & Payer-Rigo, P. (1978). Discrimination of voice versus place contrasts in aphasia. *Brain and Language, 2,* 434–450.

Miceli, G., Gainotti, G., Caltagirone, C., & Masullo, C. (1980). Some aspects of phonological impairment in aphasia. *Brain and Language, 11,* 159–169.

Miceli, G., Mazzucchi, A., Menn, L., & Goodglass, H. (1983). Contrasting cases of Italian agrammatic aphasia without comprehension disorder. *Brain and Language, 19,* 65–97.

Milberg, W., & Blumstein, S. (1981). Lexical decision and aphasia: Evidence for semantic processing. *Brain and Language, 14,* 371–385.

Milberg, W., Blumstein, S., & Dworetzky, B. (1987). Processing of lexical ambiguities in aphasia. *Brain and Language, 31,* 138–150.

Milberg, W., Blumstein, S. E., & Dworetzky, B. (1988). Phonological processing and lexical access in aphasia. *Brain and Language, 34,* 279–293.

Milberg, W., Blumstein, S. E., Katz, D., & Gershberg, F. (1995). Semantic facilitation in aphasia: Effects of time and expectancy. *Journal of Cognitive Neuroscience,* in press.

Miller, G. A., & Nicely, P. E. (1955). An analysis of perceptual confusions among some English consonants. *Journal of the Acoustical Society of America, 27,* 338–352.

Naeser, M. A., & Chan, S. W.-C. (1980). Case study of a Chinese aphasic with the Boston Diagnostic Aphasia Examination. *Neuropsychologia, 18,* 389–410.

Neville, H., Nicol, J., Barss, A., Forster, K. I., & Garrett, M. F. (1991). Syntactically based sentence processing classes: Evidence from event-related brain potentials. *Journal of Cognitive Neuroscience, 3,* 151–165.

Niemi, J., Koivuselka-Sallinen, P., & Hanninen, R. (1985). Phoneme errors in Broca's aphasia: Three Finnish cases. *Brain and Language, 26,* 28–48.

Ojemann, G. A. (1983). Brain organization for language from the perspective of electrical stimulation mapping. *Behavioral and Brain Sciences, 6,* 189–230.

Onifer, W., & Swinney, D. A. (1981). Accessing lexical ambiguities during sentence comprehension: Effects of frequency of meaning and contextual bias. *Memory & Cognition, 9,* 225–236.

Osterhut, L., & Holcomb, P. (1994). Event-related brain potentials elicited by syntactic anomaly. *Journal of Memory and Language, 31,* 785–806.

Parisi, D., & Pizzamiglio, L. (1970). Syntactic comprehension in aphasia. *Cortex, 6,* 204–215.

Petersen, S. E., Fox, P. T., Posner, M. I., Mintun, M., & Raichle, M. E. (1988). Positron emission tomographic studies of the cortical anatomy of single-word processing. *Nature (London), 331,* 585–589.

Petersen, S. E., Fox, P. T., Posner, M. I., Mintun, M., & Raichle, M. E. (1989). Positron emission tomographic studies of the processing of single words. *Journal of Cognitive Neuroscience, 1,* 153–170.

Peuser, G., & Fittschen, M. (1977). On the universality of language dissolution: The case of a Turkish aphasic. *Brain and Language, 4,* 196–207.

Posner, M., & Snyder, C. (1975). Facilitation and inhibition in the processing of signals. In P. M. A. Rabbitt & S. Dornic (Eds.), *Attention and performance V.* New York: Academic Press.

Posner, M. I., Petersen, S. E., Fox, P. T., & Raichle, M. (1988). Localization of cognitive operations in the human brain. *Science, 240,* 1627–1631.

Rinnert, C., & Whitaker, H. A. (1973). Semantic confusions by aphasic patients. *Cortex, 9,* 56–81.

Rochford, G., & Williams, M. (1962). Studies in the development and breakdown in the use of names. IV. The effects of word frequency. *Journal of Neurology, Neurosurgery, and Psychiatry, 28,* 407–413.

Rosler, F. Putz, P., Friederici, A., & Hahne, A. (1993). Event-related brain potentials while encountering semantic and syntactic constraint violations. *Journal of Cognitive Neuroscience, 5,* 345–362.

Ryalls, J. (1982). Intonation in Broca's aphasia. *Neuropsychologia, 20,* 355–360.

Ryalls, J. (1986). An acoustic study of vowel production in aphasia. *Brain and Language, 29,* 48–67.

Sasanuma, S., Tatsumi, I. F., & Fujisaki, H. (1976). Discrimination of phonemes and word accent types in Japanese aphasic patients. *International Congress of Logopedics and Phoniatrics, 16th,* pp. 403–408.

Schwartz, M. (1984). What the classical aphasia categories can't do for us, and why. *Brain and Language, 21,* 3–8.

Shewan, C. M., Leeper, H., & Booth, J. (1984). An analysis of voice onset time (VOT) in aphasic and normal subjects. In J. Rosenbek, M. McNeill, & A. Aronson (Eds.), *Apraxia of speech.* San Diego, CA: College-Hill Press.

Shiffrin, R. M., & Schneider, W. (1977). Controlled and automatic human information processing. II. Perceptual learning, automatic attending, and a general theory. *Psychological Review, 84,* 127–190.

Swinney, D. A., Zurif, E. B., & Nicol, J. (1989). The effects of focal brain damage in sentence processing: An examination of the neurobiological organization of a mental module. *Journal of Cognitive Neuroscience, 1,* 25–37.

Tanenhaus, M. K., Carlson, G., & Seidenberg, M. S. (1985). Do listeners compute linguistic representations? In D. Dowty, L. Kartunen, & A. M. Zwicky (Eds.), *Natural language processing: Psychological, computational and theoretical perspectives.* Cambridge, UK: Cambridge University Press.

Tissot, R., Lhermitte, F., & Ducarne, B. (1963). Etat intellectuel des aphasiques. *Encephale, 52,* 285–320.

Tuller, B. (1984). On categorizing aphasic speech errors. *Neuropsychologia, 22,* 547–557.

Tuller, B., & Story, R. S. (1986). Co-articulation in aphasic speech. *Journal of the Acoustical Society of America, 80*(Suppl. 1), MM17.

Tyler, L. (1985). Real-time comprehension processes in agrammatism: A case study. *Brain and Language, 26,* 259–275.

von Stockert, T. R. (1972). Recognition of syntactic structure in aphasic patients. *Cortex, 8,* 323–334.

Zangwill, O. L. (1964). Intelligence in aphasia. In A. V. S. de Reuck & M. O'Connor (Eds.), *Disorders of language.* London: Churchill.

Zatorre, R. J., Evans, A. C., Meyer, E., & Gjedde, A. (1992). Lateralization of phonetic and pitch discrimination in speech processing. *Science, 256,* 846–849.

Ziegler, W., & von Cramon, D. (1985). Anticipatory coarticulation in a patient with apraxia of speech. *Brain and Language, 26,* 117–130.

Ziegler, W., & von Cramon, D. (1986). Disturbed coarticulation in apraxia of speech: Acoustic evidence. *Brain and Language, 29,* 34–47.

Zurif, E. B., & Caramazza, A. (1976). Psycholinguistic structures in aphasia: Studies in syntax and semantics. In H. Whitaker & H. Whitaker (Eds.), *Studies in neurolinguistics* (Vol. 1). New York: Academic Press.

Zurif, E. B., Caramazza, A., & Myerson, R. (1972). Grammatical judgements of agrammatic aphasics. *Neuropsychologia, 10,* 405–417.

Zurif, E. B., Caramazza, A., Myerson, R., & Galvin, J. (1974). Semantic feature representations for normal and aphasic language. *Brain and Language, 1,* 167–187.

CHAPTER 11

Pragmatics and Discourse

Herbert H. Clark
Bridget Bly

I. INTRODUCTION

Language is an instrument people use for everything from gossip to diplomacy. It is a complicated instrument like an airplane, and just as engineers can describe the structure of an airplane, linguists can describe the structure of a language—its sounds, words, phrases, and sentences and their organization. Yet, just as we could know the structure of an airplane with little idea of how it is used, we could know the sounds, syntax, and meaning of a language with little idea of how it is used. Knowing the structure of *I am hot* does not tell us how a particular speaker used it on a particular occasion to do something—or even how speakers in general could use it for doing things. We will focus on how people use language, a field of study often called pragmatics, especially on how they use it in discourse, broad but bounded stretches of language activity.

At the heart of language use is human action, people doing things with language. At the grossest level, people transact business, gossip, plan everyday chores with each other. At a lower level, they make statements, ask questions, and apologize to each other. At a still lower level, they utter and identify words, phrases, and sentences. At an even lower level, they produce and attend to sounds, gestures, and facial expressions. People using language take actions at all of these levels simultaneously. But what actions are these, and how do they fit together to form the whole?

Speech, Language, and Communication

People take actions for particular purposes, and in language use, their purposes are fundamentally social. Some of their purposes are public, and some are private. Some of their purposes are precise, as when they ask for a telephone number, and some are vague, as when they gossip with friends. Some of their purposes are fully formed ahead of time, as in church ceremonies, and others are worked out only as they go along, as in most conversation. Some of their purposes are in the foreground of their awareness, as when they decide to ask a question, and others are only in the background, as when they try to maintain their face and not look foolish. People are always trying to satisfy multiple purposes. So what purposes do people use language for, and how?

Our review of pragmatics and discourse has five parts. In the first, we consider the traditional view of the actions people perform in using language. In the second, we consider a contrasting view about the way speakers and addressees act jointly in discourse. In the next two parts, we look at how the participants in a discourse achieve local and more extended joint projects, and in the last, how they coordinate with each other in telling stories.

II. SPEECH ACTS

Speakers do many things in uttering even a single sentence. In John Austin's (1962) account, they act at several levels at once. When Paul says to Jean, "Please sit down," he is doing these things among others:

1. *Phonetic act:* Paul is producing the noises that constitute "Please sit down."
2. *Phatic act:* Paul is uttering the vocables or words of "Please sit down."
3. *Rhetic act:* Paul is using these vocables with a certain sense and reference.
4. *Locutionary act:* Paul is saying to Jean, "Please sit down."
5. *Illocutionary act:* Paul is asking Jean to sit down.
6. *Perlocutionary act:* Paul is getting Jean to sit down.

Austin's names for these acts may be abstruse, but the acts themselves are simple in conception. They bear important relations to one another. Phonetic, phatic, and rhetic acts are parts of locutionary acts. Illocutionary acts are performed *in* performing locutionary acts, and perlocutionary acts are performed *by* performing illocutionary acts. All of these acts have come to be called *speech acts* (Bach & Harnish, 1979; Cole & Morgan, 1975; Searle, 1969). Since Austin, most of the focus has been on illocutionary and perlocutionary acts. There have been so many studies of illocutionary acts that they form the foundation of most pragmatic theories.

A. Illocutionary Acts

Paul is doing something *in* saying, "Please sit down" to Jean: he is asking her to sit down. He may also be doing something *by* asking her to sit down, namely getting her to sit down. According to Austin, to do something *in* saying something is an illocutionary act, and to do something *by* saying something is a perlocutionary act. The difference lies in what Paul expects to accomplish. He will have succeeded in asking Jean to sit down (the illocutionary act) when she recognizes what he wants. He will have succeeded in getting her to sit down (a perlocutionary act) when she actually sits down. She could recognize that he wants her to sit down (his illocutionary act would be successful) and yet refuse to sit down (his perlocutionary act would be unsuccessful). Notice that Paul can say, "I hereby ask you to sit down" as a way of asking Jean to sit down, an illocutionary act. He cannot say, "I hereby get you to sit down" as a way of getting her to sit down, a perlocutionary act. The contrast is characteristic of illocutionary and perlocutionary acts.

Illocutionary acts come in many types. They include telling, asking, warning, ordering, offering, thanking, congratulating, appointing, firing. Verschueren (1980) counted more than 150 such illocutionary verbs in English. According to John Searle (1975b), these acts differ principally in what he called their *illocutionary point,* their primary publicly intended perlocutionary effect. In making a request, speakers are trying to get their addressees to do something: the illocutionary point is to get them to do that something. For other illocutionary acts, the point is different. Searle divided illocutionary points into five main categories:

1. *Assertives.* The point of an assertive is to get addressees to form or attend to the belief that the speaker is committed to a certain belief. When Paul tells Jean, "I'm tired," he is trying to get her to accept the belief that he is tired. Assertives range from simple assertions through predictions, notifications, confessions, denials, retorts, conjectures, suppositions, and many others.

2. *Directives.* The point of a directive is to get addressees to do things. When Paul asks Jean to sit down, he is trying to get her to do something, to sit down. Directives fall into two major classes: requests for nonlinguistic actions (as with most commands and suggestions), and requests for linguistic actions (as with most questions). In asking Jean, "What time is it?" Paul is requesting a linguistic action: she is to tell him what time it is. Directives range in force from mild hints to commands, and they vary on other dimensions, too.

3. *Commissives.* The point of a commissive is to commit the speaker to some future action. The commonest commissive is the promise. When Paul

says to Jean, "I'll be there in a minute," he is committing himself to being there in a minute. A promise can be absolute or conditional, and when it is conditional, it is called an offer. When Paul says to Jean, "Can I get you a beer?" he is committing himself to getting Jean a beer, but only if she wants one.

4. *Expressives.* The point of an expressive is to express certain psychological feelings toward the addressees. When Paul steps on Jean's foot by mistake, he says, "Sorry." In doing so, he presupposes that he has caused Jean some harm and tries to get her to recognize his regret in having done so. Expressives include thanking, greeting, congratulating, apologizing, well-wishing, and many other types.

5. *Declarations.* The point of a declaration is to effect an institutional state of affairs. Declarations take place within institutions such as the law, the church, and organized games, and speakers do certain things by virtue of their institutional roles as judges, priests, or referees. In a company, a boss can appoint, promote, or fire people, and an employee can quit, simply by saying the right words at the right time: "You're fired" or "I quit." Likewise, with the right words at the right times, a judge can indict, pardon, and sentence people; a referee can start a game, call fouls, and call time-outs; a police officer can arrest people; and a priest can baptize, marry, and bless people. As Austin noted, all of these acts must be performed with the proper institutional authority or they are defective, null and void.

Like any taxonomy, this scheme has problems. Some illocutionary acts appear to belong to more than one category; for example, the order of a general or of a police officer has properties of both a directive and a declaration. The categories are not by any means mutually exclusive or exhaustive. The scheme has also been criticized for misclassifying acts (Hancher, 1979; Linell, Alemyr, & Jonsson, 1993; Linell & Markova, 1993; van Eemeren & Grootendorst, 1982) and cultural bias (Wierzbicka, 1985). Other schemes have been proposed (e.g., Austin, 1962; Ballmer & Brennenstuhl, 1981; van der Auwera, 1980), but they suffer from similar problems. Still, the scheme illustrates the range of what speakers can intend to do with respect to their addressees, and it has heuristic value for describing illocutionary acts.

B. Speaker's Meaning

An illocutionary act is an act by which the speaker means something. Although Austin and Searle focused on the act itself, one could focus instead on what the speaker means by the act. That is what H. Paul Grice (1957) did in his account of meaning.

As Grice noted, English has two different notions of meaning. Compare these two statements:

1. Those black clouds mean rain.
2. In uttering "Please sit down" Paul meant that Jean was to sit down.

Statement 1 describes a connection between certain events or states in the world and their natural consequences. Grice called this *natural meaning.* Statement 2, in contrast, describes the connection between a person's action and certain of its intended consequences, or what Grice called *nonnatural meaning.* Nonnatural meaning itself divides into subtypes. Some have to do with what signals mean, such as "The word *up* can mean 'happy' " or "The sentence *I'm up* can mean that the speaker is happy at the moment of utterance." Let us call this *signal meaning.* Other subtypes have to do with what speakers mean in using such signals, as in "In uttering 'Please sit down,' Paul meant that Jean was to sit down." This is what Grice called utterer's meaning, and what others have called speaker's or speaker meaning (e.g., Bach & Harnish, 1979). We will use the term *speaker's meaning.*

Speaker's meaning is any proposition *p* that fits the formula "In doing *x,* a speaker *S* meant for hearers *H* that *p.*" Grice and his successors have shown that the actions that fit this formula must satisfy the following condition:

In doing *x,* a speaker *S* means that *p* for hearers *H* if and only if:

(*i*) *S* intends that *H* recognize that *p* in part by recognizing that *i.*

Notice that speaker's meaning, unlike signal meaning, is really a type of intention. The intention is special because of two properties. The first is its *reflexivity.* The *i* in "recognizing that *i*" refers to the full statement labeled (*i*), namely, "*S* intends that *H* recognize that *p* in part by recognizing that *i.*" The statement refers back to itself—it is *reflexive.* So, in uttering, "Please sit down" to Jean, Paul intends her to recognize that she is to sit down in part by recognizing that he has that very intention. The second property of this intention is its *linkage.* It is an intention by one person that cannot be satisfied without the linked action of another person. Paul cannot fulfill his intention toward Jean without her coordinated action in recognizing that intention.

In Grice's account, then, the actions by which speakers mean things, the *x* in the formula for speaker's meaning, are special. They are signals and have signal meaning. Ordinarily, when we think of signals, we think of linguistic utterances, and that is what most psychological and linguistic theories concentrate on. But signals do not have to be linguistic. One of Grice's own examples was of a bus conductor (in the old British system) ringing a bell twice to tell the driver that the bus could now proceed. Nonlinguistic signals are an essential ingredient of spontaneous discourse, where they come mainly in the form of gesticulations, facial expressions, and vocal gestures (Bavelas, 1994; Bavelas, Black, Chovil, Lemery, & Mullett, 1988; Bavelas, Black, Lemery, & Mullett, 1986; Clark & Gerrig, 1990;

Ekman & Friesen, 1969; Feyereisen & de Lannoy, 1991; C. Goodwin, 1981; M. H. Goodwin & Goodwin, 1986; Kendon, 1980, 1987; McNeill, 1985, 1992; McNeill & Levy, 1982).

Discourse cannot be understood without considering all the actions by which people can mean things for their addressees. Grice's characterization of speaker's meaning takes us far beyond the simplistic view that discourse is all linguistic. Even a casual look at face-to-face conversation shows how central a role nonlinguistic signals play. In ordinary talk, communicative acts are a mix of all types of signals.

C. Implicatures

How do we decipher what speakers mean? The traditional answer is that we look at what they say. But in his 1967 William James Lectures, Grice argued that we must view what they say against the ongoing discourse and its "accepted purpose or direction." He put it this way (Grice, 1975, p. 45):

> Our talk exchanges do not normally consist of a succession of disconnected remarks, and would not be rational if they did. They are characteristically, to some degree at least, cooperative efforts; and each participant recognizes in them, to some extent, a common purpose or set of purposes, or at least a mutually accepted direction. The purpose or direction may be fixed from the start (e.g., by an initial proposal of a question for discussion), or it may evolve during the exchange; it may be fairly definite, or it may be so indefinite as to leave very considerable latitude to the participants (as in a casual conversation). But at each stage, some possible conversational moves would be excluded as conversationally unsuitable.

The participants of a conversation, Grice argued, therefore expect each other to adhere to the cooperative principle, which he expressed as an exhortation to speakers:

> *Cooperative Principle:* Make your conversational contribution such as is required, at the stage at which it occurs, by the accepted purpose or direction of the talk exchange in which you are engaged.

In Grice's view, people take for granted that actions in discourse are to be interpreted against the "accepted purpose or direction of the talk exchange." Grice's insight can be pursued in many ways. He chose to apply it to the traditional problem of what sentences are taken to mean on the occasion of their use.

To see what speakers mean, Grice argued, we generally go beyond what they actually say. He asked us to imagine A standing by an obviously immobilized car and striking up a conversation with passerby B:

A: I am out of petrol.

B: There is a garage round the corner.

All B has said is that there is a garage, a gas station, around the corner. Yet that is not all A takes him as doing. A can suppose B was trying to offer information relevant to the situation at hand, that A is stranded and has just remarked that he is out of gasoline. So B must also mean, in Grice's words, "that the garage is, or at least may be open, etc." This he called an *implicature*. In Grice's scheme, speaker's meaning divides into two parts: *saying* and *implicating*.

What is the difference? What is *said*, in Grice's sense, is what speakers mean mostly through the conventional content of the sentence they utter. In uttering "There is a garage round the corner," all B is saying is that there is a garage around the corner. The rest of what B meant is implicated. Some implicatures are conventional and, therefore, part of the sentence meaning. The ones we shall be concerned with Grice called *conversational implicatures*. One example is B's implicature that the garage may be open and selling petrol. A recognizes it not because of any conventional connection with what B said. Rather, as Grice puts it, A "works it out."

For Grice, conversational implicatures have three main properties (but see Nunberg, 1981; Sadock, 1978). (1) They are *nonconventional*. They are not conventionally associated with the words or sentence uttered. "There is a garage round the corner" does not conventionally mean that the garage is open. Yet (2) they are *calculable*. Speakers intend addressees to be able to work them out. A is to work out that B means that he believes the garage may be open. Conversational implicatures are the parts of what speakers mean that addressees can recognize only by "working them out." Finally (3) they are *defeasible:* Speakers can cancel them, rendering them null and void. B could have said, "There's a garage round the corner, but I doubt if it's open," nullifying the implicature A would otherwise work out.

How are implicatures to be worked out? Since Grice argued that every utterance "contributes" to the "accepted purpose or direction of the talk exchange," we might have expected him to develop the notions of "contribution" and "accepted purpose" and show how implicatures follow. What he did instead was offer four rules of thumb, four *maxims,* that he argued enable listeners to work out implicatures. He expressed the maxims as exhortations to speakers (Grice, 1975, pp. 45–46):

Maxim of Quantity	1. Make your contribution as informative as is required (for the current purposes of the exchange).
	2. Do not make your contribution more informative than is required.
Maxim of Quality	1. Do not say what you believe to be false.
	2. Do not say that for which you lack evidence.

Maxim of Relation   Be relevant.
Maxim of Manner   1. Avoid obscurity of expression.
                    2. Avoid ambiguity.
                    3. Be brief (avoid unnecessary prolixity).
                    4. Be orderly.

Once listeners take for granted that speakers adhere to these maxims and to the cooperative principle itself, they can work out what the speakers are implicating.

Speakers create implicatures in two main ways. The first is by direct appeal to the maxims. Take this invented exchange:

Burton: How many children do you have?

Connie: I have two children.

All Connie has said is that she has two children, which would be literally true even if she had three or four or twelve. Yet, by the maxim of quantity, Burton can assume she has been as informative as she needs to be for the current purposes of this exchange. And because in this exchange he was asking about the *total* number of children she has, she must be giving the total number. Contrast that exchange with this one:

Burton: Does anyone have two quarters I could borrow for the pay phone?

Connie: I have two quarters.

In this exchange, Burton is not trying to find out the total number of quarters Connie has, but trying merely to borrow two quarters. Connie may have three, four, or twelve quarters, but she is being "as informative as is required for the current purposes of the exchange" by saying that she has two quarters. These two circumstances contrast. In "I have two children" the "two" implicates "and no more than two," whereas in "I have two quarters" it does not. Both are meanings Connie expects Burton to work out via the maxim of quantity. Direct application of the other maxims works in similar ways.

The second main way speakers create implicatures is by blatantly violating, or *flouting,* a maxim. In the following example, Kate is describing a visit to a women's college (1.3.560)[1]:

Kate: and . um then, . a bell rang, – – and - millions of feet, . ran, . along corridors, you know, and then they . it all died away, it was like like sound effects from the Goon Show

When Kate claimed "millions" of feet ran along the corridors, she was blatantly violating the Maxim of Quality, "Do not say what you believe to be false." The violation was so blatant, indeed, that she must have intended her audience to reason: "Kate is flouting the maxim, yet is otherwise being cooperative. She must therefore intend 'millions' to be taken, not literally, but as hyperbole. It only *seemed* as if there were millions of feet." Flouting maxims also leads to meiosis, metaphor, irony, and other effects.

There may be a better account, however, for the implicatures created by the flouting of maxims. Irony is one example. When Burton fails Connie in some way, she might say, "What a fine friend you are!" In doing so, she is merely pretending to compliment Burton, and he is expected to discover that. But *pretending* to say something is not the same type of action as actually *saying* something, and it takes more than the flouting of the maxim "Be truthful" to establish that. The same goes for hyperbole and other related tropes (see Clark & Gerrig, 1984, 1990; Isaacs & Clark, 1990; Sperber & Wilson, 1981).

All things considered, the cooperative principle has offered a creditable first account for a variety of phenomena, and most investigators have accepted its basic insight. The issue is how best to formulate it. Various investigators have quibbled with the maxims, offered new versions (e.g., Horn, 1984; Kasher, 1977; Leech, 1983; Levinson, 1987), and have even tried to reduce them all to the maxim of relevance (Sperber & Wilson, 1986). But in the end, rules of thumb can never be more than just that— rules of thumb. To understand the phenomena Grice noted, we need to understand two notions from which all the maxims follow: "the accepted purpose or direction of the talk exchange," and how people "contribute" to that accepted purpose or direction. These are topics we turn to next.

III. COORDINATING ACTIONS

In Austin's and Searle's accounts, the acts of interest are performed by speakers, and listeners are passive receptacles. The acts Austin named, from phonetic to perlocutionary acts, are those performed by speakers, not listeners. Grice's account of meaning is of what speakers mean, not what addressees understand, and his maxims are exhortations to speakers, not listeners. Searle (1969, p. 16) was quite explicit about the centrality of speaking: "The unit of linguistic communication is not . . . the symbol, word, or sentence, but rather the production or issuance of the symbol, word, or sentence, in the performance of a speech act." For him, linguistic communication is like writing a letter and dropping it in a mailbox. It does not matter whether the addressee receives, reads, or understands it.

But communication can no more be done by the speaker alone than clapping can be done by the left hand alone. It requires two coordinated actions: speaking and listening.[2] Despite its name, speaker's meaning requires, depends on, certain actions by the addressees; this is the property we have called *linkage*. It is not enough for Paul to intend Jean to recognize that he wants her to sit down. To fulfill his intention, he must get her to recognize what he is doing. And to accomplish that, he must get her to attend, listen to his utterance, and try to understand him precisely as he speaks. When we view speaker's meaning this way, the speaker's and hearer's intentions index each other like this:

(1) By doing x, S intends H to recognize that p by means of (2).
(2) By identifying x, H intends to recognize (1).

Speakers cannot fulfill their intentions in (1) without the belief that the addressees are trying to fulfill their own intentions in (2), and vice versa. In Grice's formula, meaning and recognition are inherently linked, interdependent, coordinated.

When two people shake hands, play a piano duet, waltz, or make love, the pair of them are doing things that one of them could not do alone: they are performing *joint actions*. A joint action is an action performed not by an individual person but by an ensemble of people. Likewise, speakers and listeners accomplish communicative acts that neither of them could do alone. They, too, are performing joint acts.

One basic communicative act is the *contribution* (Clark & Schaefer, 1989; Clark & Wilkes-Gibbs, 1986). Take the question Alice asks Betty (8.31.1062):

Alice: well, um . he came through the British Council, did he –
Betty: sorry? .
Alice: he came through the British Council did he .
Betty: well no, it's not through the British Council, it's on a Goodman Fellowship, but it . it . it's suh- sort of in association with the British Council – –

In the first turn, Alice presents an utterance, "well, he came through the British Council, did he?" as a way of asking Betty a question. Apparently Betty does not hear the utterance to her satisfaction, for she asks Alice for a repeat with "sorry?" and Alice obliges. This time Betty understands and is willing to go on to answer "well no." The point is this. Although Alice tries to ask Betty a question with her first utterance, the two of them do not consider it complete until Betty has understood her well enough to go on. So, contributing to a conversation takes more than an illocutionary act, an *attempt* to get a listener to understand. The participants must reach the mutual belief that the act has succeeded, that the addressee has understood what the speaker meant. So, one form of contribution is an illocutionary act plus its mutual acceptance.

Contributions require actions from both speakers and their addressees. In face-to-face conversation, contributions ordinarily consist of two phases, the first initiated by the speaker and the second by the addressee:

Presentation phase. A presents B with utterance *u*.

Acceptance phase. B provides A with evidence that B has understood what A meant by *u* well enough for current purposes.

In our example, the presentation phase consists of Alice's utterance, "well, he came through the British Council, did he?" The acceptance phase consists of Betty's request for a repeat "sorry?" plus Alice's repeat plus Betty's willingness to go on to the answer "well no." The criterion A and B try to reach is this: the mutual belief that B has understood A well enough for current purposes. This is called the *grounding criterion,* and the process by which A and B reach it is called *grounding.*

Most of the time, the acceptance phase takes one of two forms. The first uses what have traditionally been called *back-channel responses,* signals like "uh-huh," "yeah," head nods, and smiles from the addressee while the speaker continues speaking (Duncan, 1973; Schegloff, 1982; Yngve, 1970). Take this example from a spontaneous British conversation (2.1.318):

Bernard: I don't quite know, but they would be worth approaching,
Alan: m
Bernard: - because that again, is a technical or unremunerative type of book, -
Alan: m
Bernard: in a sense I mean, it's - a limited *market*,
Alan: *mhm*
Bernard: and once you've sold it, [continues]

Alan punctuates Bernard's utterance three times with what Schegloff (1982) called *continuers,* "m," "m," and "mhm" (British equivalents to North American "yeah" and "uh-huh"). Alan's message, according to Schegloff, is "please continue," implying he has grasped what Bernard has said so far. Listeners like Alan tend to place continuers at or near the ends of clauses, often overlapping the ends, in order to accept each clause separately.

In a second common form of acceptance, the current addressee initiates an appropriate next turn. Take this example (3.1.174):

Ken: uh what modern poets have you been reading -
June: well I'm . I like Robert Graves very much -
Ken: who else
June: (continues)

In the first turn Ken presents an utterance in order to ask June what modern poets she has been reading. As evidence that she has understood him, she simply proceeds to answer the question. This way she shows that she believes: (1) Ken's utterance does not need clarification; (2) it is a question; and (3) it is appropriately answered by saying she likes Robert Graves very much. Her answer might actually have shown Ken that she had misunderstood him, and he would have followed up with something like "No I mean avant garde poets." In fact, he accepts her answer, affirming her interpretation, by following up with "Who else?"

Although these two forms of acceptance, acknowledging and proceeding on, are the commonest, there are many other forms as well. One is illustrated in the earlier example by Alice and Betty, when Betty follows Alice's question with a request for a repeat. The result is an exchange of turns called a *side sequence* (Jefferson, 1973) or an *insertion sequence* (Schegloff, 1972):

Betty: sorry? .
Alice: he came through the British Council did he .

Only once Betty and Alice have completed the side sequence does Betty proceed on to the answer. Other times the current addressee may accept a speaker's presentation by cutting into it, as illustrated in this exchange (7.1a.83):

Burton: wuh- what day are you going to have off or are going to have a day off or
Connie: I have a half day off, *I have*
Burton: *when*
Connie: Wednesday morning **off**
Burton: **Wednes**day morning . uh-huh

When Connie begins "I have a half day off," she is deliberately cutting into Burton's utterance after "or" to save him the trouble of offering another alternative. The current addressee may also accept a presentation by repeating part of it, as when Burton says, "Wednesday morning, uh-huh" as evidence that he has registered Connie's "Wednesday morning." Each acceptance phase is shaped by the participants working together, and its form and length depend on what the participants need to do to reach the grounding criterion. That may vary as widely as the topics of talk itself.

IV. LOCAL PROJECTS

Speakers say things not merely to get addressees to recognize their intentions, but to get things done. Take this British telephone conversation (8.11.851):

Betty: (rings C's telephone)
Cathy: Miss Pink's office - hello
Betty: hello, is Miss Pink in .
Cathy: well, she's in, but she's engaged at the moment, who is it?

Betty: oh it's Professor Worth's secretary, from Panamerican College

Cathy: m,

Betty: could you give her a message *for me*

Cathy: *certainly*

Betty: uh:m Professor Worth said that, if . Miss Pink runs into difficulties, . on Monday afternoon, . with the standing subcommittee, . over the item on Miss Panoff, - - -

Cathy: Miss Panoff?

Betty: yes, that Professor Worth would be with Mr Miles all afternoon, - so she only had to go round and collect him if she
needed him, - - -

Cathy: ah, - - - thank you very much indeed,

Betty: right

Cathy: Panoff, right *you* are

Betty: *right,*

Cathy: I'll tell her,

Betty: *thank you*

Cathy: *(2 to 3 syllables)* bye bye

Betty: bye

When Betty asks, "Is Miss Pink in?" she expects Betty to do more than recognize what she means, that she wants to know if Miss Pink is in. Locally, she wants an answer, and she gets one, "Well, she's in, but she's engaged at the moment." She also has a larger purpose, to tell Miss Pink where Professor Worth would be if she needed him. She asks her question as part of that more global project. Betty and Cathy do not stop with illocutionary acts or contributions. They use them to further the "accepted purpose or direction of a talk exchange." To see how, let us start with Austin's notion of perlocution.

A perlocutionary effect, or *perlocu.ion,* is any effect ... addressees that is caused by their understanding of what a speaker meant (Austin, 1962; Davis, 1979). Many perlocutions are intended. When Paul warns Jean, "There's a bicycle coming up behind you," he may intend to frighten her so she will jump out of the way. If she believes him, she may become frightened and jump, and if she does not, she will not jump. Other perlocutions are unintended or unexpected. When Paul tells Jean, "It's six o'clock," he may intend for her to learn what time it is, but he may not realize she will be upset because she just missed her train.

One perlocution has a privileged status, and it is the primary point of the illocutionary act. When Cathy asks Betty, "Who is it?" the primary intended perlocution (the primary thing she is trying to get Betty to do) is to tell her who is on the telephone. She would have judged Betty as having misunderstood if she had not recognized this. So, actions like these are expected to come in pairs:

> Cathy: who is it?
>
> Betty: oh it's Professor Worth's secretary, from Panamerican College

Cathy's question is expected to be followed by its primary intended per-locution, the answer. Likewise, a request is expected to be followed by compliance, a thanks by an acknowledgment, and an invitation by an accep-tance or rejection.

A. Adjacency Pairs

Pairs of utterances like these constitute what Schegloff and Sacks (1973) called *adjacency pairs*. According to them, adjacency pairs have five proper-ties:

1. Adjacency pairs consist of two utterances, a *first pair part* and a *second pair part*.
2. The two parts are spoken by different speakers.
3. The first and second pair parts belong to specific types, for exam-ple, question and answer, or thanks and acknowledgment.
4. The form and content of the second pair part depends on the type of the first pair part.
5. Given that a speaker has produced a first pair part, the second pair part is relevant and expectable as the next utterance. This property is called *conditional relevance*.

The first condition needs to be relaxed a bit to accommodate pairs of actions like these:

> Paul: Please sit down.
>
> Jean: [Sits down]

Here the second pair part is not an utterance even though it is the primary intended perlocution, the act of complying with the request. We assume that the parts of adjacency pairs may be either linguistic or nonlinguistic.

Adjacency pairs come in many types, some of which are illustrated in Betty and Cathy's conversation:

Adjency Pair	Example
Part 1. Summons	Betty: (rings)
Part 2. Response	Cathy: Miss Pink's Office
Part 1. Greetings	Cathy: hello
Part 2. Greetings	Betty: hello

Part 1. Question	Cathy: who is it?
Part 2. Answer	Betty: oh it's Professor Worth's secretary, from Panamerican College
Part 1. Assertion	Betty: oh it's Professor Worth's secretary, from Panamerican College
Part 2. Assent	Cathy: m
Part 1. Request	Betty: could you give her a message *for me*
Part 2. Promise	Cathy: *certainly*
Part 1. Promise	Cathy: I'll tell her
Part 2. Acknowledgment	Betty: thank you
Part 1. Thanks	Cathy: thank you very much indeed
Part 2. Acknowledgment	Betty: right
Part 1. Good-bye	Cathy: bye bye
Part 2. Good-bye	Betty: bye

This is only a sample of potential types.

B. Minimal Joint Projects

It is striking how much of the work in Betty and Cathy's conversation is accomplished with adjacency pairs. Every one of their utterances is a first or second pair part, and many are both. The conversation is less a sequence of *single* actions than it is a chain of *paired* actions. But why?

Adjacency pairs form units in which people achieve certain goals together, certain joint purposes (Clark, 1994). Suppose Paul asks Jean to sit down, and she does. But Jean does not just sit down. She sits down *for* Paul, *in response to* Paul's request, completing what Paul proposed that they do together. Paul's and Jean's individual actions together constitute a special type of joint action. Paul proposes what we will call a *joint project:* with his request he "projects" a joint action in which she sits down for him. Jean, with her response, takes up his proposal and completes the joint project. So it goes with each of the adjacency pairs in Betty and Cathy's conversation. Joint projects come in many sizes. Adjacency pairs are *minimal joint projects.*

Joint projects can be accomplished only by the participants working together. When Paul asks Jean to sit down, when he proposes that she sit down for him, she may understand him perfectly and yet be unable or unwilling to take up his proposal. With questions, respondents can deal with proposed joint projects in at least four ways (see Goffman, 1976; Stenström, 1984).

(1) *Full compliance.* Respondents may comply fully with the project as proposed:

Cathy: who is it?

Betty: oh it's Professor Worth's secretary, from Panamerican College

(2) *Alteration of project.* Respondents may *alter* the proposed project to something they are able and willing to comply with (1.2.349):

Reynard: Oscar is going to the States?

Charles: well, this is what I heard just before I came away - - -

Charles is not in a position to give a certain "yes" or "no," so he alters the project to one of telling Reynard what he has heard just before he went away. He signals the change in stance with "well." Alterations like this are a common feature of evasive or equivocal answers by politicians and salespeople, as in this example (Bavelas, Black, Chovil, & Mullett, 1990b, p. 149; see also Bavelas, Black, Chovil, & Mullett, 1990a):

A: Your brother told me you have a car for sale. What kind of shape is the car in?

B: Well- it *needs*—ah, a little bit of *minor* repairs—ah. Basically it *runs,* ah—I—that's what I *use* it for . . . So, ah, otherwise it's—it needs a *few* minor repairs you know, I— . . . it's not in *perfect* condition.

Here, after a telltale "well," B tries to say a lot about the car without revealing how bad it really is.

(3) *Declination of project.* When respondents are unable or unwilling to comply with the project as proposed, they can *decline* to take it up, usually by offering a reason why they are declining (1.8.40):

Jane: what happens if anybody breaks in and steals it, - are are is are we covered or .

Kate: um - I don't know quite honestly.

Jane presupposes that Kate knows whether they are covered by insurance, but Kate does not and declines with her reason.

(4) *Withdrawal from project.* Respondents can also *withdraw* entirely, for example, by ignoring the question and changing the topic.

With these four options, and there are further subtypes, people create not just adjacency pairs strictly defined (option 1, full compliance), but other paired utterances. The range of pairings results from two people trying to coordinate on a joint project and finding success (option 1), partial success (option 2), failure (option 3), or a termination of the attempt (option 4). Their form comes from what the participants are trying jointly to do and how they succeed, not vice versa.[3]

C. Turns

In carrying out local projects, people coordinate on who speaks when. The reason seems clear. For Paul to ask Jean a question, he must get her to attend to his voice, identify his phrasing, and understand what he means precisely as he is uttering what he says. He will not succeed if she is attending to something else—if, for example, she is speaking to *him*. To contribute successfully, they must ordinarily make sure that at each moment only one of them is talking and the other is listening. Likewise, for Paul and Jean to complete a minimal joint project, he must make his proposal before she takes it up, since she cannot know what to take up until she has heard his proposal. That, too, forces them to take turns. Turns emerge from coordinating on contributions and joint projects.

Turns, Sacks, Schegloff, and Jefferson (1974) noted, tend to conform to these, among other, properties of conversations:

1. Speaker change recurs, or, at least, occurs.
2. Overwhelmingly, one party talks at a time.
3. Occurrences of more than one speaker at a time are common, but brief.
4. Transitions from one turn to a next with no gap and no overlap between them are common. Together with transitions characterized by slight gap or slight overlap, they make up the vast majority of transitions.
5. Turn order is not fixed, but varies.
6. Turn size is not fixed, but varies.
7. Length of conversation is not fixed, specified in advance.
8. What parties say is not fixed, specified in advanced.
9. Relative distribution of turns is not fixed, specified in advance.

Many of these properties are illustrated in the telephone conversation between Betty and Cathy.

To account for these properties, Sacks et al. argued, we need a system of rules. In conversation, the participants speak in units that are potential turns, so-called *turn-constructional units*. These range in size from a single word (e.g., Cathy's "Certainly") to clauses filled with many embedded clauses (e.g., Betty's "uh:m Professor Worth said that, if . Miss Pink runs into difficulties, . on Monday afternoon, . with the standing subcommittee, . over the item on Miss Panoff, - - - that Professor Worth would be with Mr Miles all afternoon, - so she only had to go round and collect him if she needed him, - - -"). Each such unit ends at a *transition-relevance place*, a point at which the next speaker may begin a turn. The participants then follow a set of turn-allocation rules, to quote Sacks et al.:

(1) For any turn, at the initial transition-relevance place of an initial turn-constructional unit:
(a) If the turn-so-far is so constructed as to involve the use of a "current speaker selects next" technique, then the party so selected has the right and is obliged to take next turn to speak; no others have such rights or obligations, and transfer occurs at that place.

(b) If the turn-so-far is so constructed as not to involve the use of a "current speaker selects next" technique, then self-selection for next speakership may, but need not, be instituted; first starter acquires rights to a turn, and transfer occurs at that place.

(c) If the turn-so-far is so constructed as not to involve the use of a "current speaker selects next" technique, then current speaker may, but need not continue, unless another self-selects.

(2) If, at the initial transition-relevance place of an initial turn-constructional unit, neither 1a nor 1b has operated, and, following the provision of 1c, current speaker has continued, then the rule-set a–c reapplies at next transition-relevance place, and recursively at each next transition-relevance place, until transfer is effected. (p. 704)

The result of these rules is an orderly sequence of turns.

These rules look more complicated than they actually are. Rule 1a reflects the structure of minimal joint projects. When Cathy asks Betty, "Who is it?" she is using a "current speaker selects next" technique to oblige Betty to take the next turn, an obligation that begins at the end of Cathy's question. Rules 1b and 1c reflect the structure of contributions. For Cathy to complete the presentation phase of a contribution, she must ordinarily complete a turn construction unit, such as "Well, she's in, but she's engaged at the moment." If Betty had spoken up at that point, she would have been following Rule 1b. In fact, Cathy continues to the next turn-constructional unit—the presentation phase of the next contribution—by saying, "Who is it?"

These rules, according to Sacks et al., account for the nine properties listed earlier. Take brief overlaps (property 3). For adjacency pairs, according to rule 1a, Cathy should try to project the end of Betty's turn so she can begin her response at that point. That is, she should try to *predict* the end of Betty's turn, not merely *react* to it, as is assumed in an alternative model of turn taking (Duncan, 1972, 1973). But if Cathy's projection is off, her response may overlap. Indeed, when Betty says, "Could you give her a message. . . ," Cathy apparently projects the turn's end after "message" and responds "certainly." The trouble is, Betty happens to extend her question with "for me," which overlaps with Cathy's "certainly." The overlap was an inadvertent consequence of projecting the turn's end.

Turns at talking are not the whole story (see, e.g., Brennan, 1990; Edelsky, 1981; C. Goodwin, 1987; Houtkoop & Mazeland, 1985). Speakers quite deliberately use overlaps, interruptions, and unfinished turns as devices for completing contributions, as we have seen in earlier examples. They often deliberately produce "uh-huh" and "yeah" to overlap the ends of what they acknowledge. They sometimes interrupt with precise timing to indicate references they already understand (Jefferson, 1973). Other signals in conversation are not performed in turns at all, and these include head nods, smiles, frowns, empathetic winces, eye gaze, and unison completions of utterances (Bavelas et al., 1986, 1988; Chovil, 1991–1992; Tannen, 1983). What is important in the end are the joint actions by which the participants coordinate on the "accepted purpose or direction of the talk exchange." Some of these actions lead to turns at talk, but others do not.

Conversations, then, are ordinarily dominated by adjacency pairs, which emerge as the participants try to complete joint projects. The minimal joint project takes two utterances, the first from the person proposing the project, and the second from the person taking it up. The two utterances have to be done in sequence, and that leads to turns. The participants also have to ground what they say as they go along, and that also leads to turns. Turns are not really "turns at talk;" that would be taking only the speaker's point of view. They are "turns at who speaks and who listens," and occasionally people have reasons and the wherewithal for doing both at once.

V. EXTENDED PROJECTS

Conversations pose a paradox. On one hand, people engage in conversations, as in any joint activity, to do things with each other. On the other hand, they can never know in advance what they will actually do. Betty and Cathy's telephone conversation is a good illustration. Betty rang up to tell Miss Pink where Professor Worth would be that afternoon. When she discovered Miss Pink was busy, she recruited Cathy to pass on the information. Cathy had her own aims in answering the telephone. Her job was to take messages and keep callers from interrupting Miss Pink's meeting, but she had no idea who was calling or what they would say. Even though Betty and Cathy began with their own purposes, they could not know what they would end up doing. As Sacks et al. (1974) argued, they had to manage their conversation turn by turn. They had to adapt their actions to deal with the exigencies of each moment. In conversation, the participants' actions are *local* and *opportunistic*.

The paradox leaves us with a puzzle: how do people in conversation ever achieve their broader goals or interests. How do they engineer the large joint projects of their talk exchange? Part of the answer is by the clever use of minimal joint projects.

A. Pre-sequences

One remarkable device for achieving larger joint projects is what Schegloff (1980) and others have called *pre-sequences*. A good example is the *pre-question*, as illustrated in this sequence from an American conversation:

Adam: **Let me ask you a question off the subject though.**
Bret: **Okay.**

Adam: You're in, you're living in the Castle Park area?

Bret: That's right.

Adam: I grew up in Oak Cliff.

Bret: Did you really?

Adam: Yes, I did. Uh, just close to Methodist Hospital.

Bret: Okay, yeah.

Adam: On Candy, C A N D Y.

Bret: Right

Adam: Oh, in fact, I lived there oh, until nineteen, late nineteen fifties.

Bret: Okay, okay.

Adam: And that area, **is it changing back again?** So many people are moving back into those old houses and are restoring them.

When Adam says, "Let me ask you a question off the subject though," he is performing a pre-question. He is asking Bret to allow him to ask a question, and Bret consents with "Okay." But what does Adam do next? He does not ask what he wants to ask, Is the Castle Park area changing back again? Instead, he takes up preliminaries to that question, establishing that he and Bret both know the area. Only then does he ask, "Is it changing back again?" Pre-questions request space not just for questions, but for preliminaries to those questions. They are, as Schegloff (1980) put it, preliminaries to preliminaries. The result is a structure like this:

   I. Pre-question plus consent
  II. Preliminaries to a question plus answer
 III. Question plus answer

Locally, the pre-question and its response (I) form a minimal joint project: Adam seeks permission to ask a question and Bret grants it. But in doing that, Adam projects a larger enterprise consisting of I, II, and III, and when Bret consents, he is agreeing to that enterprise, too. Put another way, Adam and Bret use the minimal joint project (I) to initiate the larger joint project (I + II + III).

Pre-questions are only one type of pre-sequence. Just as pre-questions gain consent to ask a question, pre-announcements gain consent to make an announcement, pre-invitations to make an invitation, pre-requests to make a request, and pre-narratives to tell a story. Here are some examples:

Pre-sequence	Example
Pre-question	A. Let me ask you a question off the subject though.
Response	B. Okay.
Pre-announcement	A. tell you who I met yesterday—
Response	b. who

Pre-invitation	A. Are you doing anything tonight?
Response	B. No.
Pre-request	A. Do you have hot chocolate?
Response	B. Yes, we do.
Summons	A. Hey, Molly
Response	B. Yes?
Telephone summons	A. (rings telephone)
Response	B. Miss Pink's office
Pre-closing statement	A. Well okay
Response	B. Okay
Pre-narrative	A. I acquired an absolutely magnificent sewing machine, by foul means, did I tell you about that?
Response	B. no

For each pre-sequence, once A has got B's consent, he or she has B's permission to proceed with the question, announcement, invitation, request, conversation, closing, or narrative.

B. Indirect Speech Acts

Another type of extended project achieved with pre-sequences is the *indirect speech act*. When Jean asks Paul, "Can you reach the salt?" she appears to be asking whether or not he can reach the salt, a yes/no question. Yet she also appears to be asking him to pass the salt, a request. In traditional terminology, the question is a direct or literal speech act, or illocutionary act, and the request is an indirect speech act. In Grice's scheme, indirect speech acts are implicatures (Searle, 1975a). Jean expects Paul to see that she *knows* he can reach the salt, so she cannot be asking whether or not he can. She expects him instead to see that she is flouting the maxim of quality, "Be truthful," and to work out that she is requesting him to pass the salt. Indirect speech acts come in a great many types, though the best studied are requests, the type we will concentrate on here.

Treating indirect speech acts as implicatures has problems. One is that indirect speech acts range in how conventional they are (Clark, 1979; Morgan, 1978). "Could you pass the salt?" is a highly conventional way of requesting salt. "Are you close enough to the salt to pass it to me?" is not. Addressees view the first yes/no question ("Could you . . . ?") as *pro forma*, not to be taken seriously, but the second one ("Are you close enough . . . ?") as serious. As a result, they are more likely to answer "yes" to "Are you close enough?" than to "Could you?" before complying with the indirect request (Clark, 1979). Implicatures give us no account for these variations. Worse, they give us no account for the collaborative way in which indirect requests get taken up. Let us see how.

In conversation, requests always arise as parts of local joint projects. Requests and their uptake take at least two steps, as in this hypothetical example:

Waitress: What'll ya have? [*request for order*]
Customer: A hot dog and an order of fries. [*uptake of request*]

The waitress asks for the customer's order and gets it immediately, the two turns forming a minimal joint project. Other requests require a more complicated uptake (Merritt, 1976, p. 333):

Waitress: What'll ya have girls? [*request for order*]
Customer: What's the soup of the day?
Waitress: Clam chowder.
Customer: I'll have a bowl of clam chowder and a salad with Russian dressing. [*uptake of request*]

Again, the waitress asks for the order, but before the customer can comply, she needs to know the soup of the day, so she initiates an *embedded* joint project to find out. The embedded project is designed to satisfy a *precondition* on her uptake. Every request has preconditions, and many are dealt with in the course of local joint projects.

Prerequests are often based on such preconditions (Gordon & Lakoff, 1971; Labov & Fanshel, 1977; Searle, 1975a). Let us consider four cases. Case 1 is a spontaneous example from a notions store (Merritt, 1976, p. 324):

Customer: Do you have uh size C flashlight batteries? [*prerequest*]
Server: Yes sir. [*answer to prerequest*]
Customer: I'll have four please [*request*]
Server: (turns to get) [*uptake of request*]

The customer checks on the availability of size C flashlight batteries before he makes his request. Turn 1 queries a precondition for the request, so it is heard as a prerequest. Often, the respondent can short-cut the process by anticipating the initiator's request, as in Case 2 (Merritt, 1976, p. 337):

Customer: Do you have the pecan Danish today? [*prerequest*]
Server: Yes we do. [*answer to prerequest*] **Would you like one of those?** [*offer*]
Customer: Yes please [*uptake of offer*]
Server: O.K. (turns to get) [*uptake of request*]

Again, the customer checks on a precondition, but this time the server preempts the customer's request with an *offer* of a pecan Danish.

From here it is a short step for respondents to anticipate the request entirely, as in Case 3, a telephone call to a business (Clark, 1979, p. 441):

Caller: Do you close before seven tonight? [*prerequest + request*]

Merchant: Uh, no. [*answer to prerequest*]. We're open until nine o'clock. [*offer of information, or uptake of request*]

The merchant takes up the prerequest, but without waiting for an explicit request, he provides the information he assumed the customer wanted. Respondents can go one step further and treat the prerequest as *pro forma*, not answering it, and offer the wanted information immediately, as in Case 4 (Clark, 1979, p. 444):

Caller: Could you tell me what time you close tonight? [*prerequest + request*]

Merchant: Nine. [*offer of information, or uptake of request*]

The caller here uses a highly conventional prerequest ("Could you tell me?") that invites the merchant to treat it as *pro forma*.

Prerequests are useful precisely because they leave the respondents options for uptake, or, at least, make the appearance of doing so. In Case 1 the prerequest elicits a literal answer alone; in Case 2, a literal answer plus an offer; in Case 3, a literal answer plus compliance; and in Case 4, compliance alone. Which of these are indirect requests? This may be the wrong question because it depends on how they were construed. Cases 1, 2, and 3 were treated as questions, but Cases 2 and 3 were treated as initiating something more as well. Only case 4 was treated as a request pure and simple.

The construal of prerequests is partly in the hands of the respondents. In one study (Clark, 1979), a woman telephoned 50 restaurants and asked, "Do you accept credit cards?" The restaurant managers gave her three types of replies:

	Direct answer	Indirect compliance	Percentage
1.	Yes, we do.		44
2.	Yes.	we accept Mastercard and Visa.	38
3.		We accept Mastercard and Visa.	16

The same prerequest was treated as a direct question by 44% of the restaurant managers, as a question plus a request by 38%, and as a request alone by 16%. So, when the caller asked, "Do you accept credit cards?" was she performing an indirect request? Yes and no. She deliberately left the construal of her utterance for the manager to determine. When a manager said, "Yes, we do," it would have been odd to correct him, "Oh, but I wanted to know what credit cards you accept." He could justifiably have complained, "Then why didn't you say so?" Indirect requests are jointly determined, though only ostensibly so in the most conventional cases.

People should often give such options if they want to be practical. For many requests, it will save time to check on certain preconditions first, because if they cannot be satisfied, there is no use in going further. If the answer to "Do you have size C flashlight batteries?" had been "No," the follow-up request would have been unnecessary. Are people really that practical? If they are, they should design their prerequests to address what they think is the greatest potential obstacle to compliance by the respondent. Paul wants to borrow *Huckleberry Finn* from Jean. If he thinks she owns the book, but may be unwilling to lend it, he might ask, "Would you mind lending me *Huckleberry Finn* for a couple of days?" But if he is not sure she owns it, he might ask, "Do you happen to own a copy of *Huckleberry Finn?*" Evidence suggests that speakers choose their requests on just these grounds (Francik & Clark, 1985; Gibbs, 1986).

It is also polite to give options, as long as they are the right options (Brown & Levinson, 1987; Clark & Schunk, 1980; Lakoff, 1973; Leech, 1983). When Paul asks Jean, "Would you mind lending me *Huckleberry Finn?*" he indicates that she might mind, and that is being considerate of her. He is also giving her the chance to decline the proposed project by saying yes to the precondition, "Yes, sorry, I'm reading it myself," and that is considerate as well. In contrast, if he had asked "Won't you ever lend me *Huckleberry Finn?*" he indicates a different potential obstacle, that she will probably never want to lend him the book, and to accuse her of stinginess is a threat to her self-esteem. People have an immense range of prerequests to choose from depending on what they want to accomplish, the obstacles they see, and how polite they want to be.

C. Emergence of Conversations

Conversations are activities that individual people are "in," but never by themselves. At least two people must be "in" the same conversation at the same time, or it is not a conversation. As a result, two people trying to talk with each other must coordinate: (1) their simultaneous *entry* into the conversation; (2) what they do in it, its *body;* and (3) their simultaneous *exit* from it. How do they manage these feats? One important resource is the presequence, as we can see in Betty and Cathy's telephone conversation.

The opening of a telephone conversation is ordinarily initiated by a caller causing the recipient's telephone to ring (Schegloff, 1968, 1979, 1986), as here:

Betty: (rings C's telephone)
Cathy: Miss Pink's office - hello
Betty: hello

Betty's first action, a *summons*, is a request to enter a conversation with whoever is willing and able to answer that telephone. Cathy's *response,*

"Miss Pink's office," displays such a willingness and ability. It also identifies Cathy as speaking for Miss Pink and willing to accept calls in that role. The purpose of the summons and response is endorsed by the exchange of greetings initiated by Cathy's "hello." The summons–response exchange, then, is a presequence by which Betty and Cathy engineer joint entry into a conversation. It commits them to an extended joint project, a conversation together, even though they do not yet know what it will be about.

The body of the conversation is ordinarily initiated by the caller, too. Here Betty sets up a prerequest of a request to talk to Miss Pink:

Betty: is Miss Pink in .
Cathy: well, she's in, but she's engaged at the moment

Cathy recognizes Betty's projected request but blocks it because Miss Pink is engaged at the moment. Betty, as a result, takes an opportunistic action. After identifying herself, presumably to establish her legitimacy, she sets up a second prerequest to accomplish much the same thing as she would have accomplished with the first:

Betty: could you give her a message *for me*
Cathy: *certainly*

This time Cathy accedes, and Betty makes the request proper, allowing the two of them to complete Betty's purpose for calling.

Making a joint exit from a conversation is also a feat because the participants must pull it off simultaneously (Schegloff & Sacks, 1973). Betty cannot hang up once she is done, because a unilateral withdrawal would offend Cathy by letting her believe she was still in the conversation when she was not. So Betty initiates yet another presequence to open up the closing section of the conversation:

Betty: right
Cathy: Panoff, right you are

Betty produces a preclosing statement, "right," with which she proposes closing the conversation, and Cathy accepts that proposal with "right you are." That done, they enter the closing section proper:

Cathy: I'll tell her,
Betty: *thank you*
Cathy: *(2 to 3 syllables)* bye bye
Betty: bye

In it they review pieces of the conversation and exchange "bye bye" and "bye," all so that they can hang up simultaneously without cutting each other off.

The entry, body, and exit of a conversation are needed so the participants can get in the conversation together, do their work together, and get out together. These sections change shape depending on the number of participants (Sacks et al., 1974), the medium of communication (e.g., face-to-face vs. telephone vs. computer terminals; Clark & Brennan, 1991; Cohen, 1984; Oviatt & Cohen, 1991), the formality of the setting (Irvine, 1984), cultural expectations (Frake, 1964; Gumperz, Aulakh, & Kaltman, 1982; Keenan & Ochs, 1979; Schiffrin, 1984), whether the participants are strangers, acquaintances, or intimates (Coupland, Coupland, & Robinson, 1992; Irvine, 1974; Tannen, 1984), and other factors. Regardless of the situation, the problem to be solved is this: how to enter, carry out, and finish off extended joint projects by local means.

VI. NARRATIVES

Language is ordinarily used for greatly extended projects, global projects. Two people might plan a party, discuss a film, negotiate a contract, or gossip, or one person might buy a car from another, pass information on to others, or tell others stories. People try to establish and manage "accepted purposes and directions of a talk exchange" that are global in scope, and what emerges are the longer stretches of language use called discourse. Although the Latin *discursus* means "conversation," the term now covers any circumscribed piece of language use created for a coherent purpose, including lectures, narratives, essays, novels, newspaper articles, and many more.

Global projects are more complex than local projects. Local projects get proposed by one person and taken up, altered, or declined by another. It takes more serious social engineering to complete the sale of a car, the telling of a joke, or the negotiation of a contract. The participants also have auxiliary goals—establishing social solidarity, maintaining face, impressing each other, keeping certain information hidden, for example—and these complicate the engineering still further (Greene, Lindsay, & Hawn, 1990; Tracy & Moran, 1983; Waldron, Cegala, Sharkey, & Keboul, 1990). Still, the fundamental problem is how to initiate, carry out, and complete global projects by local means. We will consider the issue for narratives.

A. Entering Narratives

Narratives are a type of discourse in which people describe a series of events from an actual or fictional world in the past (Labov, 1972; Labov & Waletzky, 1967; Polanyi, 1989). In conversation they are common in the form of stories, jokes, and anecdotes. Narratives are special in several ways. They tend to be told, or controlled, by a single speaker. They are usually told in extended turns. And they have a special organization. These features pose two problems for the participants of a conversation. The first is how to set narrators up with the extended turn they need for their narrative. The second is how to coordinate the ideas, or mental representations, of the narrator and audience as they navigate the narrative world. Let us consider the entry problem first.

Narratives, like all joint activities, must be entered into together by all the participants, and that takes coordination. In conversation, narratives ordinarily need an occasion: (1) the participants *want* the narrator to tell the narrative; (2) they want *this* narrative in particular; and (3) they want it told *now*. These occasions can be engineered by either the narrators or their partners.

Narrators are often explicitly requested to provide narratives, as in this example (Polanyi, 1989, p. 67):

Bill: I heard second hand or whatever that you got robbed

Susan: Yeah

Bill: That's distressing. Was it near your house?

Susan: Yeah. We parked down at the hill you know (continues story)

In his first turn, Bill brings up an episode Susan could tell a story about, hinting that he would like to hear the story now. Susan could easily have construed his utterance as a request for the story, but she seems reluctant to do that. In his second turn, Bill reemphasizes his interest and indicates that he *wants* to hear *this* particular story *now*. He accomplishes that by asking her, "Was it near your house?" which forces her to start in on the story setting. So Bill initiates a global joint project, Susan's telling him the story of the robbery, through two local joint projects, the assertion and assent, and the question and answer.

It is more complicated for narrators to introduce their own stories into a conversation because they have to persuade their partners that they want to hear the story now. They accomplish this in what Sacks (1974) called the *preface*. Consider this example (Polanyi, 1989, pp. 50–51):

Livia: Do not eat on the New York Thruway

Carol: Yeah, no don't it's

     . . .

Carol: Yeah. You wouldn't believe it

Alice: I forget

Carol: I mean I mean Did I ever tell you the story about the water? I mean the coke?

The discussion about eating on the New York Thruway reminded Carol of a story she wanted to tell Alice. But she could not launch into it straightaway. She had to get her partners to agree that they wanted to hear it now. The cardinal rule of stories is, "Don't tell people a story they have already heard," so Carol's technique was to ask them, "Did I ever tell you the story about the water? I mean the coke?" This served as a prenarrative, and when no one objected, she started her story:

> Carol: I went i- . . . I always drink coke, right?
>
> Livia: Right.
>
> Carol: So, Livia is thr- . . . walking around with this gallon of spring water and I can't understand (continues story)

Conversational partners can of course decline a story, as here (2.14.600):

> Jane: did I tell you, when were in this African village, and *- they were all out in the fields, - the*
>
> Kate: *yes you did, yes, - yes*
>
> Jane: babies left alone, -
>
> Kate: yes .

Once Kate answered yes, Jane aborted the story. In all these examples, the participants negotiated the entry into a global joint project, a story, by means of local joint projects, the prenarrative and its response.

B. Situation Models

The participants in any joint activity must keep track of what the others are thinking, or the activity will collapse. When people enter an activity, they presuppose they share a certain common ground, certain mutual knowledge, mutual beliefs, and mutual assumptions (Clark & Marshall, 1981; Lewis, 1969; Schiffer, 1972). With each joint action they take, they add to this common ground (Clark & Schaefer, 1989; Clark & Wilkes-Gibbs, 1986; Stalnaker, 1978). For their additions to be orderly, the participants must each have a representation of the *current state of the activity*. They will be able to understand the next utterance only if they can figure out how it changes the current state. The point here merely echoes Grice's cooperative principle, "Make your conversational contribution such as is required, at the stage at which it occurs, by the accepted purpose or direction of the talk exchange in which you are engaged."

Suppose Jean is telling Paul how to get from San Francisco's Golden Gate Park to Fisherman's Wharf, or how an interview went, or why it is his turn to clean their apartment. In each case, they take for granted a shared representation of the situation being described and build on it. For the directions, the two of them might assume a shared mental map of San Francisco, and as Jean gives directions, Paul tries to imagine the route on his mental map. For the interview, they might assume that they both know who the interviewer is, why Jean was being interviewed, and the circumstances of the interview, and as Jean narrates, Paul tries to build a model of these agents and what they did. For cleaning the apartment, they might assume shared beliefs about the rights and responsibilities of roommates, and as they talk, they try to build a model of where they agree and disagree in their beliefs.

So people's mental representation of the current state of an activity includes what is often called a *situation model:* a representation of the situation being talked about (Perrig & Kintsch, 1985; Schmalhofer & Glavanov, 1986; van Dijk & Kintsch, 1983). Precisely what is represented in these models has been an issue of debate. Among the types of information they may represent are these:

1. *Visual information,* for example, a mental map of a city or building (Perrig & Kintsch, 1985; but see Taylor & Tversky, 1992a, 1992b).

2. *Spatial information,* for example, where one object is with respect to another (Mani & Johnson-Laird, 1982; Miller & Johnson-Laird, 1976; Morrow & Clark, 1988; Taylor & Tversky, 1992a, 1992b). Narrators and their audiences, for example, can foreground certain parts of the model or certain objects within the model (Bower & Morrow, 1990; Glenberg, Meyer, & Lindem, 1987; Morrow, Bower, & Greenspan, 1989; Morrow, Greenspan, & Bower, 1987).

3. *Scripts of routine cultural activities,* for example, what people are expected to do in a restaurant or in a doctor's office (Bower, Black, & Turner, 1979; R. C. Schank, 1975; R. Schank & Abelson, 1977).

4. *Temporal information,* for example, how one event occurs after another (Clark & Clark, 1968; Foos, 1992; Taylor, 1992; van Jaarsveld & Schreuder, 1986).

5. *Causal information,* for example, what causes a light to turn on or a person to become sad (Black & Bern, 1981; Myers, Sinjo, & Duffy, 1987; Trabasso & Sperry, 1985; Trabasso & van den Broek, 1985).

6. *Kinematic information,* for example, the way things move (Hegarty, 1992; Hegarty, Just, & Morrison, 1988).

7. *Emotional information,* for example, feelings of suspense, anger, fear (Brewer & Lichtenstein, 1981, 1982; Gerrig, 1993).

The idea is that the participants in a discourse update their situation models as the discourse progresses, adding, deleting, or changing elements to mirror changes in the situation being described (Gentner & Stevens, 1983; Johnson-Laird, 1983).

Situation models are essential if the participants are to coordinate what they are thinking. Listeners often need to keep track simply to know what speakers are referring to. In one study (Morrow, 1985), people memorized the layout of an apartment and then read brief descriptions like this:

> Bill and Kathy prepared to go for a drive to the mountains.
> Bill went outside to wait for Kathy in the car.
> Kathy freshened up before leaving.
> Suddenly Kathy noticed that she didn't have her sunglasses.
> *She walked from the study into the bedroom.*
> She didn't find the glasses in **the room.**

When asked "Which room is being referred to?" they answered "bedroom" 77% of the time and "study" 21%. When the italicized sentence was replaced with "She walked past the living room to the bedroom," they answered "living room" 73% of the time and "bedroom" only 21%. To make these assignments, readers had to do more than register the word and sentence meanings. They had to follow the narrator's focus of attention and imagine the room Kathy would be in at the moment the narrator announced she did not find her glasses. The narrator signaled the focus of attention through the use of prepositions (*into* vs. *to*), verb aspect (*walked* vs. *was walking*), deixis (*this* vs. *that, come* vs. *go*), and many other features (Clark, 1973; Fillmore, 1975; Talmy, 1975, 1983, 1988). The issue is what the narrators' and their audience's situation models represent and how, and that issue is hardly resolved.

C. Narrative Organization

Narrators and their audience know they have to coordinate situation models, and that helps dictate the way narrators organize their stories and the way their audience interprets them. As an illustration, consider what Labov (1972) called *narratives of personal experience*. These narratives, he argued, tend to divide into six parts, which we will illustrate with Susan's narrative about the robbery (Polanyi, 1989).

1. *Abstract.* Narrators usually begin with an abstract, a brief summary of the entire story. In Susan's narrative, it was expressed by Bill, "I heard secondhand or whatever that you got robbed."

2. *Orientation.* Narrators then create an orientation, a stage setting about the who, when, what, and where of the story. Susan began, "We parked down at the hill you know . . . we were walking home. It was late at night."

3. *Complicating action.* Next, narrators describe the complicating action, what happened. Susan, for example, went on, "and then this strange car pulled up and we thought 'oh,'" and continued telling what happened.

4. *Evaluation.* Narrators ordinarily describe the complicating action along with what Labov called an evaluation, "the point of the narrative, its raison d'être: why it was told, what the narrator is getting at" (Labov, 1972, p. 266). As Susan related what happened, she made remarks such as these: "You know, it was real scary cause you know at a whim he could have shot at us," "Oh God," and "It was really like a movie."

5. *Result or resolution.* Narrators finish off the complicating action, usually, with a result or resolution, how the complicating action got resolved. In Susan's narrative, she said, "And so when [the police] came they said 'Come identify them. We've caught them.' It was ridiculous. It was about five or ten minutes after."

6. *Coda.* At the end, narrators produce the coda, a signal that they have completed their narrative. In Susan's case, she turned to her audience and asked, "Has anything like that ever happened to you? Have you ever had your purse snatched?"

Narrators are really guides. They help their audience create a mental model of the narrative world, and then take them on a tour through it. The six parts of spontaneous narratives reflect their guiding strategies.

The abstract and coda mark the boundaries of the narrative world. The narrators and audience usually begin in the here-and-now, talking about people, things, and happenings around them. Susan, Bill, Livia, and Nancy might have been sitting around a kitchen table drinking coffee. For a narrative, they must leave the here-and-now together, enter the narrative world, conjure up its own people, things, and happenings, and, at the end, leave that world and return to the here-and-now. They enter the narrative world by means of the abstract, which offers a brief description of that world ("you got robbed"), and they leave it via the coda, which refocuses their attention on the here-and-now ("Has anything like that ever happened to you?").

It is the orientation that supplies the initial frame of reference for the narrative world. The idea is that narrators cannot describe a complicating action without presupposing (1) the people taking that action, (2) the time and place of the action, and (3) other background facts. Nancy's initial orientation allows her audience to imagine the place ("we parked down at the hill you know"), the time ("it was late at night"), and other circumstances ("we were walking home") to set up her vulnerability to a robbery. It gives just enough background for her to introduce the complicating action ("a strange car pulled up . . . and then this guy ran around and around to the back of it"). The audience could not know the significance of these events if they had not known Nancy was on the street alone with a friend late at night. The orientation is essential to creating a vivid model of the narrative world.

Labov's complicating action and evaluation correspond to what have sometimes been called the *foreground* and *background* of a narrative (Grimes, 1975; Hopper, 1979; Hopper & Thompson, 1980; Polanyi, 1989; Polanyi-Bowditch, 1976). Narrators treat certain events in their story—Labov called them *narrative events*—as foreground. They describe these events in strict chronological order (except in flashbacks and flashforwards), often introducing them with *and* or *and then,* in order to stake out a clear temporal path through the narrative world, as here:

and then this strange car pulled up
and we thought "oh"
and then this guy ran around and around to the back of it
and he held his gun
and said "Gimme your purse"
and I said I didn't have one
and I just gave him my wallet fast

These events define the chronological foundation of what happened. The background is everything else. It is used to comment on, evaluate, give reasons for, or otherwise situate what happened, as in these clauses:

and he had an actual gun
You know, it was real scary
cause you know at a whim he could have shot at us

Here Nancy describes relevant background about the robber's gun and her emotions.

If the foreground is intended to identify the time course of the narrative, it should describe events that resemble clock ticks, and it does. The events tend to be punctual, goal directed, volitional, affirmative, and real, such as hitting, noticing, telling, and finding. These are ideal for the foreground because they can be ordered chronologically. The background, in contrast, tends to describe states or properties that are durative, stative, passive, negative, and hypothetical, such as knowing, having, sleeping, seeing, and not finding. In English it is common to express the foreground in independent clauses (not subordinate clauses) and in the simple past or historical present tense (not in the progressive), as illustrated in Nancy's narrative clauses beginning "and then this strange car pulled up." Subordinate clauses and other tenses and verb forms are reserved for backgrounded information.

Narrators use the foreground and background to guide their audience on the paths they have chosen to take through their narrative worlds. By exploring these constructions, they can highlight protagonists against minor characters, important props against unimportant ones, essential events against inessential ones. And they get their audience to infer the right causal relations among the events, which events were the causes of which. People have been shown to recall stories around the foregrounded events and the causal relations between them (Black & Bern, 1981; Trabasso & van den Broek, 1985). The more causal connections a foregrounded event has, the better it is remembered.

Narratives, therefore, emerge with an organization shaped by the narrators' attempts to coordinate with their audience. The two must coordinate their entry and exit from the narrative world, and that leads to the abstract and coda. The two must create a starting model of the narrative world, and that requires an orientation. And the two must coordinate on the path that narrators have chosen to take through the events of the narrative world, and that separates foreground from background, the actions proper from their evaluation of them. The point of a narrative is ordinarily to create emotions—surprise, mystification, amazement, sympathy, suspense—and that cannot be ordinarily done without a vivid mental re-creation of the narrative world by both narrators and their audience (Gerrig, 1993; Walton, 1990).

VII. CONCLUSION

Whenever people use language, they are taking actions. But their individual actions are not autonomous. They are parts of joint actions in which the participants are trying to coordinate with each other. When Paul speaks to Jean, he expects her to try to attend to, identify, and understand what he is saying while he is speaking. In particular, they try to reach the mutual belief that she has understood him well enough for current purposes, and that requires coordination at all levels. Speakers and addressees cannot do without each other. Illocutionary acts cannot succeed without coordinated acts of recognition. Speaker's meaning makes no sense without the reciprocal addressee's understanding.

But people use language to do things with each other. Paul may use an utterance to propose a local project for Jean and him to accomplish together; for example, she is to tell him what time it is. She, in turn, has the choice of taking up the project as is, altering it, declining it, or withdrawing altogether. Remarkably, people can accomplish extended projects only by means of such local projects. Discourses are global joint activities that emerge from an artful and opportunistic series of local joint actions.

Acknowledgment

Preparation of this chapter was supported in part by NSF Grant SBR-9309612.

Endnotes

1. All of the examples marked with this notation come from a large corpus of spontaneous British conversations transcribed by Svartvik and Quirk (1980). Each example is identified by text number (here 1.3) and beginning line (560). In the transcription, a comma indicates the end of a tone unit, - and . indicate long short pauses, colons (:) indicate stretched vowels, and adjacent pairs of phrases in asterisks indicate overlapping speech.
2. The point has been made by investigators working in a variety of disciplines. They include: Clark and Schaefer (1989), Clark and Wilkes-Gibbs (1986), Duranti (1986), Gumperz (1982), Kochman (1986), McDermott and Tylbor (1983), Sacks, Schegloff, and Jefferson (1974), Schegloff and Sacks (1973), and Tannen (1989).
3. For a related notion, see the discussion of preferred response by Davidson (1990), Houtkoop (1987), Levinson (1983), Pomerantz (1984), and Sacks (1987).

References

Austin, J. L. (1962). *How to do things with words*. Oxford: Oxford University Press.
Bach, K., & Harnish, R. M. (1979). *Linguistic communication and speech acts*. Cambridge, MA: MIT Press.
Ballmer, T., & Brennenstuhl, W. (1981). *Speech act classification: A study in the lexical analysis of English speech activity verbs*. Berlin & New York: Springer-Verlag.
Bavelas, J. B. (1994). Gestures as part of speech: Methodological implications. *Research on Language and Social Interaction, 27*, 201–221.
Bavelas, J. B., Black, A., Chovil, N., Lemery, C. R., & Mullett, J. (1988). Form and function in motor mimicry. Topographic evidence that the primary function is communicative. *Human Communication Research, 14*, 275–299.
Bavelas, J., Black, A., Chovel, N., & Mullett, J. (1990a). *Equivocal communication*. Newbury Park, CA: Sage.
Bavelas, J., Black, A., Chovel, N., & Mullett, J. (1990b). Truths, lies and equivocations. The effects of conflicting goals on discourse. *Journal of Language and Social Psychology, 9*, 135–161.
Bavelas, J. B., Black, A., Lemery, C. R., & Mullett, J. (1986). "I show you how you feel": Motor mimicry as a communicative act. *Journal of Personality and Social Psychology, 50*, 322–329.
Black, J. B., & Bern, H. (1981). Causal coherence and memory for events in narratives. *Journal of Verbal Learning and Verbal Behavior, 20*, 276–285.
Bower, G. H., Black, J. B., & Turner, T. J. (1979). Scripts in memory for text. *Cognitive Psychology, 11*, 177–220.
Bower, G. H., & Morrow, D. G. (1990). Mental models in narrative comprehension. *Science, 247*, 44–48.
Brennan, S. E. (1990). *Seeking and providing evidence for mutual understanding*. Unpublished doctoral dissertation, Stanford University, Stanford, CA.

Brewer, W. F., & Lichtenstein, E. H. (1981). Event schemas, story schemas, and story grammars. In J. Long & A. Baddeley (Eds.), *Attention and performance IX* (pp. 363–379). Hillsdale, NJ: Erlbaum.

Brewer, W. F., & Lichtenstein, E. H. (1982). Stories are to entertain: A structural affect theory of stories. *Journal of Pragmatics, 6,* 473–486.

Brown, P., & Levinson, S. C. (1987). *Politeness.* Cambridge, UK: Cambridge University Press.

Chovil, N. (1991-1992). Discourse-oriented facial displays in conversation. *Language and Social Interaction, 25,* 163–194.

Clark, H. H. (1973). Space, time, semantics, and the child. In T. Moore (Ed.), *Cognitive development and the acquisition of language* (pp. 27–63). New York: Academic Press.

Clark, H. H. (1979). Responding to indirect speech acts. *Cognitive Psychology, 11,* 430–477.

Clark, H. H. (1994). Discourse in production. In M. A. Gernsbacher (Ed.), *Handbook of psycholinguistics.* San Diego, CA: Academic Press.

Clark, H. H., & Brennan, S. A. (1991). Grounding in communication. In L. B. Resnick, J. M. Levine, & S. D. Teasley (Eds.), *Perspective on socially shared cognition* (pp. 127–149). Washington, DC: APA Books.

Clark, H. H., & Clark, E. V. (1968). Semantic distinctions and memory for complex sentences. *Quarterly Journal of Experimental Psychology, 20,* 129–138.

Clark, H. H., & Gerrig, R. J. (1984). On the pretense theory of irony. *Journal of Experimental Psychology: General, 113,* 121–126.

Clark, H. H., & Gerrig, R. J. (1990). Quotations as demonstrations. *Language, 66,* 764–805.

Clark, H. H., & Marshall, C. R. (1981). Definite reference and mutual knowledge. In A. K. Joshi, B. L. Webber, & I. A. Sag (Eds.), *Elements of discourse understanding* (pp. 10–63). Cambridge, UK: Cambridge University Press.

Clark, H. H., & Schaefer, E. R. (1989). Contributing to discourse. *Cognitive Science, 13,* 259–294.

Clark, H. H., & Schunk, D. H. (1980). Polite responses to polite requests. *Cognition, 8,* 111–143.

Clark, H. H., & Wilkes-Gibbs, D. (1986). Referring as a collaborative process. *Cognition, 22,* 1–39.

Cohen, P. R. (1984). The pragmatics of referring, and the modality of communication. *Computational Linguistics, 10,* 97–146.

Cole, P., & Morgan, J. L. (Eds.). (1975). *Syntax and semantics: Vol. 3. Speech acts.* New York: Academic Press.

Coupland, J., Coupland, N., & Robinson, J. D. (1992). "How are you?" Negotiating phatic communication. *Language in Society, 21*(2), 207–230.

Davidson, J. A. (1990). Modifications of invitations, offers and rejections. In G. Psathas (Ed.), *Interaction competence* (pp. 149–180). Washington, DC: International Institute for Ethnomethodology and Conversational Analysis and University Press of America.

Davis, S. (1979). Perlocutions. *Linguistics and Philosophy, 3,* 225–243.

Duncan, S. D., Jr. (1972). Some signals and rules for taking speaking turns in conversations. *Journal of Personality and Social Psychology, 23,* 283–292.

Duncan, S. D., Jr. (1973). Toward a grammar for dyadic conversation. *Semiotica, 9,* 29–47.

Duranti, A. (1986). The audience as co-author: An introduction. *Text, 6*(3), 239–247.

Edelsky, C. (1981). Who's got the floor? *Language in Society, 10,* 383–423.

Ekman, P., & Friesen, W. (1969). The repertoire of nonverbal behavior: Categories, origins, usage and coding. *Semiotica, 1,* 49–98.

Feyereisen, P., & de Lannoy, J.-D. (1991). *Gestures and speech: Psychological investigations.* Cambridge, UK: Cambridge University Press.

Fillmore, C. (1975). *Santa Cruz lectures on deixis*. Bloomington: Indiana University Linguistics Club.

Foos, P. W. (1992). Constructing schemata while reading simple stories. *Journal of General Psychology, 119*(4), 419–425.

Frake, C. O. (1964). How to ask for a drink in Subanun. *American Anthropologist, 66,* 127–132.

Francik, E. P., & Clark, H. H. (1985). How to make requests that overcome obstacles to compliance. *Journal of Memory and Language, 24,* 560–568.

Gentner, D., & Stevens, A. (Eds.). (1983). *Mental models*. Hillsdale, NJ: Erlbaum.

Gerrig, R. J. (1993). *Experiencing narrative worlds*. New Haven, CT: Yale University Press.

Gibbs, R. W. (1986). What makes some indirect speech acts conventional? *Journal of Memory and Language, 25*(2), 181–196.

Glenberg, A. M., Meyer, M., & Lindem, K. (1987). Mental models contribute to foregrounding during text comprehension. *Journal of Memory and Language, 26*(1), 69–83.

Goffman, E. (1976). Replies and responses. *Language in Society, 5,* 257–313.

Goodwin, C. (1981). *Conversational organization: Interaction between speakers and hearers*. New York: Academic Press.

Goodwin, C. (1987). Forgetfulness as an interactive resource. *Social Psychology Quarterly, 50*(2), 115–131.

Goodwin, M. H., & Goodwin, C. (1986). Gesture and coparticipation in the activity of searching for a word. *Semiotica, 62,* 51–75.

Gordon, D., & Lakoff, G. (1971). Conversational postulates. In *Papers from the seventh regional meeting of the Chicago Linguistic Society*. (pp. 63–84). Chicago: Chicago Linguistic Society.

Greene, J. O., Lindsey, A. E., & Hawn, J. J. (1990). Social goals and speech production: Effects of multiple goals on pausal phenomena. *Journal of Language and Social Psychology, 9*(1–2), 119–134.

Grice, H. P. (1957). Meaning. *Philosophical Review, 66,* 377–388.

Grice, H. P. (1975). Logic and conversation. In P. Cole & J. L. Morgan (Eds.), *Syntax and semantics: Vol. 3. Speech acts* (pp. 113–128). New York: Seminar Press.

Grimes, J. E. (1975). *The thread of discourse*. The Hague: Mouton.

Gumperz, J. J. (1982). *Discourse strategies*. Cambridge, UK: Cambridge University Press.

Gumperz, J. J., Aulakh, G., & Kaltman, H. (1982). Thematic structure and progression in discourse. In J. J. Gumperz (Ed.), *Language and social identity*. Cambridge, UK: Cambridge University Press.

Hancher, M. (1979). The classification of cooperative illocutionary acts. *Language in Society, 8,* 1–14.

Hegarty, M. (1992). Mental animal: Inferring motion from static displays of mechanical systems. *Journal of Experimental Psychology: Learning, Memory, and Cognition, 18*(5), 1084–1102.

Hegarty, M., Just, M. A., & Morrison, I. R. (1988). Mental models of mechanical systems: Individual differences in qualitative and quantitative reasoning. *Cognitive Psychology, 20*(2), 191–236.

Hopper, P. J. (1979). Aspect and foregrounding in discourse. In T. Givon (Ed.), *Syntax and semantics: Vol. 12. Discourse and syntax* (pp. 213–241). New York: Academic Press.

Hopper, P. J., & Thompson, S. (1980). Transitivity in grammar and discourse. *Language, 56,* 251–299.

Horn, L. R. (1984). Toward a new taxonomy for pragmatic inference: Q-based and R-based implicature. In D. Schiffrin (Ed.), *Meaning, form and use in context: Linguistic application*. Washington, DC: Georgetown University Press.

Houtkoop, H. (1987). *Establishing agreement: An analysis of proposal-acceptance sequences*. Providence, RI: Dordrecht.

Houtkoop, H., & Mazeland, H. (1985). Turns and discourse units in everyday conversation. *Journal of Pragmatics, 9,* 595–619.

Irvine, J. T. (1974). Strategies of status manipulation in the Wolof greeting. In R. Bauman & J. Scherzer (Eds.), *Explorations in the ethnography of speaking*. Cambridge, UK: Cambridge University Press.

Irvine, J. T. (1984). Formality and informality in communicative events. In J. Baugh & J. Scherzer (Eds.), *Language in use: Readings in sociolinguistics*. Englewood Cliffs, NJ: Prentice-Hall.

Isaacs, E. A., & Clark, H. H. (1990). Ostensible invitations. *Language in Society, 19,* 493–509.

Jefferson, G. (1973). A case of precision timing in ordinary conversation: Overlapped tag-positioned address terms in closing sequences. *Semiotica, 9,* 47–96.

Johnson-Laird, P. N. (1983). *Mental models*. Cambridge, UK: Cambridge University Press.

Kasher, A. (1977). Foundations of philosophical pragmatics. In R. Butts & J. Hintikka (Eds.), *Basic problems in methodology and linguistics*. Dordrecht: Reidel.

Kennan, E. L., & Ochs, E. (1979). Becoming a competent speaker of Malagasy. In T. E. Shopen (Ed.), *Languages and their speakers* (pp. 113–160). Philadelphia: University of Pennsylvania Press.

Kendon, A. (1980). Gesticulation and speech: Two aspects of the process of utterance. In M. R. Key (Ed.), *Relationship of verbal and nonverbal communication*. Amsterdam: Mouton de Gruyter.

Kendon, A. (1987). On gesture: Its complementary relationship with speech. In A. W. Siegman & S. Feldstein (Eds.), *Nonverbal communication and language* (2nd ed., pp. 65–97). Hillsdale, NJ: Erlbaum.

Kochman, T. (1986). Strategic ambiguity in Black speech genres: Cross-cultural interference in participant-observation research. *Text, 6*(2), 153–170.

Labov, W. (1972). The transformation of experience in narrative syntax. In W. Labov (Ed.), *Language in the inner city: Studies in the Black English vernacular* (pp. 354–396). Philadelphia: University of Pennsylvania Press.

Labov, W., & Fanshel, D. (1977). *Therapeutic discourse*. New York: Academic Press.

Labov, W., & Waletzky, J. (1967). Narrative analysis: Oral versions of personal experience. In J. Helms (Ed.), *Essays on the verbal and visual arts*. Seattle: University of Washington Press.

Lakoff, R. (1973). The logic of politeness; or, Minding your p's and q's. In *Papers from the ninth regional meeting of the Chicago Linguistics Society* (pp. 292–305). Chicago: Chicago Linguistics Society.

Leech, G. N. (1983). *Principles of pragmatics*. London: Longman.

Levinson, S. C. (1983). *Pragmatics*. Cambridge, UK: Cambridge University Press.

Levinson, S. C. (1987). Minimization and conversational inference. In J. Verschueren & M. Bertuccelli-Papi (Eds.), *The pragmatic perspective* (pp. 61–130). Amsterdam: John Benjamins.

Lewis, D. K. (1969). *Convention: A philosophical study*. Cambridge, MA: Harvard University Press.

Linell, P., Alemyr, L., & Jonsson, L. (1993). Admission of guilt as a communicative project in judicial settings. *Journal of Pragmatics, 19*(2), 153–176.

Linell, P., & Markova, I. (1993). Acts in discourse: From monological speech acts to dialogical inter-acts. *Journal for the Theory of Social Behavior, 23*(2), 173–195.

Mani, K., & Johnson-Laird, P. N. (1982). The mental representation of spatial descriptions. *Memory & Cognition, 10,* 181–187.

McDermott, R. P., & Tylbor, H. (1983). On the necessity of collusion in conversation. *Text, 3*(3), 277–297.

McNeill, D. (1985). So you think gestures are nonverbal? *Psychological Review, 92,* 350–371.

McNeill, D. (1992). *Hand and mind*. Chicago: University of Chicago Press.

McNeill, D., & Levy, E. (1982). Conceptual representations in language activity and gesture. In R. Jarvella & W. Klein (Eds.), *Speech, place, and action: Studies in deixis and related topics* (pp. 271–295). Chichester: Wiley.

Merritt, M. (1976). On questions following questions (in service encounters). *Language in Society, 5,* 315–357.

Miller, G. A., & Johnson-Laird, P. N. (1976). *Language and perception.* Cambridge, MA: Belknap Press.

Morgan, J. L. (1978). Two types of convention in indirect speech acts. In P. Cole (Ed.), *Syntax and semantics: Vol. 9. Pragmatics* (pp. 261–280). New York: Academic Press.

Morrow, D. G. (1985). Prepositions and verb aspect in narrative understanding. *Journal of Memory and Language, 24,* 390–404.

Morrow, D. G., Bower, G. H., & Greenspan, S. L. (1989). Updating situation models during narrative comprehension. *Journal of Memory and Language, 28*(3), 292–312.

Morrow, D. G., & Clark, H. H. (1988). Interpreting words in spatial descriptions. *Language and Cognitive Processes, 3,* 275–291.

Morrow, D. G., Greenspan, S. E., & Bower, G. H. (1987). Accessibility and situation models in narrative comprehension. *Journal of Memory and Language, 26,* 165–187.

Myers, J. L., Sinjo, J., & Duffy, S. (1987). Degree of causal relatedness and memory. *Journal of Memory and Language, 26,* 453–465.

Nunberg, G. (1981). Validating pragmatic explanations. In P. Cole (Ed.), *Radical pragmatics* (pp. 199–222). New York: Academic Press.

Oviatt, S. L., & Cohen, P. R. (1991). Discourse structure and performance efficiency in interactive and noninteractive speech modalities. *Computer Speech and Language, 5,* 297–326.

Perrig, W., & Kintsch, W. (1985). Propositional and situational representations of text. *Journal of Memory and Language, 24*(5), 503–518.

Polanyi, L. (1989). *Telling the American story.* Cambridge, MA: MIT Press.

Polanyi-Bowditch, L. (1976). Why the whats are when: Mutually contextualized realms of narrative. In *Proceedings of the second annual meeting of the Berkeley Linguistics Society* (pp. 59–78). Berkeley, CA: Berkeley Linguistics Society.

Pomerantz, A. (1984). Agreeing and disagreeing with assessments: Some features of preferred/dispreferred turn shapes. In J. M. Atkinson & J. Heritage (Eds.), *Structures of social action: Studies in conversation analysis* (pp. 57–101). Cambridge, UK: Cambridge University Press.

Sacks, H. (1974). An analysis of the course of a joke's telling in conversation. In R. Bauman & J. Sherzer (Eds.), *Explorations in the ethnography of speaking* (pp. 337–353). Cambridge, UK: Cambridge University Press.

Sacks, H. (1987). On the preference for agreement and contiguity in sequences in conversation. In G. Button & J. R. E. Lee (Eds.), *Talk and social organization* (pp. 54–69). Clevedon, UK: Multilingual Matters.

Sacks, H., Schegloff, E. A., & Jefferson, G. (1974). A simplest systematics for the organization of turn-taking in conversation. *Language, 50,* 696–735.

Sadock, J. M. (1978). On testing for conversational implicature. In P. Cole (Ed.), *Syntax and semantics: Vol. 9: Pragmatics* (pp. 281–297). New York: Academic Press.

Schank, R. C. (1975). The structure of episodes of memory. In D. G. Bobrow & E. A. Collins (Eds.), *Representation and understanding: Studies in cognitive science* (pp. 237–272). New York: Academic Press.

Schank, R., & Abelson, R. P. (1977). *Scripts, plans, goals, and understanding.* Hillsdale, NJ: Erlbaum.

Schegloff, E. A. (1968). Sequencing in conversational openings. *American Anthropologist, 70*(4), 1075–1095.

Schegloff, E. A. (1972). Notes on a conversational practice: Formulating place. In D. Sudnow (Ed.), *Studies in social interaction* (pp. 75–119). New York: Free Press.

Schegloff, E. A. (1979). Identification and recognition in telephone conversational openings. In

G. Psathas (Ed.), *Everyday language: Studies in ethnomethodology* (pp. 23–78). New York: Irvington.

Schegloff, E. A. (1980). Preliminaries to preliminaries: "Can I ask you a question?" *Sociological Inquiry, 50,* 104–152.

Schegloff, E. A. (1982). Discourse as an interactional achievement: Some uses of "uh huh" and other things that come between sentences. In D. Tannen (Ed.), *Analyzing discourse: Text and talk. Georgetown University Roundtable on Languages and Linguistics 1981* (pp. 71–93). Washington, DC: Georgetown University Press.

Schegloff, E. A. (1986). The routine as achievement. *Human Studies, 9,* 111–152.

Schegloff, E. A., & Sacks, H. (1973). Opening up closings. *Semiotica, 8,* 289–327.

Schiffer, S. R. (1972). *Meaning.* Oxford: Oxford University Press.

Schiffrin, D. (1984). Jewish argument as sociability. *Language in Society, 14,* 311–335.

Schmalhofer, F., & Glavanov, D. (1986). Three components of understanding a programmer's manual: Verbatim, propositional, and situational representations. *Journal of Memory and Language, 25*(3), 279–294.

Searle, J. R. (1969). *Speech acts.* Cambridge, UK: Cambridge University Press.

Searle, J. R. (1975a). Indirect speech acts. In P. Cole & J. L. Morgan (Eds.), *Syntax and semantics: Vol. 3. Speech acts* (pp. 59–82). New York: Seminar Press.

Searle, J. R. (1975b). A taxonomy of illocutionary acts. In K. Gunderson (Ed.), *Minnesota studies in the philosophy of language* (pp. 334–369). Minneapolis: University of Minnesota Press.

Sperber, D., & Wilson, D. (1981). Irony and the use-mention distinction. In P. Cole (Ed.), *Radical pragmatics* (pp. 295–318). New York: Academic Press.

Sperber, D., & Wilson, D. (1986). *Relevance.* Cambridge, MA: Harvard University Press.

Stalnaker, R. C. (1978). Assertion. In P. Cole (Ed.), *Syntax and semantics: Vol. 9. Pragmatics* (pp. 315–332). New York: Academic Press.

Stenström, A. B. (1984). *Questions and responses in English conversation.* Lund, Sweden: Gleerup.

Svartvik, J., & Quirk, R. (Eds.). (1980). *A corpus of English conversation.* Lund, Sweden: Gleerup.

Talmy, L. (1975). Semantics and syntax of motion. In J. Kimball (Ed.), *Syntax and semantics.* New York: Academic Press.

Talmy, L. (1983). How language structures space. In H. Pick & L. Acredolo (Eds.), *Spatial orientation: Theory, research, and application.* New York: Plenum Press.

Talmy, L. (1988). Force dynamics in language and cognition. *Cognitive Science, 12*(1), 49–100.

Tannen, D. (1983). When is an overlap not an interruption? One component of conversational style. In R. DiPietro, W. Frawley, & A. Wedel (Eds.), *The First Delaware Symposium on Language Studies* (pp. 119–129). Newark: University of Delaware Press.

Tannen, D. (1984). *Conversational style: Analyzing talk among friends.* Norwood, NJ: Ablex.

Tannen, D. (1989). *Talking voices: Repetition, dialogue and imagery in conversational discourse.* Cambridge, UK: Cambridge University Press.

Taylor, H. A. (1992). *Who did what when? Memory organization of event descriptions.* Doctoral dissertation, Stanford University, Stanford, CA.

Taylor, H. A., & Tversky, B. (1992a). Descriptions and depictions of environments. *Memory & Cognition, 20*(5), 483–496.

Taylor, H. A., & Tversky, B. (1992b). Spatial mental models derived from survey and route descriptions. *Journal of Memory and Language, 31*(2), 261–292.

Trabasso, T., & Sperry, L. L. (1985). Causal relatedness and importance of story events. *Journal of Memory and Language, 24,* 595–611.

Trabasso, T., & van den Broek, P. (1985). Causal thinking and the representation of narrative events. *Journal of Memory and Language, 24,* 612–630.

Tracy, K., & Moran, J. P., III. (1983). Conversation relevance in multiple-goal settings. In

Herbert H. Clark and Bridget Bly

R. T. Craig & K. Tracy (Eds.), *Conversational coherence: Form, structure and strategy*. Beverly Hills, CA: Sage.

van der Auwera, J. (1980). On the meaning of basic speech acts. *Journal of Pragmatics, 4*(3), 253–264.

van Dijk, T. A., & Kintsch, W. (1983). *Strategies of discourse comprehension*. New York: Academic Press.

van Eemeren, F. H., & Grootendorst, R. (1982). The speech acts of arguing and convincing in externalized discussions. *Journal of Pragmatics, 6*, 1–24.

van Jaarsveld, H. J., & Schreuder, R. (1986). Implicit quantification of temporal adverbials. *Journal of Semantics, 4*, 327–339.

Verschueren, J. (1980). *On speech act verbs* Amsterdam: John Benjamins.

Waldron, V. R., Cegala, D. J., Sharkey, W. F., & Keboul, B. (1990). Cognitive and tactical dimension of conversational goal management. *Journal of Language and Social Psychology, 9*(1-2), 101–118.

Walton, K. L. (1990). *Mimesis as make-believe: On the foundations of the representational arts*. Cambridge, MA: Harvard University Press.

Wierzbicka, A. (1985). A semantic metalanguage for a cross-cultural comparison of speech acts and speech genres. *Language in Society, 14*(4), 491–513.

Yngve, V. H. (1970). On getting a word in edgewise. In *Papers from the sixth regional meeting of the Chicago Linguistic Society* (pp. 567–578). Chicago: Chicago Linguistic Society.

Index